Date Due

M

I

Monoclonal Antibodies: Principles and Practice

Second Edition

Monoclonal Antibodies: Principles and Practice

Production and Application of
Monoclonal Antibodies in Cell Biology,
Biochemistry and Immunology

Second Edition

JAMES W. GODING

*Department of Pathology and Immunology,
Monash University, Alfred Hospital,
Prahran, Victoria, Australia*

1986

ACADEMIC PRESS
Harcourt Brace Jovanovich, Publishers

London   Orlando
New York   San Diego   Austin
Boston   Tokyo   Sydney   Toronto

ACADEMIC PRESS INC. (LONDON) LTD.
24/28 Oval Road
London NW1

United States Edition published by
ACADEMIC PRESS
Orlando, Florida 32887

British Library Cataloguing in Publication Data

13334375   3.13.87 Ac

Goding, James W.
  Monoclonal antibodies: principles and
  practice: production and application of
  monoclonal antibodies in cell biology,
  biochemistry and immunology. — 2nd ed.
  1. Immunoglobulins   2. Gammopathies,
  Monoclonal
  I. Title
  599.02'93   QR186.7
  ISBN 0-12-287021-2

Typeset at the Alden Press
Oxford London and Northampton

Preface

Ever since the beginnings of experimental immunology at the end of the nineteenth century, scientists have exploited the specificity of antibodies to detect, isolate and analyse biological material. The power of antibodies as probes for biological structure underwent a quantum increase in 1975, when Köhler and Milstein published their classic paper on the production of monoclonal antibodies of predefined specificity. Paradoxically, the very success of monoclonal antibodies has generated a literature which is now so vast and scattered that it has become difficult for the non-specialist to obtain a perspective.

I believe that the need has arisen for an integrated text which treats the application of monoclonal antibodies as a subject in its own right. In any field, the best results cannot be achieved until the basic principles are understood. I have therefore tried to integrate theory and practice, and to write in such a way that the reader will be able to adapt and change procedures to suit individual needs and resources. One of the recurring themes in the history of scientific discovery is the improvement in precision and scope of analytical systems. I have therefore emphasized the factors which set the limits to the performance of each system, and indicated ways in which these limits might be extended or bypassed.

I am deeply indebted to many people for help in various aspects of this book. In particular, I want to thank Leonard and Leonore Herzenberg, in whose laboratory I was first introduced to monoclonal antibodies, and to Vernon Oi, Jeff Ledbetter and Israel Pecht, from whom I learned so much. Many people helped by discussions, critical comments and reading portions of the manuscript. I am grateful to Gustav Nossal, Donald Metcalf, Alan

Harris, Grant Morahan, Nick Gough, Suzanne Cory, Roland Scollay and Richard Haugland for many helpful suggestions, and to Jenny Taylor for patient, accurate and cheerful help with typing and word processing. The illustrations were drawn by Richard Mahoney and Peter Maltezos, and were photographed by Sonya Belan.

I would welcome suggestions, criticism or correction from readers of this book, so that any future editions might be as accurate and useful as possible.

James W. Goding   *Melbourne, April 1983*

Preface to Second Edition

It has been very pleasing to see the acceptance of the first edition of this book. However, almost as soon as the manuscript had been sent to the publishers, I found myself compiling a list of ways in which it could be improved. These involved clarification of detail, the discovery of exceptions to generalizations, the rapid advance of knowledge, and correction of errors.

It is said that the best way to neutralize a scientific opponent is to make sure he or she writes a book. I have therefore chosen to update the book selectively, concentrating on areas of practical importance, rather than attempting to give the last word on each of the many topics covered.

Once again, I ask the reader of this book to offer suggestions, criticism or correction.

James W. Goding   *Melbourne, January 1985*

Contents

List of Abbreviations

Å	angstrom unit
AP	ammonium persulphate
Bis	N,N′-methylenebisacrylamide
BLOTTO	5% nonfat powdered milk in PBS
BSA	bovine serum albumin
cpm	counts per minute
DATD	N,N′ diallyltartardiamide
DEAE	diethylaminoethyl
DME	Dulbecco's modified Eagle's medium
DMSO	dimethyl sulphoxide
DTT	dithiothreitol
EDTA	ethylenediamine tetra-acetic acid
ELISA	enzyme-linked immunosorbent assay
FACS	fluorescence-activated cell sorter
FCS	fetal calf serum
FITC	fluorescein isothiocyanate
h	hours
HAT	hypoxanthine, aminopterin, thymidine
HEPES	N-2-hydroxyethylpiperazine-N′-2 ethane sulphonic acid
HGPRT	hypoxanthine guanosine phosphoribosyl transferase
HT	hypoxanthine, thymidine
IEF	isoelectric focusing
Ig	immunoglobulin
M	moles per litre

2ME	2-mercaptoethanol
MEM	minimal Eagle's medium
min	minute
mM	millimoles per litre
M_r	relative molecular mass; molecular weight
NEM	N-ethyl maleimide
NEPHGE	non-equilibrium pH gradient electrophoresis
nm	nanometre
PAGE	polyacrylamide gel electrophoresis
PBS	phosphate-buffered saline
PEG	polyethylene glycol
PMSF	phenylmethylsulphonyl fluoride
RIA	radioimmunoassay
SDS	sodium dodecyl sulphate
TCA	trichloracetic acid
TEMED	N,N,N′,N′-tetramethylene-ethylenediamine
Tris	Tris (hydroxymethyl) aminoethane
TRITC	tetramethylrhodamine isothiocyanate
XRITC	a derivative of rhodamine isothiocyanate

1   Introduction

The last ten years have witnessed the birth and development of genetic engineering. It is now possible to study, control and manipulate genes in ways which continue to amaze even those working in the field. As a result, we have seen a quantum leap in our understanding of biological problems. The development of a technique for the production of monoclonal antibodies was an integral part of this revolution. By combining the nuclei of normal antibody-forming cells with those of their malignant counterparts, Köhler and Milstein (1975) developed an unprecedentedly powerful way of analysing and purifying individual molecules within the enormously complex mixtures encountered in biological material. They were awarded the Nobel Prize in Physiology and Medicine for this work in 1984.

It is important to appreciate that Köhler and Milstein's monumental achievement was the culmination of many seemingly unrelated discoveries by other workers (Table 1.1). Of particular importance were the proof of the clonal selection theory (Nossal and Lederberg, 1958), the development of cell fusion techniques (Okada, 1962; Littlefield, 1964), the artificial induction of plasmacytomas (Potter and Boyce, 1962), and their adaptation to tissue culture (Horibata and Harris, 1970). Finally, the demonstration that it was possible to fuse two different plasma cell tumour lines with retention of both antibody products (Cotton and Milstein, 1973) paved the way for subsequent developments.

In order to appreciate the revolutionary impact of monoclonal antibodies, it is necessary to understand the problems and limitations of conventional serology. Suffice it to say that prior to 1975, the production of antibodies was considered by some to be a black art practised by immunologists. While the

1

Table 1.1 Landmarks in the history of antibody research

1847	Urinary protein in myeloma	Bence Jones
1890	Discovery of antibodies	von Behring and Kitazato
1900	"Side-chain" theory formulated	Ehrlich
	Discovery of ABO blood groups	Landsteiner
1955–6	Allotypes	Grubb, Oudin
1956	Classification of Bence-Jones proteins into two groups (now called κ and λ in honour of their discoverers)	Korngold and Lipari
1957	Clonal selection theory	Burnet
1958	One cell; one antibody	Nossal and Lederberg
	Cell fusion by Sendai virus	Okada
1959	Elucidation of disulphide-bonded chain structure of antibodies	Edelman
1960	Discovery of spontaneous cell fusion	Barski
1962	Demonstration that Bence-Jones proteins are antibody light chains	Edelman and Gally
	Induction of plasmacytomas by mineral oil	Potter and Boyce
1962–3	Controlled proteolytic cleavage of IgG, identification of Fab and Fc; topographic relationship between light and heavy chains	Porter, Fleischman, Pain and Press
1964	Use of mutant cells and selective media to isolate hybrids	Littlefield
1965	Amino acid sequencing reveals that N-terminal half of light chains is variable; C-terminal constant	Hilschmann and Craig
	Postulate of two genes; one polypeptide	Dreyer and Bennett
1969	First complete amino acid sequence of an immunoglobulin; concept of domains	Edelman and colleagues
1970	Hypervariable regions	Wu and Kabat
	Growth of plasmacytomas in continuous culture	Horibata and Harris
1973	Fusion of mouse and rat myeloma cells with preservation of secretion of both immunoglobulins sets the stage for production of monoclonal antibodies	Cotton and Milstein
1975	Construction of hybridomas secreting antibody of predefined specificity	Köhler and Milstein
1976	Demonstration of DNA rearrangements in antibody-forming cells	Tonegawa and colleagues
	Use of polyethylene glycol for cell fusion	Pontecorvo
1977	Cloning and sequencing λ genes; J segments	Tonegawa and colleagues
1977–80	Multiple germ-line genes for V regions	Many authors
	Discovery of D segments	Group of L. Hood
1980	Mechanism of insertion of membrane Ig	Groups led by L. Hood and R. Wall
1982	Discovery that a chromosome translocation in plasma cell tumors involves the oncogene *myc*	Many authors

Table 1.1 cont.

1983	Discovery of "enhancer" elements in Ig genes	Many authors
	Identification of the T cell receptor protein	Group of Marrack
1984	Cloning of genes for T cell receptor	Groups of M. Davis and T. Mak

specificity of antibodies provided a way of overcoming the enormous complexity of biological material, the production of highly specific antisera was difficult and unreliable. It required highly purified antigen. The uncertainties about the specificity of individual antisera led to many prolonged and acrimonious debates. All that has now changed. It is now possible to produce unlimited quantities of exquisitely specific antibodies against virtually any molecule, regardless of the purity of the immunizing antigen. The fine specificity, degree of cross-reaction, affinity, and physical properties of antibodies may be selected to suit individual needs.

It would be wrong to think that monoclonal antibodies will completely replace conventional serology. The production of monoclonal antibodies involves a great deal of work, and a high level of commitment. There will often be occasions when the effort required may not be justified. Fortunately, a wide range of monoclonal antibodies is becoming available commercially. Polyclonal antibodies may be preferred when the antigen to be recognized is denatured or altered in some other way. It would be unwise to use monoclonal antibodies for the detection of molecules in genetically diverse species without thorough testing to ensure that some molecules do not escape detection due to genetic polymorphism. For all these reasons, the book concludes with a chapter on the production of conventional antibodies.

I have written this book because I believe that previous accounts of the production, and particularly the usage, of monoclonal antibodies have been too dogmatic and inflexible. "Recipes" have been given which work if followed to the letter, but little attention has been given to the underlying principles. In the real world, one has to adapt each procedure to an individual biological problem.

I have therefore tried to emphasize the important variables which make for success or failure in the use of antibodies, and those points of refinement which allow the capabilities of a system to be pushed to the limit. I have also tried to point out areas in which the literature gives misleading impressions, and a few situations in which published procedures are unreliable.

This book thus represents the distillation and critical evaluation of many hundreds of publications relating to the production and use of antibodies, together with some of my own experience. Immunochemistry also has an oral tradition, and a surprising number of key elements of knowledge are not easily accessible from the literature. I have incorporated some of these elements where appropriate; in many cases no citation is possible.

It is not possible to cover all possible applications of antibodies in one book, nor would it be wise to attempt to do so. I have therefore restricted the book to the "core" techniques of production and handling of antibodies, and their use in studies of antigen analysis, purification and localization. Similarly, it is neither possible nor desirable to cite all the literature. I have chosen references which explain basic principles, or illustrate the use of these principles in practical situations.

Finally, I have tried to write a book that would be useful to a wide range of biologists. The use of antibodies is becoming increasingly important in botany, cell biology, embryology, endocrinology, enzymology, forensic studies, genetics, haematology, medicine, microbiology, molecular biology, neurobiology and parasitology. It is not realistic to expect workers in these fields to be intimately acquainted with the minutiae of immunochemistry, and yet it is very likely that they will need to use antibodies at some point in their research.

Increasingly, success in the biological sciences is achieved by those individuals who refuse to accept the artificial boundaries between fields. It is to them that this book is dedicated.

References

Cotton, R. G. H. and Milstein, C. (1973). Fusion of two immunoglobulin-producing myeloma cells. *Nature* **244**, 42–43.

Horibata, K. and Harris, A. W. (1970). Mouse myelomas and lymphomas in culture. *Exp. Cell Res.* **60**, 61–77.

Köhler, G. and Milstein, C. (1975). Continuous cultures of fused cells secreting antibody of predefined specificity. *Nature* **256**, 495–497.

Littlefield, J. W. (1964). Selection of hybrids from matings of fibroblasts *in vitro* and their presumed recombinants. *Science* **145**, 709–710.

Nossal, G. J. V. and Lederberg, J. (1958). Antibody production by single cells. *Nature* **181**, 1419–1420.

Okada, Y. (1962). Analysis of giant polynuclear cell formation caused by HVJ virus from Ehrlich's ascites tumor cells. I. Microscopic observation of giant polynuclear cell formation. *Exp. Cell Res.* **26**, 98–107.

Potter, M. and Boyce, C. R. (1962). Induction of plasma cell neoplasms in strain BALB/c mice with mineral oil adjuvants. *Nature* **193**, 1086–1087.

2   Theory of Monoclonal Antibodies

In this chapter, the cellular and genetic mechanisms of antibody formation will be described, leading up to the mechanisms of antibody assembly and secretion. The major physical and biological properties of the various immunoglobulin classes will be discussed. Finally, the consequences of the heterogeneity of immune responses will be explored, and the concept of monoclonal serology introduced.

2.1 The Clonal Selection Theory

The problem of antibody diversity is one of the central themes of immunology. Prior to the 1950s it was widely believed that antigen must somehow "instruct" the specificity of antibodies by providing some sort of template. However, the clear demonstration that proteins had defined sequences (Sanger and Thompson, 1953), and the gradual realization that the primary amino acid sequence was sufficient to specify all the biological activity of a protein (reviewed by Anfinsen, 1973) created great difficulties for instructionist theories. Even more importantly, the elucidation of the structure of DNA, the genetic code, the mechanism of protein synthesis and the realization that the flow of sequence information from DNA to protein was essentially one-way, provided the final nails in the coffin of instructionist theories.

The clonal selection theory (Burnet, 1957) avoided all these difficulties by postulating that each lymphocyte had a unique receptor specificity, and was thus precommitted to making only one antibody after appropriate stimulation (Fig. 2.1). The theory was able to explain the specificity of the immune response within the general framework of modern genetics, although it took

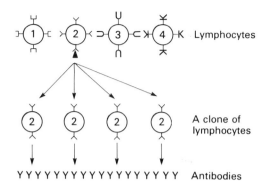

Fig. 2.1. *The clonal selection theory. Interaction of antigen (solid triangle) with specific receptor immunoglobulins on the surface of clone 2 leads to proliferation and differentiation into cells which secrete antibody of the same specificity as the receptor.*

a further quarter of a century before the precise mechanisms of diversity generation were understood.

Evidence in support of the clonal selection theory was first provided by Nossal and Lederberg (1958), who showed that single antibody-forming cells from rats immunized with two different antigens made antibody to one or other antigens, but never both. However, the clonal selection theory remained controversial until the mid-1960s, and it was not until the Cold Spring Harbor Conference of 1967 that it was generally accepted (Burnet, 1968).

Since the clonal selection theory was enunciated, it has been found that lymphocytes can be divided into two families. B lymphocytes, which are the precursors of antibody-forming cells, are formed in the bone marrow and bear "receptor" forms of antibody on their surfaces. T lymphocytes arise in the thymus, and do not make conventional antibodies, although their receptor for antigen is clearly related to antibodies in structure (Chien *et al.*, 1984). The main function of T cells is regulation of the immune response of B cells via "help" and "suppression". In addition, a subset of T cells is capable of differentiating into cytotoxic killer cells, which may be important in the elimination of virally infected cells and foreign grafts. It is now well established that clonal selection applies to both T and B families.

The clonal selection theory provides the conceptual framework for all that follows in this book. We will return to clonal selection towards the end of this chapter.

2.2 Structure of Antibodies

As a general rule, antibodies are symmetrical molecules made up of two identical glycosylated heavy chains of M_r (relative molecular mass, or molecular weight) 50 000–75 000, and two identical nonglycosylated light chains of $M_r \sim 25\,000$. The heavy chains are joined by disulphide bonds to each other, and each light chain is joined by a disulphide bond to one heavy chain (Fig. 2.2). Proteins which have the general structural features of antibodies, but which do not have known antigen-bonding properties, are known as *immunoglobulins*. Although disulphide bonding between chains is characteristic of immunoglobulins, the exact number and location of such bonds is somewhat variable (Nisonoff *et al.*, 1975).

Immunoglobulins may be grouped into five main *classes*: IgM, IgD, IgG, IgE and IgA. Individual classes of immunoglobulins have distinctive structural and biological properties (Table 2.1). The class of an immunoglobulin molecule is determined by its heavy chains. Thus IgM, IgD, IgG, IgE and IgA possess μ, δ, γ, ε and α heavy chains respectively.

In addition, IgG may be subdivided into four *subclasses* (G1–4 in humans; G1, G2a, G2b and G3 in the mouse; G1 G2a, G2b and G2c in the rat). It is important to appreciate that the IgG subclass nomenclature in one species

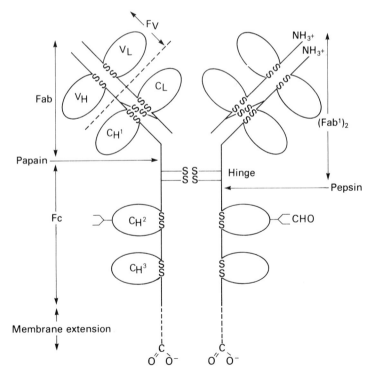

Fig. 2.2. Structure of an IgG molecules. Each chain is made up of a series of homology units of approximately 110 amino acids. The sites of proteolytic cleavage usually lie between the homology units. Membrane forms possess a hydrophobic C-terminal extension, but are otherwise identical in sequence to the secretory forms.

Table 2.1 Properties of mouse immunoglobulin classes (isotypes)

	IgM	IgD	IgG	IgE	IgA
Serum concentration	0.1–1.0 mg/ml	1–10 µg/ml	3–20 mg/ml	0.1–1 µg/ml	1–3 mg/ml
M_r	900 000	180 000	160 000	190 000	170 000–500 000
Heavy chains	µ	δ	γ	ε	α
Heavy chain M_r					
Secretory	80 000	65 000	55 000	80 000	70 000
Membrane	84 000	70–75 000	65 000	?	
Light chains	κ or λ	κ or λ	κ or λ	κ or λ	κ or λ
Subclasses	1	1	4	1	1
Stoichiometry (secreted form)	(µ2 κ2)5 (µ λ2)5	(δ2 κ2)2 (δ2 κ2)	γ2 κ2 γ2 λ2	ε2 κ2 ε2 λ2	(α2 κ2)1–3 (α2 λ2)1–3
Stoichiometry (receptor form)	µ2 κ2 µ2 λ2	δ2 λ2, δ1 κ1 δ2 λ2, δ1 λ1	γ2 κ2 γ2 λ2	?	α2 κ2 α2 λ2
Carbohydrate	9–12%	12–15%	2–3%	12%	7–11%
Prosthetic groups (secreted form)	J Chain	—	—	—	J Chain Secretory piece
Complement-mediated cytotoxicity	+	—	G1 weak or − others +	—	—
Placental passage	—	—	+ (All subclasses)	—	—
Protein A binding	—	—	See text	—	—
E_{280} 0.1% 1 cm	Absorbance at 280 nm largely reflects tryptophan content, and will vary depending on variable region sequence. Typical values are 1.3–1.5. For a rough estimate, assume a value of 1.4.				
Serum half-life	1 day	Short (probably less than 1 day)	G1, G2a, G3 4 days G2b 2 days	Short (probably less than 1 day)	1 day
Special properties	First antibody in most responses	Major class on lymphocyte surface. Minor class in serum.	Major class in serum. IgG-bearing lymphocytes are rare.	Minor class in serum. Binds to mast cells. Responsible for allergic reactions, histamine and serotonin release.	Major class in secretions (e.g. tears, saliva, bile, gut)

bears no particular relationship to that of another species. For example, rat IgG2c is similar to mouse IgG3 and human IgG2 (Der Balian *et al.*, 1980; Nahm *et al.*, 1980). The evolutionary relationship between the IgG subclasses is still far from clear.

There are two types of light chains, κ or λ. Each immunoglobulin class contains molecules with either κ or λ light chains. Individual molecules may possess either κ or λ light chains, but never both.

In the mouse and rat, over 95% of light chains are κ. In the mouse, there is only one κ light chain class, but paradoxically there are four λ chain subclasses (λ_I–λ_{IV}). In humans the κ:λ ratio is about 60:40, but the exact number of subclasses is unknown; there are certainly several λ subclasses.

Both κ and λ light chains appear to be able to take part in all biological functions of antibodies although in some special circumstances and for poorly understood reasons, one light chain may predominate. The light chains play an important part in determining the specificity of antibodies, but all known 'effector' functions of antibodies (e.g. complement-mediated lysis of cells) are determined by the heavy chains.

Each light and heavy chain is made up of a series of *homology units* of ~ 110 amino acids (Fig. 2.2). The amino acid sequences of individual homology units are sufficiently similar to suggest that they arose by gene duplication from a common primordial gene. Each homology unit characteristically contains one intra-chain disulphide bond between cysteine residues situated about 20 amino acids from each end.

Each homology unit is folded into a *domain*, which is a compact, globular structure containing large amounts of β-pleated sheet (Poljak *et al.*, 1972). Individual domains are rather resistant to proteolytic attack (Fig. 2.2). In contrast, the short linking sequences joining individual domains are often susceptible to proteolysis. Some classes of antibody contain an extra *hinge* region (Fig 2.2) which has a more open structure, and is especially susceptible to proteolysis.

The amino acid sequence of the N-terminal homology units varies greatly between molecules, and is therefore known as the *variable* (V) region. The N-terminal homology units of heavy and light chains are designated V_H and V_L respectively. Within each variable region lie three *hypervariable* segments. The V_H and V_L domains are folded in such a way that brings the hypervariable regions together to create an *antigen-combining site*, the specificity of which is determined by both heavy and light chains. Each antibody molecules has two identical antigen-combining sites, except for polymeric IgM, which has ten (see later). The mechanisms of generation of the diverse combining sites will be discussed in a subsequent portion of this chapter.

The heavy and light chains of immunoglobulin molecules remain tightly associated with each other after reduction of all inter-chain disulphide bonds. The reduced chains can only be separated after denaturation in urea, guanidine or acid, indicating the presence of strong noncovalent interactions between chains. X-ray analysis shows that the V_H and V_L domains are in intimate contact with each other, as are C_L and C_H1, and pairs of C_H3 (Huber *et al.*, 1976). On the other hand, interaction between pairs of C_H1, or pairs of C_H2, do not occur (Huber *et al.*, 1976; Deisenhofer *et al.*, 1976).

The affinity of interacting domains is such a prominent feature of antibody structure that some authors define a domain as a *pair* of corresponding homology units folded together (Fig. 2.2). However, the term "domain" is more commonly used to describe the globular structure made up by a single homology unit. The term "domain" is also used in a looser way which is virtually synonymous with "homology unit".

2.2.1 Nature of the Antigen–Antibody Bond

In some cases where detailed crystallographic studies have been performed, the antigen-combining site has been found to consist of a narrow non-polar groove. The bond between antigen and antibody involves multiple weak noncovalent interactions, including electrostatic, hydrogen bonding, van der Waals and hydrophobic effects. Typical dissociation constants are 10^{-5}–10^{-10}M.

Antigen–antibody bonds are usually stable over a pH range of 4–9 and a wide range of salt concentrations (0–1.0 M NaCl), although occasional monoclonal antibodies may be dissociated from their antigen under these mild conditions (Herrman and Mescher, 1979). Dissociation of antigen–antibody bonds more usually requires the use of strong denaturing conditions, such as a pH of less than 3.0 or greater than 10.0, or high concentrations of thiocyanate (3.5 M), guanidine-HCl (6 M) or urea (9 M). Usually, but not always, antibody activity is restored once the denaturing conditions are removed. The question of dissociation of antigen–antibody interactions will be discussed in detail in Chapter 6.

2.2.2 Membrane Immunoglobulins

The heavy chains of membrane bound receptor forms of antibody are identical to the secreted forms over most of their sequence, but contain an extension at their C-terminus which is responsible for membrane attachment (Rogers and Wall, 1984). The C-terminal membrane extension can be divided into three segments. The first is a highly charged ~ 15 amino-acid sequence rich in acidic amino acids, and is followed by an uninterrupted stretch of ~ 25 uncharged and predominantly hydrophobic amino acids which presumably span the lipid bilayer. Finally, there is a basic triplet (lys-val-lys), which probably marks the entry into the cytoplasm. The C-terminal lysine may be removed post-translationally. Membrane IgM and IgD terminate at this point (Rogers *et al.*, 1980; Cheng *et al.*, 1982), while membrane IgG has an additional cytoplasmic "tail" of ~ 28 amino acids (Tyler *et al.*, 1982).

2.2.3 Proteolytic Fragmentation of Immunoglobulins

Controlled proteolysis of immunoglobulins often generates large fragments, with the cleavage sites usually lying between domains. Proteolytic attack of IgG by papain at neutral pH cleaves at the hinge, generating two identical Fab fragments, each containing one intact light chain disulphide-bonded to a fragment of the heavy chain (Fd) containing the V_H and C_H1 domains (Fig. 2.2). The Fab fragments each contain one antigen-combining site. The remaining portion of the IgG molecule consists of a dimer of C_H2 and C_H3, and is called Fc, because in some cases it can be crystallized. The Fc portion is homogeneous, and contains no antigen-binding activity.

In a few very special cases, it is possible to generate an even smaller antigen-binding fragment (Fv) by proteolysis (Fig. 2.2). The Fv fragment contains only the noncovalently associated V_H and V_L domains (Inbar *et al.*,1972; Kakimoto and Onoue, 1974).

Another proteolytic reaction of major importance is the attack of antibodies by pepsin at pH ~ 4. Like papain, pepsin cleaves IgG at the hinge, but the pepsin cleavage site lies on the carboxy side of the inter-heavy chain disulphide bond(s) (Fig. 2.2). The divalent antigen-binding fragment so produced is known at $F(ab')_2$. The heavy chain fragment in $F(ab')_2$ is a little longer than the papain Fd fragment, and is known as Fd'. Pepsin cleavage usually results in the breakdown of the C_H2 domain into small peptides, although under certain circumstances, a fragment approximating a dimer of C_H3 (pFc') may be recovered.

Controlled proteolysis of immunoglobulins is useful in many practical situations, and also illustrates some of the basic principles and nomenclature of antibody structure. However, the rate and nature of fragmentation depends greatly on the species and class of antibody. The "classical" recipes which work well for human or rabbit IgG may fail completely when applied to the mouse or rat, or to classes other than IgG. We will return to this important subject in Chapter 4.

2.3 Properties of the Individual Immunoglobulin Classes

The physical and biological properties of the individual classes of immunoglobulin are summarized in Table 2.1.

2.3.1 IgM

IgM is phylogenetically the oldest immunoglobulin, and is also the first to appear in ontogeny. The μ heavy chain has four constant region domains (Kehry *et al.*, 1979, 1982). Homology considerations suggest that the "extra" domain over IgG is $C_\mu 2$, which is located between $C_\mu 1$ and the first inter-heavy chain disulphide bonds. IgM lacks a well-defined hinge, although the preferred site of proteolytic attack is usually the region of the $C_\mu 2$ domain (Shimizu *et al.*, 1974). Overall, IgM is rather resistant to proteolysis. Fragmentation of IgM will be discussed in Chapter 4.

In mammals, secretory IgM consists of a pentamer (M_r 900 000) of $\mu_2\kappa_2$ or $\mu_2\kappa_2$ subunits ("monomers") with an M_r of 180 000. The membrane receptor form of IgM is a monomer in which the heavy chains possess a hydrophobic C-terminal extension. Subunits of pentameric murine IgM are held together be easily reduced disulphide bonds, most likely at Cys 575 in the $C_\mu 4$ domain (Milstein *et al.*, 1975).

Pentameric IgM also contains a single J chain, a very acidic non-immunoglobulin polypeptide of $M_r \sim 15\,000$, which is rich in carbohydrate and cysteine residues. J chain is somehow involved in the polymerization of IgM, and is probably added in the endoplasmic reticulum (Tartakoff and Vassalli, 1979). It is disulphide bonded to the Cys 575 residues of two adjacent IgM monomers. The function of J chain will be discussed in Section 2.3.5.

IgM consitutes roughly 5% of total serum immunoglobulins, although the levels vary depending on the degree of antigenic stimulation. Catabolism of IgM is rapid. The serum half-life in the mouse is approximately 1 day (Spiegelberg, 1974).

IgM is the first antibody to appear in most immune responses. In some cases, particularly for autoantibodies, it may be the only class represented. IgM antibodies are usually of relatively low affinity, and their affinity does not seem to rise (i.e. "mature") with time (Gearheart *et al.*, 1981). However, the relatively low affinity of IgM antibodies is compensated for by multi-valency. If all sites are available for binding to antigen, the functional affinity or "avidity" might theoretically be equal to the affinity of one combining site raised to the power of the number of sites involved. Because pentameric IgM has ten antigen-binding sites (Nisonoff *et al.*, 1975), its functional avidity may be extremely large, and it may thus perform well in an initial response to infection. IgM is also very effective in complement-mediated cell lysis, perhaps because of the close proximity of multiple Fc units in the pentamer.

2.3.2 IgD

In marked contrast to all the other immunoglobulins classes, IgD is rarely secreted, and its main function seems to be as a receptor for antigen (Blattner and Tucker, 1984). The murine δ chain has an M_r of $\sim 68\,000$, and contains only two constant region domains (Cδ1 and Cδ3) and an extended hinge (Liu *et al.*, 1980). The rat δ chain has a similar structure. The human δ chain is somewhat larger, containing three constant region domains (Cδ1, Cδ2 and Cδ3), and also has an extended hinge (Takahashi *et al.*, 1982).

The great majority of mature B lymphocytes have IgD on their surface, usually in combination with IgM, and on any one B cell the two classes of receptor have the same specificity for antigen (Goding and Layton, 1976). Immature B lymphocytes possess only IgM on their surface, and IgD is acquired with maturation. Most splenic B cells have approximately 10 times as much IgD as IgM on their surface (Havran *et al.*, 1984). After stimulation of the B cell with mitogen, IgD is rapidly lost (Bourgois *et al.*, 1977). This orderly appearance and disappearance thus suggests a unique physiological role for IgD, but so far none has been found.

Unlike IgM, IgD is highly susceptible to proteolytic cleavage at the hinge (Vitetta and Uhr, 1975; Goding, 1980; Takahashi *et al.*, 1982). Membrane IgM and IgD both contain a hydrophobic C-terminal segment which ends in lys-val-lys. The terminal tripeptide presumably marks the entry into the cytoplasm. The amino acid sequences of the transmembrane segments and cytoplasmic tails of IgM and IgD are highly homologous, and it has been suggested that any difference in signalling function must arise from their extracellular portions, which are very dissimilar (Cheng *et al.*, 1982).

Secretory forms of IgD also exist, and very rarely IgD myelomas are found (Finkelman *et al.*, 1981). In contrast to membrane IgD, the secretory form has a hydrophilic C-terminus (Takahashi *et al.*, 1982; Cheng *et al.*, 1982).

There is some variation in inter-heavy chain disulphide bonds in murine IgD. The membrane form sometimes lacks an inter-heavy chain disulphide bond (Pollock *et al.*, 1980) while the secretory form appears to be a disulphide-bonded dimer of the basic $\delta_2 L_2$ structure (Finkelman *et al.*, 1981).

The levels of secretory IgD in serum are very low (of the order of $1-10\,\mu g/$ml). Secretory IgD does not appear to fix complement, cross the placenta, cause mast cell degranulation, or localize in secretions. So far its role is completely unknown.

2.3.3 IgG

IgG is by far the most abundant immunoglobulin in serum. It consists of two heavy chains of M_r of $\sim 160\,000$. The constant regions of γ chains have three regular domains (Cγ1, Cγ2 and Cγ3) and a short hinge. In the mouse and rat, there are four IgG subclasses (Table 2.2).

The four IgG subclasses have heavy chains with virtually identical molecular weights, and cannot be distinguished with certainty by electrophoretic mobility in agarose or cellulose acetate under non-denaturing conditions

(Section 2.3.7). In general, $\gamma 1$ antibodies have a "faster" (i.e. more anodal) mobility than $\gamma 2$, although there is considerable overlap. It is virtually impossible to separate mouse or rat IgG subclasses by classical procedures such as ion exchange chromatography or zone electrophoresis. The heavy chains of murine IgG2b run as a double band on SDS-polyacrylamide gel electrophoresis (Köhler *et al.*, 1978; Parham, 1983; Lo *et al.*, 1984).

In spite of their virtually identical size and overlapping electrophoretic mobilities, the murine $\gamma 1$, $\gamma 2a$, $\gamma 2b$ and $\gamma 3$ subclasses have rather dissimilar amino acid sequences, and apart from $\gamma 2a$ and $\gamma 2b$ show little serological cross-reaction. In fact, they are so different that some authors have considered them to be different classes (named IgF, IgG, IgH and IgI respectively; see Potter and Lieberman, 1967).

The $C_H 1$ homology units of mouse $\gamma 1$, $\gamma 2a$ and $\gamma 2b$ are $\sim 85\%$ homologous. The $C_H 2$ domains of $\gamma 2a$ and $\gamma 2b$ are 94% homologous, but only 67% homologous to $\gamma 1$, while the $C_H 3$ domains of $\gamma 2a$ and $\gamma 2b$ are only 61% homologous to each other and $\sim 55\%$ homologous to $\gamma 1$ (Sikorav *et al.*, 1980). Hinge region homology varies from 18% ($\gamma 1 : \gamma 2b$) to 64% ($\gamma 2a : \gamma 2b$). In this context, it is interesting to note that there is a correlation between hinge region flexibility and ability to fix complement. IgG1 has a rigid hinge

Table 2.2 Properties of IgG subclasses

Species	Subclass	Complement-mediated Cytotoxicity	Protein A[a] Binding	Comments
Mouse	G1	−	pH > 8 (weak)	Fast electrophoretic mobility. Major subclass.
	G2a	+ +	pH > 4.5	Major subclass.
	G2b	+ + +	pH > 3.5	Tends to precipitate in low salt concentrations.
	G3	+	pH > 4.5	Minor subclass; associated with anti-carbohydrate activity. Tends to precipitate in low salt concentrations.
Rat	G1	−	−	Minor subclass. Sometimes binds to protein A.
	G2a	±	±	Major subclass.
	G2b	+	−	Major subclass.
	G2c	+	+	Minor subclass; associated with anti-carbohydrate activity. Tends to precipitate in low salt concentrations.

[a]See Chapter 4.

and cannot fix complement, while IgG2b has a flexible hinge and is very efficient in complement fixation (Oi *et al.*, 1984).

The IgG subclasses of the mouse and rat have quite distinct biological properties (Table 2.2). It is important to note that the similar names of the mouse and rat IgG subclasses do not imply homology in structure or function. The properties of the mouse subclasses are characterized with more certainty than those of the rat, where some controversy still exists (Bazin *et al.*, 1974; Medgyesi *et al.*, 1978; Ledbetter and Herzenberger, 1979). Part of the confusion has probably resulted from the use of artificially aggregated myeloma proteins to assess complement fixation, rather than "real" antibody binding and cytotoxicity assays (see Neuberger and Rajewsky, 1981; Hirayama *et al.*, 1982). It may be anticipated that as the number of well characterized hybridoma proteins increases, we will have a much clearer picture.

All of the IgG subclasses are relatively stable in solution, although they can be cleaved at the hinge by proteolytic enzymes under appropriate conditions (see Chapter 4 for details). Murine IgG2b and IgG3 and rat IgG2c are inclined to precipitate in low salt concentrations (< 50 mM), and are rather prone to aggregation upon freezing.

From a practical point of view, one of the most useful properties of IgG is its interaction with staphylococcal protein A (Goding, 1978; Surolia *et al.*, 1982). Affinity chromatography on protein A-agarose is a very simple and efficient way of purifying IgG, and differential elution from protein A with stepwise pH gradients is capable of separating most mouse IgG subclasses (Ey *et al.* 1978; Seppälä *et al.*, 1981). The protein A-binding region has been localized to the junction of the C_H2 and C_H3 domains (Lancet *et al.*, 1978). Purification of IgG by affinity chromatography on protein A-agarose is discussed in detail in Chapter 4.

One very important property of IgG is the binding of its Fc portion to "Fc receptors" present on many cell types (Dickler, 1976). This binding is relatively low affinity, and is mainly observed when aggregation of IgG increases the strength of interaction. Nonetheless, some cell types (especially macrophages) possess relatively high affinity for monomeric IgG (Unkeless, 1979).

Binding of antibody to Fc receptors is important from a practical viewpoint because it may cause artefactual 'nonspecific' binding to tissues. This artefact has probably been responsible for many misleading observations in the literature (Vitetta and Uhr, 1975; Winchester *et al.*, 1975). Although there are reports indicating that certain subclasses of IgG bind to certain types of Fc receptors, no safe generalizations can be made at present. Controls for Fc receptor binding should include use of a control antibody of the *same subclass* but different specificity to the active antibody. It is wise to deaggregate IgG antibodies by high speed centrifugation (100 000 **g**) just before each use. The Beckmann Airfuge is ideal for this purpose, because only 5–10 min at 100 000 **g** are required. Alternatively, Fab or F(ab')$_2$ fragments may be used to prevent binding to Fc receptors (Chapter 4).

2.3.4 IgE

IgE is a quantitatively very minor immunoglobulin class (serum concentration $\sim 0.3\,\mu g/ml$). It consists of two light chains and two ε chains of M_r $\sim 70\,000$ (Liu *et al.*, 1980). Sequence studies indicate the presence of four constant region domains (Dorrington and Bennich, 1978; Ishida *et al.*, 1982).

IgE is responsible for hypersensitivity and allergic reactions, which are mediated by binding of IgE to mast cells, followed by degranulation upon antigenic stimulation. Binding of IgE to mast cells occurs via a specific receptor for $Fc(\varepsilon)$, and the signal for degranulation involves antigen-mediated cross-linking of these receptors (Metzger, 1978).

IgE myelomas are very rare in man, and so far none have been reported in the mouse. However, a number of rat IgE myelomas have been described (Bazin *et al.*, 1973). IgE-secreting hybridomas with specificity against ovalbumin and dinitrophenyl have been constructed (Böttcher *et al.*, 1978; Liu *et al.*, 1980; Eshhar *et al.*, 1980). The biological advantage of IgE is not known, although it is suspected to be an important defense against parasitic infestation (Mitchell, 1979).

2.3.5 IgA

IgA is the main immunoglobulin of body fluids, such as saliva, tears, colostrum and intestinal secretions (Tomasi and Grey, 1972; Lamm, 1976), and is also present at low concentrations in serum. The molecular weight of the α heavy chain is approximately $68\,000-75\,000$, (the range is due to carbohydrate heterogeneity), and there are three constant region homology units (Tucker *et al.*, 1981).

In serum IgA consists mainly of an $\alpha_2 L_2$ tetramer of $M_r \sim 180\,000$, but also as disulphide-bonded polymers of this basic structure (Nisonoff *et al.*, 1975). IgA myeloma proteins show similar heterogeneity. The disulphide bond between polyer subunits is easily reduced. In IgA myelomas of BALB/c mice, the light chains are not disulphide bonded to the heavy chains. The disposition of the disulphide bonds in mouse IgA is somewhat variable (Stanisz *et al.*, 1983) and will be discussed in Section 2.3.6.

In contrast to the serum form, IgA in secretory fluids is mostly a disulphide-bonded dimer of the basic $\alpha_2 L_2$ structure. Secretory IgA also contains J chain disulphide bonded to the Fc piece (Koshland, 1975), and a second non-immunoglobulin component known as "secretory piece" or "secretory component". Secretory component is attached to α chains by strong noncovalent forces, and also by disulphide bonding in some species (Tomasi and Grey, 1972).

It has recently been shown that secretory piece is a proteolytic fragment of the receptor for IgA on epithelial cells. The complete amino acid sequence of the receptor for transepithelial transport of IgA is now known. It contains five extracellular domains which are strikingly homologous to each other and to antibody variable regions (Mostov *et al.*, 1984). The function of J chain in dimeric IgA and pentameric IgM appears to involve the creation of a binding site for the receptor for these antibodies on epithelial cells (i.e. secretory piece) (Brandtzaeg and Prydz, 1984). It appears that transport of IgA from serum into bile involves binding to secretory piece, endocytosis via coated vesicles, transport through the cell, and exocytosis at the luminal side of the cell with part of the receptor (the "secretory piece") still attached (Kühn and Kraehenbuhl, 1981; Mullock and Hinton, 1981). In addition to its transport function, secretory piece may protect IgA from proteolysis.

IgA has two subclasses (IgA1 and IgA2) in man, goats, monkeys and rabbits (Nisonoff *et al.*, 1975) but only one in rats and mice. IgA2 constitutes about 10% of IgA in serum, but about 50% in secretory fluids (Grey *et al.*, 1968). The α_1 and α_2 chains are encoded by separate genes.

IgA does not mediate complement-dependent cell lysis by the direct pathway. Its main role is probably to neutralize viruses and bacteria, and to mediate excretion of antigen via the bile (Peppard *et al.*, 1981; Russell *et al.*, 1981). The increased valency of secretory IgA polymers may aid viral neutralization, and its great resistance to proteolysis probably improves its survival in the gut (Underdown and Dorrington, 1974).

2.3.6 Immunoglobulin Allotypes

The products of allelic forms of the same gene are known as *allotypes*. Allotypes are now known for all mouse heavy chains (Lieberman, 1978; Herzenberg and Herzenberg, 1977; Borges *et al.*, 1981; Huang *et al.*, 1984; Amor *et al.*, 1984). There are no known serologically detectable allotypes of mouse κ chains. The constant regions of $\lambda 1$ chains of mice show a single amino acid difference between BALB/c and SJL mice (Arp *et al.*, 1982). In the rat, the κ chains show extensive polymorphism (Sheppard and Gutman, 1981a,b), and variants have also been described for α and $\gamma 2b$ heavy chains (Gasser, 1977).

Immunoglobulin allotypes are important for several reasons. They allow genetic linkage studies to be carried out, and the origin of immunoglobulins to be determined in cell transfer experiments. They were central in demonstrating allelic exclusion (see later), in showing that variable and constant region genes were linked, and in showing that all the heavy chain genes are linked to each other. However, a detailed account of the esoteric world of immunoglobulin allotypes is beyond the scope of this book. A comprehensive review of mouse immunoglobulin allotypes is given by Herzenberg and Herzenberg (1977).

The heavy chain locus in the mouse is designated *Igh*, and the constant

Table 2.3 Locus symbols for mouse immunoglobulin heavy chains

Constant region	*Igh-C*
Constant region loci	*Igh-1* (γ2a)
	Igh-2 (α)
	Igh-3 (γ2b)
	Igh-4 (γ1)
	Igh-5 (δ)
	Igh-6 (μ)
	Igh-7 (ε)
	Igh-8 (γ3)

region loci are designated *Igh-C*. The genes are named in order of discovery *Igh-1* to *Igh-8* (Table 2.3). [Note that the order of the genes on the chromosome (Fig. 2.4) is completely different]. Alleles at each locus are designated by superscripts (e.g. *Igh-1^b*). The *combination* of *Igh-C* alleles in a particular mouse strain is known as a *haplotype*, and in many cases the haplotype designation is the same letter as the allele for that strain at the *Igh-1* (γ2a) locus (Table 2.4).

The structural bases of these variations are still being elucidated. In many cases, there are multiple amino acid substitutions at several different regions of the chain (Sheppard and Gutman, 1981a,b; Ollo and Rougeon, 1983). Allotypic variation can affect physical properties such as solubility, binding to staphylococcal protein A (Seppälä *et al.*, 1981) and electrophoretic mobility (Herzenberg *et al.*, 1967). Mouse IgG of the *b* allotype (i.e. from C57Bl and related strains) is less soluble than IgG of the *a* allotype (from BALB/c).

One particularly interesting allotypic difference concerns IgA. In BALB/c mice, the light chains of myeloma IgA are disulphide bonded to each other and not to the heavy chains, while the conventional IgA structure is seen in myelomas from NZB mice (Warner and Marchalonis, 1972). A similar genetic variation is seen in human IgA2 (Grey *et al.*, 1968). Until recently, it was thought that the different arrangement of disulphide bonds seen in BALB/c and NZB IgA myeloma proteins reflected the known allotypic difference. However, it has now been shown that each strain produces both forms of IgA, and that in each strain, both forms share the serological allotypic characteristics of that strain (Stanisz *et al.*, 1983). It would therefore appear that the myeloma proteins are not necessarily typical of the structure of all IgA molecules produced by these strains. It would appear that these mouse strains have a single α chain gene (Tucker *et al.*, 1981), so the dimorphism in mouse IgA structure is probably not a consequence of the known allotypic differences in α chain (see Stanisz *et al.*, 1983, for further discussion).

Table 2.4 Distribution of alleles of the Igh-C loci in the Igh-C haplotypes

Haplotype	Prototype Strain	Locus and Chain							
		Igh-1 γ2a	Igh-2 α	Igh-3 γ2b	Igh-4 γ1	Igh-5 δ	Igh-6 μ	Igh-7 ε	Igh-8[a] γ3
a	BALB/c	a	a	a	a	a	a	a	a
b	C57B1	b	b	b	b	b	b	b	a
c	DBA/2	c	c	a	a	a	—	—	a
d	AKR	d	d/e	d	d	d	d	a	a
e	A/J	e	d/e	e	a	e	e	a	a
f	CE	f	f	f	a	a	—	—	a
g	RIII	g	c	g	a	a	—	—	a
h	SEA	h	a	a	a	a	a	a	a
j	CBA/H	j	a	a	a	a	a	a	a
k	KH-1	k	c	a	a	—	—	—	a
l	KH-2	l	c	a	a	—	—	a	a
m	Ky	m	b	b	b	d	—	—	a
n	NZB	e	d/e	e	d	d	d	—	a
o	AL/N	d	d/e	d	a	e	e	—	a

[a] Allelic forms of γ3 chains have only been found in wild mice and the SPE strain of Mus spretus (Huang et al., 1984; Amor et al., 1984).

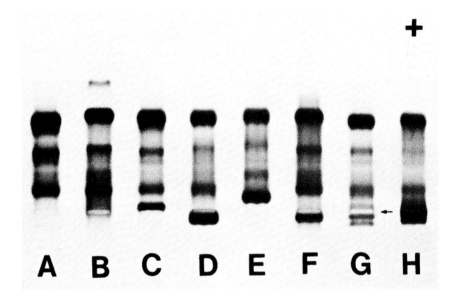

Fig. 2.3. *Agarose gel electrophoresis of serum from mice. The anode is at the top, and the origin is marked with an arrow. A: Specific pathogen-free mice. Note the virtual absence of gamma globulins. B: Mice infected with the parasite M. corti. These mice have very high levels of polyclonal IgG1, and raised levels of a protein which migrates more rapidly than albumin. C: Mice bearing the IgG1 myeloma MOPC-21. D: Mice bearing the IgG2a myeloma MOPC-173. E: Mice bearing the IgG2b myeloma MPC-11. F: Mice bearing the IgG3 myeloma Y5606. G: Mice bearing the hybridoma MAR-18-5 (Lanier et al., 1982), which contains γ1 chains from MOPC-21 and γ2a chains from spleen. Note the three "spikes" in the gamma globulin region, due to γ1/γ1, γ1/γ2a and γ2a/γ2a hybrid molecules. H: Mice bearing the IgM myeloma HPC-76.*

2.3.7 Serum Electrophoresis

Serum is a complex mixture of several hundred proteins. The total protein concentration is about 70 mg/ml; by far the most abundant single protein is albumin ($\approx$ 40 mg/ml). When analysed by electrophoresis in agarose or cellulose acetate at pH 8.3–8.6, albumin is visible as a single intense band at the anodal end (Fig. 2.3), consistent with its small size and acidic nature (pI $\approx$ 4.9). Most of the remaining bands in normal serum electrophoresis consist of mixtures of several different components, although some are identifiable as distinct proteins (Jeppsson *et al.*, 1979).

Proteins with the general structure of antibodies are referred to as *immunoglobulins* or the virtually obsolete term *gamma globulins*. They migrate as a broad band situated close to the origin (Fig. 2.3). Depending on the pH and the degree of electro-endomosis in the supporting matrix, they may move slightly towards the cathode, remain near the origin, or move slightly towards the anode. Typical immunoglobulin levels in normal mouse serum range from 1–10 mg/ml, depending on the degree of antigenic stimulation. In specific pathogen-free mice, the immunoglobulin levels may be virtually undetectable.

As a general rule, IgG1 and IgA antibodies have a more anodal ("faster") mobility than IgG2, but there is considerable overlap. IgM antibodies tend to stay close to the origin because of retardation by sieving effects.

2.4 Biosynthesis and Assembly of Immunoglobulins

The biosynthesis of immunoglobulins follows the same general pathway as other secretory and membrane glycoproteins (reviewed by Wall and Kuehl, 1983). Nascent chains are formed on polyribosomes bound to the cytoplasmic surface of the endoplasmic reticulum, and their N-terminal hydrophobic "leader sequence" guides them through the membrane and into the lumen (Milstein *et al.*, 1972; Walter and Blobel, 1982). As the nascent chain appears on the luminal side, its leader sequence is proteolytically removed and glycosylation occurs (Tartakoff and Vassalli, 1979). Secretory forms of heavy chains pass into the lumen, while membrane forms remain embedded in the membrane via their hydrophobic C-terminus (Vassalli *et al.*, 1980). Membrane and secretory forms are assembled in the same intracellular compartment (Goding, 1982).

Carbohydrate is added to the nascent heavy chains via preformed dolichol phosphate donor, and is initially of the "high mannose" endoglycosidase H-sensitive type containing N-acetyl glucosamine and mannose, but lacking galactose and sialic acid (Tartakoff and Vassalli, 1979; Goding and Herzenberg, 1980). In most cases, the carbohydrate of immunoglobulins is attached to asparagine. Glycosylation of serine and threonine is uncommon in immunoglobulins, but is known to occur in IgA and IgD. The light chains are usually not glycosylated.

Shortly after synthesis, pairing of heavy and light chains commences. In some cases the order of assembly is H → HH → HHL → LHHL, while in others it is H → HL → LHHL (Baumal and Scharff, 1973; Bergman and Kuehl, 1979). Assembly appears to depend on random collision and follow the law of mass action (Goding, 1982). Formation of inter-chain disulphide bonds probably requires a disulphide exchange enzyme (Roth and Koshland, 1981a,b). Most immunoglobulin-secreting cells make an excess of light chains, and these are usually secreted (Parkhouse, 1971; Goding and Herzenberg, 1980). Isolated heavy chains without light chains are thought to be toxic to the cell (Köhler, 1980; Argon *et al.*, 1983).

Following initial glycosylation and assembly, immunoglobulins are transported to the Golgi apparatus, probably via coated vesicles. In the Golgi, the carbohydrate chains are trimmed and galactose and sialic acid added, producing modified carbohydrates which are generally resistant to endoglycosidase H (Tartakoff and Vassalli, 1979; Goding and Herzenberg, 1980). Polymerization of IgM to the pentameric form and addition of J chain occur in the endoplasmic reticulum (Tartakoff and Vassalli, 1979).

The role of carbohydrate in immunoglobulins is still poorly understood (Wall and Kuehl, 1983). Treatment of cells with tunicamycin (an antibiotic which blocks addition of N-linked sugars) reduces IgM secretion but does not affect IgG secretion (Blatt and Haimovitch, 1981). Glycosylation is not essential for membrane insertion or secretion, and there are as yet no general differences in glycosylation between membrane and secretory forms (Vassalli *et al.*, 1980). Nonglycosylated forms of glycoproteins from tunicamycin-treated cells are often very sensitive to proteolysis, and one function of glycosylation may be to protect membrane and secretory proteins from extracellular proteases (Olden *et al.*, 1982). Nose and Wigzell (1983) found that IgG2b antibodies lacking N-linked glycans bound antigen normally (a feature of the Fab region), and still bound to staphylococcal protein A (dependent on integrity of the C_H2/C_H3 junction). However, they lost the ability to bind to Fc receptors on macrophages, to activate complement and to induce antibody-dependent cellular cytotoxicity. Antigen–antibody complexes failed to be rapidly removed from circulation. It has been suggested that IgG2b may possess an O-linked glycan on one chain (Parham, 1983), which would not be eliminated by tunicamycin. Nonetheless, the results of Nose and Wigzell point to an important role for N-linked sugars.

2.5 Antibody Genes

2.5.1 Three Clusters of Genes

Antibody genes exist in three clusters; κ light chains, λ light chains, and heavy chains (Gally and Edelman, 1972). In the mouse, the κ group lies on chromosome 6, and the heavy chain group on chromosome 12. Mouse λ chain genes are situated on chromosome 16 (D'Eustachio *et al.*, 1981). In each case, the genes for the variable region are linked to the constant region genes.

In recent years, studies using recombinant DNA technologies have given an extremely detailed picture of mouse immunoglobulin genes (reviewed by Early and Hood, 1981a). A simplified picture is given in Fig. 2.4. The overall organisation of the DNA is best thought of as a series of discrete coding segments separated by variable distances.

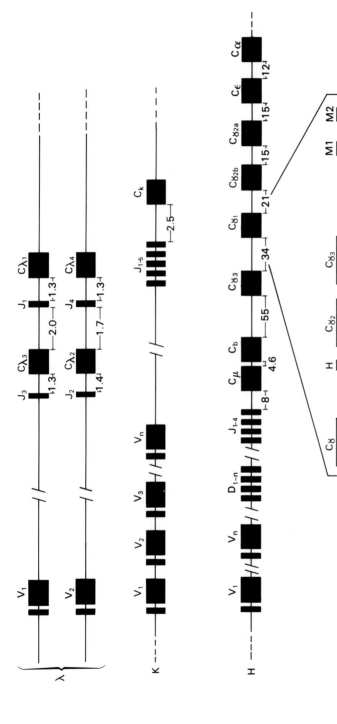

Fig. 2.4. Organization of immunoglobulin genes. There are three clusters, situated on different chromosomes, encoding λ light chains and heavy chains. The light chain genes contain segments encoding the hydrophobic leader sequence, the variable region, the joining (J) region, and the constant region. The heavy chain complex possesses in addition a number of "D" (diversity) segments between V and J. The constant region domains of the heavy chains are encoded by discrete segments (open boxes). Downstream from the last constant domain of each heavy chain lie two segments (M1 and M2) which encode the membrane extension.

2.5.2 The κ Complex

The mouse κ complex has only one constant region gene, but has a few hundred variable region genes (Cory *et al.*, 1981). Each variable region (V) gene consists of two separate coding segments, one encoding the N-terminal leader sequence, and the other encoding the body of the variable region (Fig. 2.4). The variable region genes are situated an unknown but large distance upstream (i.e. on the 5′ side) of the constant region genes. (By convention, DNA sequences are written the same way as RNA, with the 5′ end to the left.)

Approximately 2500 bases upstream from the κ constant region gene is a cluster of five "J" or joining genes, each of some 39 nucleotides, which encode the last few amino acids of the variable region. It is likely that only four J genes are expressed. In lymphoid cells expressing κ light chains, one V_κ gene is joined directly onto one J gene, and the intervening DNA is excised (Fig. 2.5). The J genes downstream from the chosen J are retained, but the upstream J genes are deleted.

2.5.3 The λ Complex

In many respects, the λ complex is the simplest. There are now known to be four λ constant region genes, but paradoxically there are only two variable region genes (Fig. 2.4). As for κ and heavy chains, each variable region gene has its own leader sequence separated from the main portion. Approximately 1000 bases upstream from each λ constant region gene is a single J gene. A functional λ chain gene is formed in a similar way to the κ genes. In lymphoid cells expressing λ chains, one V_λ gene is joined onto a J gene, and the intervening DNA excised (see Fig. 2.5).

Very early in the development of the B lymphocyte (shortly after μ heavy chain synthesis begins), each cell attempts to produce a functional κ light chain gene. If this succeeds, the cell and all its progeny are committed to κ.

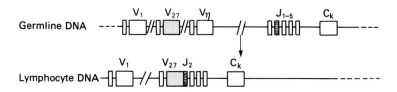

Fig. 2.5. Rearrangements of DNA encoding κ light chains in the mouse. In the germline, there are several hundred variable region genes (each with its own leader sequence slightly upstream), five J genes and one constant region gene. Expression of light chains in lymphocytes involves movement of a particular V gene such that it becomes contiguous with a particular J gene. The intervening DNA (containing V and J genes) is deleted, but the J genes and DNA between the chosen J and C_κ remain unchanged.

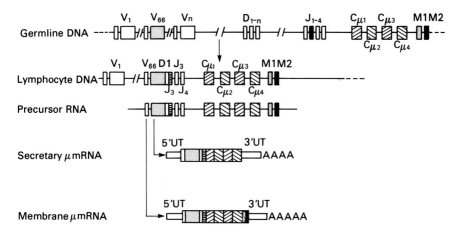

Fig. 2.6. DNA rearrangements in heavy chain genes, and subsequent RNA processing. Commitment of stem cells to the B lymphocyte series involves somatic recombination making an individual V gene contiguous with a D gene, and the D gene contiguous with a J gene. However, the J gene does not become contiguous with a constant region gene. Transcription into precursor RNA is apparently a faithful copy of the rearranged DNA. The RNA is then spliced to remove all intervening sequences, but untranslated sequences persist at both ends. Finally, a poly A tail is added. Membrane and secretory heavy chains are directed by separate RNA species, which result from alternate splicing at the 3' end.

If the κ gene rearrangement is nonfunctional, the cell then attempts to produce a functional λ chain gene. If successful at this stage, the cell and its progeny are committed to λ.

2.5.4 The Heavy Chain Complex

The heavy chain complex is by far the most complicated in its organisation (Fig. 2.6). There are a few hundred variable region genes (Kemp *et al.*, 1981), four J genes, and one constant region gene for each immunoglobulin class. The pool of V_H genes is shared by all heavy chain classes. Each constant region gene is divided into a series of segments, each coding for one domain or functional polypeptide segment. The hinge region of γ and δ chains are encoded by discrete segments, while the hinge region of α chains is encoded as a 5' extension of the $C_\alpha 2$ segment (Tucker *et al.*, 1981).

In additional to the J genes, there are ~ 12 "diversity" (D) genes, each of some 10–20 nucleotides (Sakano *et al.*, 1981). The D segments are situated between the V_H and J_H genes (Fig. 2.6), and encode much of the third hypervariable region of the heavy chains. An "enhancer" element that apparently increases transcription of immunoglobulin genes is present between J_H and C_μ (or, to be more precise, between J_H and S_μ) (Gillies *et al.*, 1983). Enhancer elements are also present between J_K and C_K.

A functional heavy chain gene is formed by joining a particular V_H gene to a particular D gene, and by joining that D gene to a particular J gene. As for κ, the J genes downstream from the chosen J gene are retained (Fig. 2.6).

Allelic exclusion

In any one lymphocyte, either the maternal or paternal light and heavy chain genes are expressed, but never both. This phenomenon is termed *allelic exclusion*, and superficially resembles the random inactivation of the X chromosome in females (Lyon, 1961). If a lymphocyte expresses more than one heavy chain class, they are always encoded by the same chromosome (*haplotype exclusion*). However, a lymphocyte may express either maternal and paternal light chains in conjunction with either maternal of paternal heavy chains. Allelic exclusion is often associated with incorrect joining in the excluded chromosome (Early and Hood, 1986), but recent work suggests a more active regulatory mechanism in which correct joining on one chromosome suppresses further rearrangement of the other (Ritchie *et al.*, 1984).

2.5.5 RNA Processing

The precise details of immunoglobulin RNA processing are still unknown (see Rogers and Wall, 1984). Transcription begins a short distance 5' to the initiation codon (ATG) of the active V gene, and continues through the various D, J and constant region segments. The final stopping point is not known, and may vary with individual circumstances. The initial very long nuclear transcript is processed in a series of poorly defined stages, until all the sequences which intervene between coding segments are excised (Fig. 2.6; see Coleclough and Wood, 1984). Segments of untranslated sequence persist at the 5' and 3' ends. The putative poly A addition signal (AAUAAA) lies 20–30 bases from the start of the poly A tail of the final messenger RNA (mRNA). The poly A tail is not encoded in the DNA. It appears to stabilize the mRNA.

In addition to excision of intervening sequences, heavy chain RNA may undergo differential splicing at its 3' end to generate distinct mRNAs, one coding for the membrane form and the other coding for the secretory form (Fig. 2.6).

2.5.6 Generation of Antibody Diversity

The diversity of antibody-combining sites depends on a large number of genetic mechanisms (Tonegawa, 1983). The number of variable region genes for heavy and κ light chains is of the order of a few hundred each. As mentioned previously, the degree of diversity of λ light chain genes is extremely limited. The random association of p light chains with q heavy chains potentially generates $p \times q$ antibody specificities. If p and q both are around 100, we already have 10 000 combining sites. This mechanism is known as 'combinational association'.

The introduction of D and J segments introduces a very large additional amount of diversity, because they lie in or close to the third hypervariable region and thus contribute to the specificity of the antigen-combining site. Variation in the precise splicing points generates additional diversity. There is now good evidence that additional diversity arises as a result of variable trimming and random re-extension of the 5' and 3' ends of the D segments of heavy chains, probably via the enzyme terminal transferase (Desiderio *et al.*, 1984). Finally, a large amount of additional diversity is generated by somatic mutation (Tonegawa, 1983). This is particularly apparent in IgG antibodies, and may account for the gradual rise in antibody affinity seen after immunization (Gearhart *et al.*, 1981; Perlmutter *et al.*, 1984; Griffiths *et al.*, 1984). The number of different antibodies is therefore virtually infinite.

2.5.7 Immunoglobulin Class Switches

Most mature but unstimulated B lymphocytes express both IgM and IgD on their surface, and the specificity of these two receptors is the same (Goding and Layton, 1976). Co-expression of IgM and IgD is probably achieved by differential splicing of a long primary transcript through the μ and δ genes (see Fig. 2.4).

Following antigenic stimulation, B cells mature into antibody-secreting cells. Production of immunoglobulin secretory mRNA is increased several hundredfold, and membrane mRNA synthesis reduced. The first antibody-secreting cells in most immune responses secrete IgM. Perhaps because the Cδ gene lacks the switching mechanisms available to other heavy chain genes (see below), IgD-secreting cells are rare at all stages in the immune response. Days or weeks after the initial response, there is a shift towards secretion of other classes, particularly IgG.

The switch from IgM to IgG, IgA or IgE secretion involves further recombination events which translocate a particular V gene onto successive C genes, via short "switch" sequences located on the 5' side of each constant region gene (Fig. 2.7). The intervening DNA is removed, either by excision or by sister chromatid exchange (Davis *et al.*, 1980).

The factors which control B-cell class switching are still poorly understood, but it is very probable that T cells are involved. It appears that a typical mature B cell expressing IgM and IgD receptors has the potential to switch to any other subclass, although it is clear that switching is essentially a "one-way" event. In other words, once a cell has switched to IgA, it usually

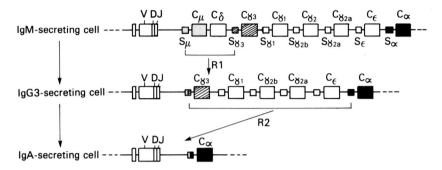

Fig. 2.7. *Immunoglobulin class switching in lymphocytes. On the 5′ side of each constant region gene lies a switch (S) sequence. Recombination in the switch sequences mediates class switching, which is virtually always in the order of the genes and irreversible.*

loses the potential to express IgG or IgE (Fig. 2.7). The light chain type and antibody specificity remain the same during class switches.

2.6 Control of the Immune Response

2.6.1 Features of the Antigen Controlling Antigenicity

The immune response to most antigens involves hundreds or thousands of clones of lymphocytes, and the products of these clones may recognize many different sites on the antigen molecule. The small site on the antigen to which the antibody-combining site binds is known as an *antigenic determinant*. If an antigenic determinant is of a known structure, it is sometimes known as an *epitope*.

A typical immune response is shown in Fig. 2.8. The immunizing antigen consists of a heterogeneous mixture of entities, and the antibody response is directed at multiple sites on each antigen molecule. Largely as a result of the work of Atassi, the concept has arisen that the antigenicity of particular proteins is restricted to a limited number of sites (Atassi, 1975). Support for this notion comes from the study of the antigenic determinants of the influenza virus spike proteins, where certain regions appear to be "immunodominant" (Wiley *et al.*, 1981). Nonetheless, much recent work has cast doubt on the original interpretation of Atassi's work, and it now appears likely that in most cases the great majority of the exposed surface of proteins is antigenic (Benjamin *et al.*, 1984).

As a general rule, the greater the phylogenetic distance between antigen and recipient, the more vigorous the immune response. Responses against

Immunization   Response

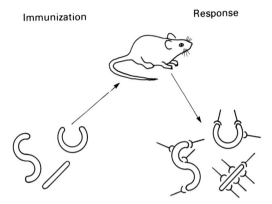

Fig. 2.8. A typical immune response. Antigen consists of a mixture of molecules, and the antibody response is directed against many different regions (determinants) on each molecule. However, some regions provoke a more vigorous response than others.

highly conserved mammalian proteins are usually weak, and are often of the IgM class. However, it is often possible to generate antibodies against substances that are not normally antigenic (e.g. hormones, small molecules, "self" component) by coupling them onto a strongly immunogenic carrier protein (e.g. keyhole limpet haemocyanin; Chapter 8) and using adjuvants (see below). It is clear that not all proteins are equally immunogenic, and it is frequently found that very minor impurities in an antigen may evoke strong antibody responses.

As a broad generalization, an array of repeating identical determinants or a high state of aggregation favours a strong antibody response. Antigens presented on cell surfaces or membrane fragments are thus particularly immunogenic, while water-soluble monomeric proteins often evoke feeble responses unless adjuvants are used.

2.6.2 Antibodies Against Synthetic Peptides Often Recognize the Native Protein

Antigenic determinants have been traditionally viewed as being capable of subdivision into two broad classes. The first has been called *linear* or *continuous*, consisting of a short stretch of perhaps 5–8 contiguous amino acids, reflecting the size of the antibody-combining site. The second major class has been named *conformational* or *discontinuous*, consisting of residues that are not contiguous in the primary structure, but are brought together by protein folding (Arnon, 1973; Crumpton, 1974).

When isolated peptides were used to inhibit the reaction of antibodies against the corresponding native antigen, very large molar ratios (10^3–10^4)

were required. Because peptides of less than ~ 20 amino acids are usually incapable of forming a well-defined three-dimensional structure, the concept emerged that their poor performance as competitive inhibitors reflected the requirement for the native antigen to be held in a particular conformation by the remainder of the protein, and that the fraction of the time that the isolated peptide was in this conformation was very small.

A considerable body of knowledge accumulated indicating that there was little cross-reactivity between the native and denatured forms of the molecule (Arnon, 1973; Crumpton, 1974). However, it should be pointed out that much of the experimental evidence for this idea came from "one-way" tests, in which the antibodies against the *native* protein were tested against the native versus the denatured antigen. The converse (antibodies against the denatured antigen or peptide tested on the native protein) was less thoroughly explored.

More recently, the interpretation of these earlier experiments has come under radical challenge. It gradually became clear that antibodies against the native antigen could be generated by immunizing with the denatured antigen (for references, see Section 8.1.4). Conversely, it was widespread experience that at least a subpopulation of polyclonal antibodies against native proteins were capable of reacting with denatured proteins (Burnette, 1981).

Subsequent work by the groups of Doolittle (Walter *et al.*, 1980) and Lerner (Lerner, 1982) showed that antibodies against short synthetic peptides were frequently capable of recognizing the native protein. These observations have now been extended to hundreds of other cases (reviewed by Lerner, 1982). Peptides from the N- and C-termini of proteins tended to have higher than average antigenicity, perhaps because they are often located on the protein surface, but a high percentage of antisera against peptides from more or less randomly chosen parts of the protein also recognized the native protein.

These results raised a major problem in understanding the nature of antigenic determinants. How could antibodies against a relatively unstructured peptide react with a highly ordered protein, when the requirement for order was so well documented?

Several hypotheses were suggested. A simple explanation would have been that the anti-peptide antibodies that reacted with native antigen were merely a very small subset of the total antibodies of the peptide. This explanation was challenged by the finding that a very high proportion of monoclonal antibodies against peptides reacted with the native antigen (Niman *et al.*, 1983), although the generality of these observations remains controversial.

More recently, evidence has been obtained that offers a reasonably satisfactory explanation of the data, and gives increased insight into the nature of the interaction between antigen and antibody. It was found that the ability of anti-peptide antibodies to recognize an antigenic determinant on a native protein correlates very well with the segmental or atomic mobility of that region of the protein (Westhof *et al.*, 1984). This correlation was considerably better than that with hydrophilicity (i.e. probability of location on the protein surface). In particular, the N- and C-regions of proteins tend to have a high relative flexibility, as do loops and turns. The mobility of the epitope in the native protein may make it easier for it to adjust to fit the anti-peptide antibody-combining site.

Conversely, it is possible that a certain degree of movement in the *antibody*-combining site might help "fine tune" the interaction with antigen. In other words, the antigen and antibody may mould to fit each other. In this context, it is interesting to note that there is also a strong correlation between segmental flexibility and an effector function of antibodies, namely their ability to fix complement (Oi *et al.*, 1984).

It should be noted that the arguments given apply only to *continuous* determinants. Discontinuous or conformational determinants are probably much more numerous (Benjamin *et al.*, 1984), and monoclonal antibodies raised against the intact protein may have a marked bias towards them. Although it will be much harder to test, it seems likely that a high degree of mobility may also be favoured in this case.

The foregoing has many practical implications. It may be possible to generate monoclonal antibodies to short synthetic peptides and find that a significant fraction of antibodies will recognize the native protein. This is likely to be of considerable use in identifying proteins encoded by cloned genes, the product of which is not yet known. (However, polyclonal antibodies may do the trick just as well, and with much less work.

On the negative side, it is not easy to predict the regions of the protein that are likely to have high mobility. Some guidelines may be used to predict turns and loops (Schulz and Schirmer, 1978), and the choice of N- or C-termini would seem to favour mobility and success with anti-peptide antibodies.

If the foregoing arguments are correct, it would seem likely that the kinetics of binding of polyclonal anti-peptide antibodies to native proteins may be highly dependent on temperature. They may proceed much more rapidly at higher temperatures, because the degree of movement of the protein will be greater.

Before concluding this discussion on anti-peptide antibodies, a few words of caution may be in order. While it is undeniable that anti-peptide antibodies may be extremely useful, there are many instances in which this approach has failed. The discrepancy between the enthusiasm of some workers for this approach and the frequent failures in other laboratories probably reflects the properties of individual proteins, the failure to appreciate that a nominally "native" antigen may have been partially denatured, and the selective publication of only those experiments that worked.

2.6.3 Adjuvants

An adjuvant is a substance which augments immune responses in a non-specific manner. The most commonly used adjuvants are *Freund's complete adjuvant* (a water-in-oil emulsion in which killed and dried *M. tuberculosis* bacteria are suspended in the oil phase) and *Freund's incomplete adjuvant* (omitting the bacteria) (Herbert, 1973).

Other adjuvants include aluminium compounds such as aluminium hydroxide gel and alums such as potassium alum ($K_2SO_4Al_2SO_4$) which strongly adsorb protein antigens from solution to form a precipitate. Alum-precipitated proteins are often administered together with killed *B. pertussis* organisms (whooping cough vaccine) (Munzo, 1964).

The mechanisms of action of adjuvants are complex (Freund, 1956). They probably include slow, prolonged release of antigen in a highly aggregated form, together with pharmacologically active substances from the mycobacteria (muramyl dipeptide; Chedid *et al.*, 1976) and *B. pertussis* ("pertussigen"; Munoz and Bergman, 1977; Munoz and Sewell, 1984; Sewell *et al.*, 1984). The use of adjuvants may alter the class of antibody produced, as well as the amount. There is some evidence that *B. pertussis* promotes IgE responses (Hirashima *et al.*, 1981).

Adjuvants are especially useful in enhancing the immune response to weak antigens such as water-soluble monomeric proteins, especially if they are closely related in structure to their mouse homologues. Cell membrane antigens are often sufficiently immunogenic without adjuvants. Practical details of adjuvant use will be discussed in Chapters 3 and 8.

2.6.4 Genetic Control of the Immune Response

In a few special cases, particularly those involving carbohydrate, synthetic peptides and "weak" antigens closely related to self, single genes controlling the ability to respond have been found (reviewed by Benacerraf and McDevitt, 1972). In almost all these cases, the loci have been mapped to the *I* (immune response gene) region of the major histocompatibility complex (Klein *et al.*, 1981) or to the immunoglobulin heavy chain complex. In the latter case, the relevant genes appear to be the antibody variable region coding sequences (Perlmutter *et al.*, 1984).

The mode of action of the histocompatibility-linked immune response genes is still unknown, although the following points seem reasonably firmly established:

(1) The functional defect in the histocompatibility-linked nonresponders is expressed at the level of T-cell help, and can often be overcome by coupling the antigen onto an immunogenic "carrier" molecule (Green *et al.*, 1966).

(2) Helper T lymphocytes do not "see" antigen alone, but rather in conjunction with products of the major histocompatibility complex (Paul and Bencerraf, 1977).

(3) The *I* (immune response gene) region of the major histocompatibility complex codes for a small number of $M_r \sim 30\,000$ polypeptides called Ia antigens. The Ia antigens are expressed on the surface of B cells, macrophages and a limited number of other cell types (Uhr *et al.*, 1979).

(4) Mutations in *Ia* genes can alter specific immune responses, indicating that the *Ia* genes and the immune response genes are one and the same thing (Michaelides *et al.*, 1981).

From a practical point of view, the main importance of the immune response gene lies in the fact that occasionally it may be necessary to try more than one mouse strain to obtain one that is capable of responding to a given antigen. It is important, however, to keep the issue in its proper perspective. While immune response genes have provided endless fascination for immunologists, the great majority of randomly chosen antigens will elicit a strong response in any mouse strain.

Genetic factors are also important in controlling the immune response in a nonspecific way. While hard data are scarce, there is a general feeling amongst immunologists that SJL and A/J mice are particularly good responders, while C57Bl mice are poorer responders. BALB/c mice are probably somewhere in between.

All mouse myeloma cells commonly used for hybridoma production are of BALB/c origin, and it is generally easiest to use BALB/c mice as the spleen donor. If an adequate response cannot be obtained, consideration should be given to varying the strain. However, strain variation is one of the least likely causes of failure of hybridoma production.

2.7 Myeloma

The tumour caused by malignantly transformed antibody-secreting cells is known as *plasmacytoma* or *myeloma*. Spontaneous myelomas are rare in mice (Potter, 1972), but are quite common in the LOU/C strain of rats (Bazin *et al.*, 1973). Myeloma occasionally occurs in other species, and is not uncommon in man.

In 1959, it was accidentally discovered that peritoneal irritants could cause development of myelomas in BALB/c mice (see Merwin and Redmon, 1963). Subsequently, it was found that mineral oil or pristane were potent inducers of myeloma in BALB/c mice (Potter and Boyce, 1962; Potter, 1972). Approximately 40% of BALB/c mice will develop myeloma within one year of a series of three intraperitoneal injections of mineral oil (Warner, 1975). The only other laboratory strain of mouse where plasmacytomas can be induced is NZB. F_1 hybrids between NZB and BALB/c are also susceptible (Warner, 1975).

The development of plasmacytomas in mice is usually associated with a chromosome translocation between chromosome 15, which bears the oncogene *c-myc*, and the heavy chain locus on chromosome 12. The translocation causes activation of the *c-myc* gene, and is an important step in the malignant transformation of the cell. In a few cases, a variant translocation involves the κ locus on chromosome 6 instead of the heavy chain on chromosome 12 (reviewed by Cory, 1983).

The development of a large number of well-characterized mouse myelomas (Potter, 1972, 1977) has been responsible for much of our current knowledge of immunoglobulin structure, biosynthesis and genetics. The number of murine myelomas that have been studied is in the thousands, and a few of these have been successfully adapted as continuous tissue culture lines (Horibata and Harris, 1970).

The immunoglobulin classes found in mouse and rat myelomas do not precisely reflect the abundance of classes in serum. BALB/c myelomas are ~ 30–50% IgA, 30% IgG and 3% IgM, while NZB myelomas are ~ 20% IgA, 50% IgG and 2% IgM (Hood *et al.*, 1976). Two IgD myelomas have been found in the mouse (Finkelman *et al.*, 1981), but no IgE myelomas. In the rat, the corresponding figures are 0.6% IgA, 47% IgG, 3% IgM, 2% IgD and 34% IgE (Bazin *et al.*, 1973, 1978).

In the great majority of cases, the antigen-binding specificity of myeloma proteins is not known, and attempts to generate antigen-specific myelomas by intense antigenic stimulation prior to tumour induction have failed. However, extensive screening programmes have turned up a number of antigen-binding myelomas, and these have been very useful in studies of the antigen-combining site (reviewed by Potter, 1977). The most common specificities have been for carbohydrate antigens and phosphoryl choline, presumably reflecting antigenic stimulation by micro-organisms in the gut.

The precise rates of immunoglobulin synthesis by myelomas are somewhat controversial. Early figures indicated that IgG could account for 30–50% of total protein synthesis (Baumal and Scharff, 1973), but more recent experience suggests that these figures are too high (Word and Kuehl, 1981). The synthesis of light chains is usually somewhat greater than that of heavy chains, possibly because isolated heavy chains may be toxic to the cell (Köhler, 1980; Argon *et al.*, 1983). The excess light chains are usually secreted. Providing the cells do not die and release their cytoplasmic contents during labelling with radioactive amino acids, immunoglobulin will be by far the major labelled protein in myeloma supernatants (Chapter 4).

2.7.1 Mutations and Deletions in Myeloma Cells

Compared with other gene products, there is a rather high frequency of variants and deletions in immunoglobulin synthesis by cultured myeloma cells (Adetugbo *et al.*, 1977). Particularly common is the loss of heavy chain production (Cotton *et al.*, 1973; Scharff, 1974). Isolated loss of light chain production without loss of the heavy chain is extremely rare, perhaps indicating that such cells cannot survive (Köhler, 1980; Argon *et al.*, 1983). Isolated heavy chains are usually rather insoluble in physiological buffers, and might be expected to form large polymers via their cysteine thiol groups (see Argon *et al.*, 1983). In almost all the cases where heavy chains are secreted alone ("heavy chain disease"), there has been a substantial deletion of part of the chain (Franklin and Frangione, 1971). Mutation in the variable region is also at a relatively high level. Cook and Scharff (1977) found a variant frequency of 0.2–2% in the phosphorylchlorine-binding myeloma S-107, although this figure is much larger than seen by other workers (Adetugbo *et al.*, 1977).

2.8 Cell Fusion and Selection of Hybrids

When cells are treated with Sendai virus or high concentration of polyethylene glycol (PEG), their membranes fuse and multinucleate cells called *heterokaryons* are formed (Ringertz and Savage, 1976). At the next cell division, the nuclei of heterokaryons fuse, and the daughter cells possess a more or less equal share of the genetic material. The mechanism of fusion is still poorly understood. It is probable that both the PEG itself and an unidentified contaminant in the PEG are required for fusion (Wojciezsyn *et al.*, 1983).

For reasons which are poorly understood, the resulting hybrid cells are not genetically stable, and there is a strong tendency for loss of chromosomes. This loss is not completely random. Depending on the species and perhaps on the individual cell types, there is usually a preferential loss of chromosomes from one or other cell. By comparing the retained functions with the retained chromosomes, it has been possible to map a large number of genes to individual chromosomes (Ruddle, 1981).

2.8.1 Selection Procedures

When a cell mixture is subjected to reagents which promote fusion, the fusion events are poorly controlled. In addition to A-B fusions, it is to be expected that many fusions will be A-A or B-B, or even higher multiples of these. Thus, if it is desired to produce a long-term hybrid cell line from two cell types, a selection procedure is required.

By far the most common selection procedure is that devised by Littlefield in 1964. Littlefield's procedure depends on the fact that when the main biosynthetic pathway for guanosine is blocked by the folic acid antagonist

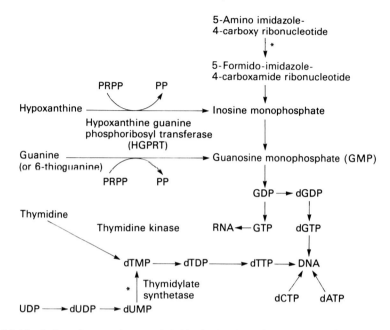

Fig. 2.9. *Metabolic pathways relevant to hybrid selection in medium containing hypoxanthine, aminopterin and thymidine (HAT medium). When the main synthetic pathways are blocked with the folic acid analogue aminopterin (*), the cell must depend on the "salvage" enzymes HGPRT and thymidine kinase. HGPRT⁻ cells can be selected by growth in medium containing the toxic base analogues 6-thioguanine or 8-azaguanine, which are incorporated into the cell via HGPRT. Only HGPRT⁻ cells survive. HGPRT⁻ cells cannot grow in HAT medium unless they are fused with HGPRT⁺ cells.*

aminopterin, there is an alternative "salvage" pathway in which the nucleotide metabolites hypoxanthine or guanine are converted to guanosine monophosphate via the enzyme *hypoxanthine guanine phosphoribosyl transferase* (HGPRT or HPRT; Fig. 2.9). Cells lacking HGPRT die in a medium containing hypoxanthine, aminopterin and thymidine (HAT medium), because both the main and the salvage pathways are blocked. However, an HGPRT⁻ cell can be made to grow in HAT medium if it is provided the missing enzyme by fusion with an HGPRT⁺ cell.

Selection of HGPRT⁻ cells is performed by use of the toxic base analogues 8-azaguanine or 6-thioguanine, which are incorporated into DNA via HGPRT. Because the salvage pathway is not normally essential for cell survival, "mutants" which lack HGPRT will continue growing, while cells which possess HGPRT will die.

Selection of HGPRT⁻ variants is usually easy because the enzyme is coded for by the X-chromosome. There is normally only one active copy of the X-chromosome per cell (Lyon, 1961). Selection of variants lacking thymidine kinase (an autosomal enzyme) is more difficult, because two simultaneous rare events are required. [This simplified description does not take into account the many complexities of the HGPRT locus (Caskey and Kruh, 1979), nor does it consider the fact that most cultured myeloma cells are sub-tetraploid rather than diploid (Ohno *et al.*, 1979).]

2.9 Hybridomas

For decades, immunologists have sought ways of producing homogeneous antibodies of defined specificity (see Krause, 1970). Some limited successes were achieved by screening myeloma proteins for antigen binding (see Potter, 1977), but a general method did not become available until Köhler and Milstein (1975, 1976) used cell hybridization to produce continuous cell lines secreting antibody of predefined specificity.

Milstein had been interested in the genetic control of antibody synthesis. In a study designed to examine the basis of allelic exclusion, hybrids between rat and mouse myeloma cells were constructed, and it was shown that the synthesis of both species of immunoglobulin was retained but mixed molecules were formed (Cotton and Milstein, 1973).

Cotton and Milstein were also interested in the rate of somatic mutation in antibody genes, and had been studying the mutation rate in the cultured mouse myeloma MOPC-21 (Cotton *et al.*, 1973). These experiments indicated a high degree of instability in immunoglobulin synthesis, but a general way of constructing continuous cell lines secreting antibody of known specificity was still needed.

In 1975, Köhler and Milstein took the bold step of extending the previous experiments by fusing a HAT-sensitive variant of MOPC-21 myeloma cells with spleen cells from mice immunized with sheep red cells. The fusion was mediated by Sendai virus, and hybrids were selected by growth in HAT medium. It was known that normal spleen cells could only survive a few days in culture, but it was hoped that they would "complement" the missing HGPRT in the myeloma cells, and that the myeloma cells would provide the "immortality" needed for continuous culture (Figs. 2.9, 2.10).

The experiment worked exactly as planned, and a number of cloned hybrid lines secreting anti-sheep erythrocyte antibodies were produced. The cell lines were capable of forming tumours when injected into mice, and these tumours are now known as "hybridomas". The serum of myeloma or hybridoma-bearing mice contains large amounts of homogeneous antibody (Fig. 2.3). The use of Sendai virus has been superseded by polyethylene glycol (Pontecorvo, 1976; Galfrè and Milstein, 1981), but apart from this modification, the basic procedure is essentially unchanged.

The implications of Köhler and Milstein's discovery were revolutionary. For the first time, unlimited quantities of absolutely specific and uniform

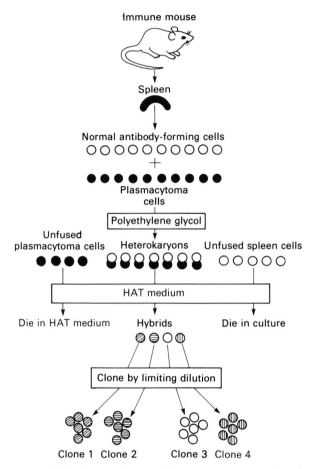

Fig. 2.10. Production of hybridomas. Spleen cells from immune mice are fused with HGPRT⁻ myeloma (plasmacytoma) cells using polyethylene glycol. The binucleate fusion products are known as heterokaryons. At the next division, the nuclei fuse, generating hybrid cells, which grow in HAT medium. Unfused myeloma cells die in HAT medium (Fig. 2.9), and unfused spleen cells can only survive a few days in culture. Hybrids are tested for production of antibody of the desired specificity, and cloned by limiting dilution.

antibodies recognizing only one antigenic site could be produced, even if the immunizing antigen was weakly immunogenic or grossly impure. All that was needed was an appropriate way of screening for antibody with the desired properties.

2.9.1 Cloning

Because of the high probability of chromosome loss in the hybrids, and to ensure that the antibodies were indeed monoclonal, it was essential to clone the hybrid cell lines. Köhler and Milstein used soft agar cultures to grow discrete colonies, and detected clones secreting anti-erythrocyte antibodies by overlaying with sheep red cells and complement. Colonies secreting anti-erythrocyte antibodies were surrounded by a zone of haemolysis.

Hybridoma lines should be cloned at least twice to make absolutely certain that each is a true clone, and also because of the relatively high probability of growth of nonproducer variants due to chromosome loss. After two cycles of cloning, the rate of chromosome loss is small, although the risk of over-growth by nonproducer cells never ceases completely.

Cloning in soft agar has the disadvantage that unless an overlay technique is available, colonies need to be plucked out and regrown in liquid culture prior to testing for antibody production. For this reason, many workers now prefer to clone by limiting dilution. If cells are grown in small numbers, the fraction of wells with growth should follow the Poisson distribution (see Lefkovits and Waldemann, 1979):

$$f(0) = e^{-\lambda}$$

where $f(0)$ is the fraction of wells with no growth, and λ is the *average* number of clones per well.

If $\lambda = 1, f(0) = 0.37$. In other words, to obtain a reasonable probability that wells with growth contain single clones, more than 37% of wells should have no growth. [This analysis assumes a cloning efficiency of 100%, and that there is no clumping of cells. Cloning should always be carried out twice.]

2.9.2 Nature of the Fusing Cell in Spleen

In a certain sense, the original experiments worked *too* well. Although only about 1% of spleen cells actively secrete immunoglobulin, about 10% of the hybrid cell lines secreted antibody. There may be two explanations. First, there seems to be a preference for myeloma cells to fuse with activated B cells. It appears that the spleen cells which fuse with myeloma cells are larger than average, and have recently undergone antigen stimulation and blast trans-formation (Andersson and Melchers, 1978). The other possible explanation may be that myeloma cells have the ability to activate non-secreting B cells to rapid secretion (Eshhar *et al.*, 1979).

It is probable that the myeloma cells also fuse with T cells and other non-B cells in the spleen. However, fusion of cells of different lineages usually results in extinction of differentiated function, and it is unlikely that these fusions would result in antibody-secreting hybrids (Köhler *et al.*, 1977).

2.9.3 Nonproducer Variants of Myeloma Cells for Fusion

The original cell line used by Köhler and Milstein secreted IgG1 with κ light chains. As expected from the earlier experiments involving rat–mouse fusions (Cotton and Milstein, 1973), mixed molecules of IgG containing light and heavy chains from both MOPC-21 and the spleen cells were found. Milstein and Köhler have proposed that the MOPC-21 heavy chain be designated G and its light chain K, while the heavy chain of the spleen cell should be designated H and the light chain L. The product of the myeloma would then be GK, the spleen cell HL, and the mixed molecules HLGK.

If the association of chains were random, only a small minority of IgG molecules would be derived entirely from the spleen. A combining site with the myeloma light or heavy chains (or both) would not be expected to bind antigen. Thus, many secreted IgG molecules would be completely inactive, while some would possess only one active antigen-binding site. Only a minority of molecules would have two combining sites (Figs. 2.3, 2.11). Fusion of two different antibody-forming cells allows the formation of mixed antibodies of dual specificity (Milstein and Cuello, 1983).

In 1976, Köhler *et al.* described a variant of MOPC-21 (P3-NS1-Ag4-1; abbreviated NS-1) which lacked heavy chain synthesis. Although NS-1 continued to make κ light chains, they were degraded intracellularly and were not secreted. Fusion of NS-1 with spleen cells resulted in the production of active antibody-secreting hybrids. The immunoglobulins secreted by NS-1 bore only spleen cell heavy chain, but had light chains derived from both spleen and MOPC-21 (i.e. HLK).

If the light and heavy chain pairing were random and the rates of synthesis of spleen and MOPC-21 light chains equal, one would expect 25% of molecules to possess only the spleen cell heavy chains (and therefore have two functional combining sites), 50% to have one spleen cell light chain and one MOPC-21 light chain (one functional site) and 25% to have both light chains from MOPC-21 (no functional combining sites). The use of NS-1 as fusion partner thus allows $\sim$ 75% of the secreted immunoglobulin to have antibody activity.

Subsequently, several cell lines have been produced which synthesize neither heavy or light chains, but which allow the production of antibody-secreting hybridomas when fused with spleen cells. These include Sp 2/0-Ag-14 (Shulman *et al.*, 1978), X63-Ag8.653 (Kearney *et al.*, 1979) and NSO/1 (Galfrè and Milstein, 1981). Of these, X63-Ag8.653 is probably the cell of choice, because it is widely available, has a high fusion frequency and is easy to grow.

In addition, several rat lines have been shown to be suitable for fusion. Y3-Ag1.2.3 (abbreviated Y3) is an azaguanine resistant derivative of the LOU/C strain myeloma R210.RCY3, and secretes κ chains (Galfrè *et al.*,

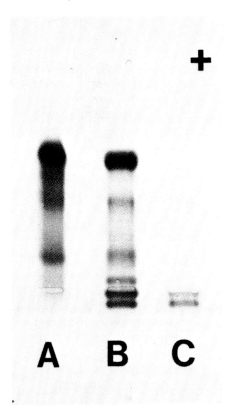

Fig. 2.11. Agarose electrophoresis of serum from normal mice (A); from mice bearing the hybridoma MAR-18.5 (lane B; see Fig. 2.3); and MAR-18.5 antibody purified by affinity chromatography on its antigen (lane C). Note that in lane B there are three "Spikes" in the gamma globulin region, but only two of these contain material which binds antigen (lane C). The most anodal spike has both heavy chains from MOPC-21 ($\gamma1/\gamma1$), the middle spike has one MOPC-21 $\gamma1$ chain and one spleen $\gamma2a$ chain, while the most cathodal spike has two spleen has both heavy chains from spleen ($\gamma2a/\gamma2a$). Because of their size, the heavy chains dominate the charge of the IgG molecule, and hence its mobility.

1979). Fusion of spleen cells with Y3 usually results in HLK antibodies. More recently, a total nonproducer line YB2/0 (Kilmartin et al., 1982; Galfrè and Milstein, 1981) was derived from a fusion between Y3 myeloma cells and spleen cells from an A0 rat. Bazin (1982) has also developed a total non-producer rat line suitable for fusion (IR 983F).

There have been several claims for human myeloma cell lines suitable for fusion. These include SK-007, which is a derivative of the human IgE myeloma U266 (Olsson and Kaplan, 1980), ARH-77 (Edwards et al., 1982) and GM1500 (Croce et al., 1980). The latter two cell lines are probably not true myelomas and may be Epstein–Barr virus transformed lymphoblastoid lines

(Karpas *et al.*, 1982). At the time of writing, there is still a need for cultured human myeloma lines suitable for fusion.

Vigorous efforts are still being made in many laboratories in attempts to overcome this problem, but so far with only limited success (Abrams *et al.*, 1983). Miller *et al.* (1982) have described a new cultured human myeloma cell line, but it has not yet been widely used for cell fusion. Kozbor *et al.* (1984) have generated somatic cell hybrids between human myeloma cells and a B lymphoblastoid line, and then re-introduced HAT sensitivity. This line grows rapidly, has a high fusion frequency and supports the production of human monoclonal antibodies. Growth in irradiated nude mice allowed the production of 1–8 mg/ml human immunoglobulin in ascites fluid.

Another approach to the production of human monoclonal antibodies involves splicing mouse variable region genes onto human constant region genes, and transfecting into mouse myeloma cells (Morrison *et al.*, 1984). The transformed lines remained tumorigenic in mice, and the hybrid molecules were present in serum and ascites fluid. Presumably, whole human antibodies will soon be produced by this method. However, the procedure is fairly laborious, and would only be attractive for antibodies that have already been shown to have important specificity. Nonetheless, the technique points the way to the future, and could be very important for the large-scale industrial production of human monoclonal antibodies.

2.10 Differences Between Conventional and Monoclonal Serology

The discovery of hybridoma antibodies has done much to put serology on a firm scientific basis. The old uncertainties of specificity and reproducibility have been replaced by the promise of unlimited supplies of standardized, monospecific antibodies. Terms like "titre" and "avidity" have become virtually obsolete. We can now talk about mass and affinity of antibody in a very precise way. However, the successful use of monoclonal antibodies requires a firm understanding of the differences between conventional and monoclonal serology.

2.10.1 Cross-reactions Due to Structural Relatedness Between Antigens

Cross-reaction may be defined as the reaction of an antiserum against an antigen molecule not present in the immunizing preparation. It is usually a manifestation of structural similarities between the immunizing antigen and the cross-reacting antigen (Fig. 2.12). An obvious practical point concerning cross-reaction is that it places some limits on the specificity of antibodies.

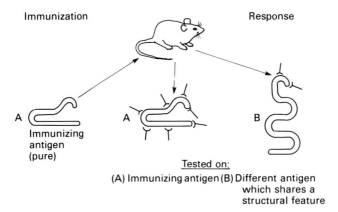

Fig. 2.12. Cross-reaction due to a shared structural feature between the immunizing antigen (A) and the test antigen (B).

For example, consider an antiserum containing antibodies against the carbohydrate moieties of a particular glycoprotein. Carbohydrate structures are widely shared between different glycoproteins, and such an antiserum is thus very likely to cross-react with other glycoproteins, even if the poly-peptide portions are totally unrelated. In other words, antibodies may have lectin-like properties due to carbohydrate cross-reactions.

The proportion of antibodies in a polyclonal antiserum which will cross-react in a given situation will depend on a number of factors. Particularly important is the degree of structural relatedness between the two antigens. Thus, a sheep anti-mouse IgG antiserum will cross-react very extensively with rat IgG, with perhaps half or more of the total mass of antibodies binding both antigens. On the other hand, cross-reaction of the same antiserum with human IgG may be weak or undetectable. The cross-reacting antibody subpopulation may be removed from an antiserum by absorption with the cross-reacting antigen coupled to agarose beads, implying that within the total antibody population there exists a cross-reacting subset and a non-cross-reacting subset.

Let us now consider the situation at the level of the individual clone. Figure 2.13 shows a simplified model of the immune response of a mouse to three antigens. Clones 1 and 4 recognize a determinant which is only present on antigen A. However, clone 5 recognizes a determinant on the same portion of A as clones 1 and 4, but it also recognizes a structure on antigen B which is *not* recognized by clones 1 and 4. By definition, then, the determinant recognized by clone 5 must be different to that recognized by clones 1 and 4.

It is crucial to understand that the determinant on antigen B which is recognized by clone 5 is *not necessarily identical* with the determinant recog-nized by the same antibody on antigen A. It is quite possible to have a similar, but non-identical determinant which allows detectable binding, perhaps of

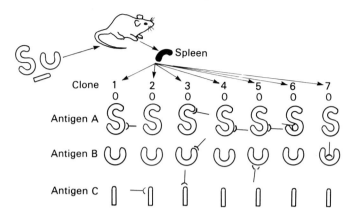

Fig. 2.13. Cross-reaction at the level of the individual clone. Clones 1, 2, 4, 6 and 7 show no cross-reaction, while clones 3 and 5 cross-react because of a shared structural feature in antigens A, B and C. Note that this structural feature does not need to be absolutely identical in A, B and C. The affinities of binding of clone 3 to A, B and C may be quite different.

lower affinity (see Birnbaum and Kourilsky, 1981, for an example). Depending on the desired application, the specificity of clone 1 and 4 or of clone 5 may be preferred.

2.10.2 Cross-reactions Due to Multiple Specificity of Individual Clones

The problem of unexpected cross-reactions of monoclonal antibodies has been reviewed by Lane and Koprowski (1982), who cited several examples where a monoclonal antibody bound two apparently quite unrelated antigens. For example, a rat anti-mouse Thy-1 monoclonal antibody also bound to a determinant on the variable region of κ light chains of the myeloma TEPC-15 (Pillemer and Weissman, 1981). Similarly, some monoclonal antibodies cross-react with two cytoskeletal proteins, tropomyosin and vimentin (Blose *et al.*, 1982).

Lane and Koprowski suggested two possible explanations for these unexpected cross-reactions. The "classical" explanation is that the cross-reacting antibodies detect a structural similarity between the two antigens, although its nature may be hard to determine. The second possibility is that the antigen-combining site of an individual antibody molecule could combine with unrelated antigens in quite different ways. In other words, combining sites might be multispecific, and recognize two or more entirely different epitopes. Richards *et al.* (1975) obtained direct evidence for such a proposal.

[One should not be too surprised at the concept of multispecificity of monoclonal antibodies. A stable antigen–antibody complex will result whenever there is sufficient number and strength of short-range interactions, and this might be achieved in many different ways. Considering the enormous number of different biological macromolecules, it is to be expected that occasionally there will be high-affinity interactions between functionally unrelated molecules. For example, tubulin has a high affinity for lactoperoxidase (Rousert and Wolff, 1980) and actin has a high affinity for deoxyribonuclease I (Hitchcock, 1980).]

These types of odd cross-reactions are seldom, if ever, seen in polyclonal sera. The specificity of a conventional polyclonal antiserum is the result of a consensus of thousands of different clones, and the likelihood is that cross-reactions due to multispecificity will be random, and therefore diluted out. Thus, an antiserum against an absolutely pure antigen A may contain clones which react with A, C, P, Z; other clones that react with A, B, D, E; and other clones that react with A, Q, R, Y etc. The only common reactivity is that against A, and the other specificities will be too dilute to be detected.

The specificity of a given monoclonal antibody is therefore unlikely to be absolute. Given a large enough panel of unrelated test antigens, sooner or later a cross-reaction will be found. Unexpected cross-reactions as cited by Lane and Koprowski are uncommon, but it is important to realize that they can and do occur.

2.10.3 Sometimes, a Monoclonal Antibody May Be Too Specific

The specificity of conventional polyclonal antisera depends on a consensus of hundreds or thousands of clonal products, which bind to antigenic determinants covering most or all of the external surface of the antigen (Benjamin et al., 1984). As a result, small changes in the structure of the antigen due to genetic polymorphism, heterogeneity of glycosylation or slight denaturation will usually have little effect on polyclonal antibody binding. Similarly, a larger or smaller subset of antibodies from a polyclonal antiserum will usually bind to antigens which have been modified or denatured (see Burnette, 1981).

In contrast, monoclonal antibodies usually bind to one single unique site on the antigen molecule. If for any reason this site is altered, the antibody may or may not continue to bind. Whether this is seen as a problem or an advantage will obviously depend on the individual circumstances. If the monoclonal antibody is used in a radioimmunoassay for a human serum protein, a minor genetic polymorphism (known or unknown) in that protein could cause gross errors. Similarly, if monoclonal antibodies were used for classification of micro-organisms, they might not give exactly the same reactivity patterns as conventional antisera.

It is therefore essential that monoclonal antibodies be tested and characterized *in the assay system in which they are to be used.* In future years, one may anticipate that commercial preparations of antibodies will be pools of several different clonal products, such that their nominal specificity will be maintained in all circumstances.

2.10.4 Affinity of Polyclonal and Monoclonal Antibodies

Most polyclonal antisera contain antibodies of a wide range of affinities, with equilibrium constants from less than 10^6 to more than 10^9 litres/mole (Mason and Williams, 1980; Dower *et al.*, 1984). Antibodies with affinities of less than about 10^6 litres/mole are not usually detected by the standard methods, and the higher affinity antibodies tend to dominate the specificity in most practical situations. These very high affinity antibodies may comprise only a small fraction of the total. It is therefore to be expected that extremely high affinity monoclonal antibodies will be less common than lower affinity ones.

The extreme heterogeneity of polyclonal antibodies has a number of other important practical consequences. It allows the antibody population to be covalently modified (e.g. with fluorochromes or ^{125}I) with the expectation that although some antibodies will no longer bind, enough reactivity will be preserved to allow the experiment to proceed. Binding may still be detected even if more than 95% of the antibodies are destroyed.

Monoclonal antibodies may behave quite differently under these conditions. In some cases, it may be possible to alter antigen or antibody quite extensively without destruction of binding. In others, it may be found that seemingly minor modifications to antibody or antigen may abolish binding completely (Nussenzweig *et al.*, 1982).

The homogeneity of monoclonal antibodies means that each clonal product will have a well-defined affinity. The use of antibodies for affinity chromatography or immunofluorescence usually involves extensive washing to remove unbound antibody. If a monoclonal antibody has a low affinity, excessive washing may dissociate the antigen–antibody complexes.

The binding of polyclonal antibodies to their antigen is usually stable over a wide range of pH ($\sim$ 4–9) and salt concentration (0–1 M NaCl). In contrast, some monoclonal antibodies may be very susceptible to minor changes. Herrmann and Mescher (1979) found that the monoclonal antibody 11–4 bound its antigen at pH 7.0 and at salt concentrations of less than 100 mM, but at pH 8.0 and 200 mM NaCl, binding was virtually abolished. However, the low affinity of certain monoclonal antibodies or their sensitivity to environmental changes is not necessarily a disadvantage. Indeed, it may facilitate affinity chromatography by allowing very gentle elution conditions. Other monoclonal antibodies may have extremely high affinities, and may require very harsh conditions (e.g. pH 2.0, 3.5 M KSCN or 7 M guanidine-HCl) before the antigen–antibody bond is disrupted (see Chapter 6).

The desired affinity of a monoclonal antibody, its binding to modified or denatured antigen, and its sensitivity to environmental conditions, may be taken into account when designing hybridoma screening protocols. If high affinity antibodies are desired, one might keep the incubation times short. Similarly, if it is vital that the antibody recognize the denatured antigen, or the antigens in a particular ionic environment, these conditions might be used during the screening assay.

2.10.5 Kinetics of Binding of Monoclonal Antibodies

A further practical consequence of the mobility of antigenic determinants (Section 2.6.2) concerns the kinetics of antibody binding (Mason and Williams, 1980; Dower *et al.*, 1984). Some monoclonal antibodies take longer than others to reach equilibrium binding to their antigen (Mason and Williams, 1980). The binding of individual monoclonal antibodies to the cell surface may reach saturation in as little as 15 min, or as long as 90 min (J. Goding, unpublished data). It seems clear that the rate of association is sometimes limited by more than simple diffusion. These results might be understood in terms of the need for an individual antigenic determinant recognized by a given monoclonal antibody to be in a particular (transient) conformation before the antibody can bind. One might expect the rate of such slow reactions to be highly dependent on temperature.

The highly individual kinetics of binding of monoclonal antibodies to their antigen makes it strongly advisable to keep incubation times constant from one experiment to another. Failure to do so may lead to errors in quantitation and poor reproducibility in cases where the kinetics of binding are slow.

2.10.6 Differences Due to Failure of Cross-linking

Many important immunological assays depend on cross-linking of antigen by antibody. Monoclonal antibodies would only be expected to cross-link antigen molecules with two or more antibody-binding sites. Thus, monoclonal antibodies would only be expected to form precipitates in gel diffusion (Ouchterlony) assays when the antigen is dimeric or multimeric. Because of their multivalency, IgM antibodies are more likely to cause cell agglutination than IgG. Whether or not a monoclonal antibody will agglutinate cells will also depend on the density and orientation of the relevant antigenic sites. However, mere binding *per se* will not guarantee agglutination.

The activation of complement also depends on the close proximity of the Fc portions of antibodies, and it is to be expected that some monoclonal IgG antibodies may fail to activate complement. Neuberger and Rajewsky (1981) have studied the relative effectiveness of monoclonal mouse antibodies in initiating complement-mediated lysis of erythrocytes. IgM, IgG2a, IgG2b and IgG3 were cytotoxic, while IgD and IgA were not. IgG1 was weakly cytotoxic in some cases. Howard *et al.* (1979) found that certain mixtures of monoclonal antibodies to different determinants were highly cytotoxic, while the individual antibodies on their own were weakly cytotoxic or not cytotoxic at all.

2.10.7 Physico-chemical Idiosyncrasies of Monoclonal Antibodies

In addition to their highly individual binding specificity and affinity, mono-clonal antibodies may have highly individual physical or chemical properties unrelated to antigen binding. As mentioned earlier in this chapter, IgM, murine IgG2b and IgG3, and rat IgG2c often precipitate in solutions of low ionic strength ("euglobulin precipitation"). The proteins will usually (but not always) redissolve upon raising the salt concentration. Euglobulin precipita-tion is often exploited in the purification of monoclonal antibodies (Chapter 4).

Occasionally, monoclonal antibodies will precipitate in the cold, and redissolve upon warming. Immunoglobulins with this property are known as "cryoglobulins" (reviewed by Grey and Kohler, 1973). The precise structural features which cause precipitation in the cold are not clear. If a monoclonal antibody is a cryoglobulin, its usefulness may be greatly diminished, because many immunological procedures are carried out in the cold. Unexpected cryoglobulin properties of a monoclonal antibody could cause significant experimental artefacts.

References

Abrams, P.G., Knost, J.A., Clarke, G., Wilburn, S., Oldham, R.K. and Foon, K.A. (1983). Determination of the optimal human cell lines for development of human hybridomas. *J. Immunol.* **131**, 1201–1204.

Adetugbo, K., Milstein, C. and Secher, D. S. (1977). Molecular analysis of spon-taneous somatic mutants. *Nature* **265**, 299–304.

Amor, M., Bonhomme, F., Guenet, J-L., Petter, F. and Cazenave, P-A. (1984). Polymorphism of heavy chain immunoglobulin isotypes in the *Mus* subgenus. I. Limited polymorphism revealed by antibodies raised in SPE wild-derived inbred strain. *Immunogenetics* **20**, 577–581.

Andersson, J. and Melchers, F. (1978). The antibody repertoire of hybrid cell lines obtained by fusion of X63-Ag8 myeloma cells with mitogen-activated B-cell blasts. *Current Topics Microbiol. Immunol.* **81**, 130–139.

Anfinsen, C. B. (1973). Principles that govern the folding of protein chains. *Science* **181**, 223–230.

Argon, Y., Burrone, O. R. and Milstein, C. (1983). Molecular characterization of a nonsecreting myeloma mutant. *Eur. J. Immunol.* **13**, 301–305.

Arnon, R. (1973). Immunochemistry of enzymes. *In* "The Antigens" (M. Sela, ed.), Vol. 1, pp. 88–159. Academic Press, New York.

Arp, B., McMullen, M. D., and Storb, U. (1982). Sequences of immunoglobulin $\lambda 1$ genes in a $\lambda 1$ defective mouse strain. *Nature* **298**, 184–187.

Atassi, M. Z. (1975). Antigenic structure of myoglobin: the complete immunochemical anatomy of a protein and conclusions relating to antigenic structures of proteins. *Immunochemistry* **12**, 423–438.

Baumal, R. and Scharff, M. D. (1973). Synthesis, assembly and secretion of mouse immunoglobulin. *Transplant Rev.* **14**, 163–183.

Bazin, H. (1982). Production of rat monoclonal antibodies with the LOU rat nonsecreting IR983F myeloma cell line. *In* "Protides of the Biological Fluids" (H. Peeters, ed), 29th Colloquium, pp. 615–618. Pergamon Press, Oxford and New York.

Bazin, H., Beckers, A., Deckers, C. and Moriamé, M. (1973). Transplantable immunoglobulin-secreting tumors in rats. V. Monoclonal immunoglobulins secreted by 250 ileocecal immunocytomas in LOU/WsI rats. *J. natn. Cancer Inst.* **51**, 1359–1361.

Bazin, H., Beckers, A. and Querinjean, P. (1974). Three classes and four sub(classes) of rat immunoglobulins: IgM, IgA, IgE and IgG1, IgG2a, IgG2b, IgG2c. *Eur. J. Immunol.* **4**, 44–48.

Bazin, H., Beckers, A., Urbain-Vansanten, G., Pauwels, R., Bruyns, C., Tilkin, A. F., Platteau, B. and Urbain, J. (1978). Transplantable IgD immunoglobulin-secreting tumors in rat. *J. Immunol.* **121**, 2077–2082.

Benacerraf, B. and McDevitt, H. O. (1972). Histocompatibility immune response genes. *Science* **175**, 273–279.

Benjamin, D. C., Berzofsky, J. A., East, I. J., Gurd, F. R. N., Hannum, C., Leach, S. J., Margoliash, E., Michael, J. G., Miller, A., Prager, E. M., Reichlin, M., Sercarz, E. E., Smith-Gill, S. J., Todd, P. E., and Wilson, A. C. (1984). The antigenic structure of proteins: a reappraisal. *Ann. Rev. Immunol.* **2**, 67–101.

Bergman, L. W. and Kuehl, W. M. (1979). Formation of intermolecular disulfide bonds on nascent immunoglobulin polypeptides. *J. biol. Chem.* **254**, 5690–5694.

Birnbaum, D. and Kourilsky, F. M. (1981). Differences in the cell binding affinity of a crossreactive monoclonal anti-Ia alloantibody in mice of different H-2 haplotypes. *Eur. J. Immunol.* **11**, 734–738.

Blatt, C. and Haimovitch, J. (1981). The selective effect of tunicamycin on the secretion of IgM and IgG produced by the same cells. *Eur. J. Immunol.* **11**, 65–66.

Blattner, F. R. and Tucker, P. W. (1984). The molecular biology of immunoglobulin D. *Nature* **307**, 417–422.

Blose, S. H., Matsumura, F. and Lin, J. J. C. (1982). Structure of vimentin 10-nm filaments probed with a monoclonal antibody that recognizes a common antigenic determinant on vimentin and tropomyosin. *Cold Spring Harbor Symp. quant. Biol.* **46**, 455–463.

Borges, M. S., Kumagai, Y., Okumura, K., Hirayama, N., Ovary, Z. and Tada, T. (1981). Allelic polymorphism of murine IgE controlled by the seventh immunoglobulin heavy chain allotype locus. *Immunogenetics* **13**, 499–507.

Böttcher, I., Hämmerling, G. and Kapp, J-F. (1978). Continuous production of monoclonal IgE antibodies with known allergenic specificity by a hybrid cell line. *Nature* **275**, 761–762.

Bourgois, A., Kitajima, K., Hunter, I. R. and Askonas, B. A. (1977). Surface immunoglobulins of lipopolysaccharide stimulated spleen cells. The behaviour of IgM, IgD and IgG. *Eur. J. Immunol.* **7**, 151–153.

Brandtzaeg, P. and Prydz, H. (1984). Direct evidence for an integrated function of J chain and secretory component in epithelial transport of immunoglobulins. *Nature,* **311**, 71–73.

Burnet, F. M. (1957). A modification of Jerne's theory of antibody production using the concept of clonal selection. *Austral. J. Sci.* **20**, 67–69.

Burnet, F. M. (1968). "Changing Patterns: An Atypical Autobiography." William Heinemann, London.

Burnette, W. N. (1981). "Western blotting": Electrophoretic transfer of proteins from sodium dodecyl sulfate-polyacrylamide gels to unmodified nitrocellulose and radiographic detection with antibody and radioiodinated protein A. *Anal. Biochem.* **112**, 195–203.

Caskey, C. T. and Kruh, G. D. (1979). The HPRT locus. *Cell* **16**, 1–9.

Chedid, L., Audibert, F., Lefrancier, P., Choay, J. and Lederer, E. (1976). Modulation of the immune response by a synthetic adjuvant and analogs. *Proc. natn. Acad. Sci. U.S.A.* **73**, 2472–2475.

Cheng, H-L., Blattner, F. R., Fitzmaurice, L., Mushinski, J. F. and Tucker, P. W. (1982). Structure of genes for membrane and secreted murine IgD heavy chains. *Nature* **296**, 410–415.

Chien, Y., Becker, D. M., Lindsten, TR., Okamura, M., Cohen, D. I. and Davis, M. (1984). A third type of murine T-cell receptor gene. *Nature,* **321**, 31–35.

Coleclough, C. and Wood, D. (1984). Introns excised from immunoglobulin premRNAs exist as discrete species. *Mol. Cell. Biol.* **4**, 2017–2022.

Cook, W. D. and Scharff, M. D. (1977). Antigen-binding mutants of mouse myeloma cells. *Proc. natn. Acad. Sci. U.S.A.* **74**, 5687–5691.

Cory, S. (1983). Oncogenes and B lymphocyte neoplasia. *Immunol. Today* **4**, 205–207.

Cory, S., Tyler, B. M. and Adams, J. M. (1981). Sets of immunoglobulin V_K genes homologous to ten cloned V_K sequences: implications for the number of germline V_K genes. *J. Mol. Appl. Genet.* **1**, 103–116.

Cotton, R. G. H. and Milstein, C. (1973). Fusion of two immunoglobulin-producing myeloma cells. *Nature* **244**, 42–43.

Cotton, R. G. H., Secher, D. S. and Milstein, C. (1973). Somatic mutation and origin of antibody diversity. Clonal variability of the immunoglobulin produced by MOPC-21 cells in culture. *Eur. J. Immunol.* **3**, 135–140.

Croce, C. M., Linnenbach, A., Hall, W., Steplewski, Z. and Koprowski, H. (1980). Production of human hybridomas secreting antibodies to measles virus. *Nature* **288**, 488–489.

Crumpton, M. J. (1974). Protein antigens: The molecular bases of antigenicity and immunogenicity. *In* "The Antigens" (M. Sela, ed), Vol. 2, pp. 1–78. Academic Press, New York.

Davis, M., Kim, S. K. and Hood, L. (1980). Immunoglobulin class switching: developmentally regulated DNA rearrangements during differentiation. *Cell* **22**, 1–2.

Deisenhofer, J., Colman, P. M., Epp, O. and Huber, R. (1976). Crystallographic structural studies of a human Fc fragment. II. A complete model based on a Fourier map at 3.5 Å resolution. *Hoppe-Seyler's Z. physiol. Chem.* **357**, 1421–1433.

Der Balian, G. P., Slack, J., Clevinger, B. L., Bazin, H. and Davie, J. M. (1980). Subclass restriction of murine antibodies. III. Antigens that stimulate IgG3 in mice stimulate IgG2c in rats. *J. exp. Med.* **152**, 209–218.

Desidero, S. V., Yancopoulos, G. D., Paskind, M., Thomas, E., Boss, M. A., Landau, N., Alt, F. W. and Baltimore, D. (1984). Insertion of N regions into heavy-chain genes is correlated with expression of terminal transferase in B cells. *Nature,* **311**, 752–755.

D'Eustachio, P., Bothwell, A. L. M., Takaro, T. K., Baltimore, D. and Ruddle, F. H. (1981). Chromosomal location of structural genes encoding murine immunoglobulin λ light chains. *J. exp. Med.* **153**, 793–800.

Dickler, H. B. (1976). Lymphocyte receptors for immunoglobulin. *Adv. Immunol.* **24**, 167–214.

Dorrington, K. J. and Bennich, H. H. (1978). Structure-function relationships for human immunoglobulin E. *Immunol. Rev.* **41**, 3–25.

Dower, S. K., Ozato, K. and Segal, D. M. (1984). The interaction of monoclonal antibodies with MHC class I antigens on mouse spleen cells. I. Analysis of the mechanism of binding. *J. Immunol.* **132**, 751–758.

Early, P. and Hood, L. (1981a). Mouse immunoglobulin genes. *In* "Genetic Engineering 3" (J. K. Setlow and A. Hollaender, eds), pp. 157–188. Plenum Press, New York.

Early, P. and Hood, L. (1981b). Allelic exclusion and nonproductive immunoglobulin gene rearrangements. *Cell* **24**, 1–3.

Edwards, P. A. W., Smith, C. M., Neville, A. M. and O'Hare, M. J, (1982). A human–human hybrid myeloma (hybridoma) system based on a fast-growing mutant of the ARH-77 myeloma line. *Eur. J. Immunol.* **12**, 641–648.

Eshhar, Z., Blatt, C., Bergman, Y., and Haimovitch, J. (1979). Induction of secretion of IgM from cells of the B cell line 38C-13 by somatic cell hybridisation. *J. Immunol.* **122**, 2430–2434.

Eshhar, Z., Ofarim, M. and Waks, T. (1980). Generation of hybridomas secreting murine reaginic antibodies of anti-DNP specificity. *J. Immunol.* **124**, 775–780.

Ey, P. L., Prowse, S. J. and Jenkin, C. R. (1978). Isolation of pure IgG1, IgG2a and IgG2b immunoglobulins from mouse serum using protein A-Sepharose. *Immunochemistry* **15**, 429–436.

Finkelman, F. D., Kessler, S. W., Mushinski, J. F. and Potter, M. (1981). IgD-secreting murine plasmacytomas: identification and partial characterization of two IgD myeloma proteins. *J. Immunol.* **126**, 680–687.

Franklin, E. C. and Frangione, B. (1971). The molecular defect in a protein (CRA) found in γ1 heavy chain disease, and its genetic implications. *Proc. natn. Acad. Sci. U.S.A.* **68**, 187–191.

Freund, J. (1956). The mode of action of immunologic adjuvants. *Adv. Tuberc. Res.* **7**, 130–148.

Galfrè, G. and Milstein, C. (1981). Preparation of monoclonal antibodies: strategies and procedures. *Meth. Enzymol.* **73**, 3–46.

Galfrè, G., Milstein, C. and Wright, B. (1979). Rat × rat hybrid myelomas and a monoclonal anti-Fd portion of mouse IgG. *Nature* **277**, 131–133.

Gally, J. A. and Edelman, G. M. (1972). The genetic control of immunoglobulin synthesis. *A. Rev. Genet.* **6**, 1–46.

Gasser, D. L. (1977). Current status of rat immunogenetics. *Adv. Immunol.* **25**, 93–139.

Gearhart, P. J., Johnson, N. D., Douglas, R. and Hood, L. (1981). IgG antibodies to phosphorylcholine exhibit more diversity than their IgM counterparts. *Nature* **291**, 29–34.

Gillies, S. D., Morrison, S. L., Oi, V. T. and Tonegawa, S. (1983). A tissue-specific transcription enhancer element is located in the major intron of a rearranged immunoglobulin heavy-chain gene. *Cell* **33**, 717–728.

Goding, J. W. and Layton, J. E. (1976). Antigen-induced co-capping of IgM and IgD-like receptors on murine B cells. *J. exp. Med.* **144**, 852–857.

Goding, J. W. (1978). Use of staphylococcal protein A as an immunological reagent. *J. immunol. Methods* **20**, 241–253.

Goding, J. W. (1980). Structural studies of murine lymphocyte surface IgD. *J. Immunol.* **124**, 2082–2088.

Goding, J. W. (1982). Asymmetrical surface IgG on MOPC-21 plasmacytoma cells contains one membrane heavy chain and one secretory heavy chain. *J. Immunol.* **128**, 2416–2421.

Goding, J. W. and Herzenberg, L. A. (1980). Biosynthesis of lymphocyte surface IgD in the mouse. *J. Immunol.* **124**, 2540–2547.

Green, I., Paul, W. E. and Bencerraf, B. (1966). The behaviour of hapten-poly-L-lysine conjugates as complete antigens in genetic responder and as haptens in nonresponder guinea pigs. *J. exp. Med.* **123**, 859–879.

Grey, H. M. and Kohler, P. F. (1973). Cryoimmunoglobulins. *Semin. Hematol.* **10**, 87–112.

Grey, H. M., Abel, C. A., Yount, W. J. and Kunkel, H. G. (1968). A subclass of human γA-globulins (γA2) which lacks the disulfide bonds linking heavy and light chains. *J. exp. Med.* **128**, 1223–1236.

Griffiths, G. M., Berek, C., Kaartinen, M. and Milstein, C. (1984). Somatic mutation and the maturation of immune response to 2-phenyl oxazalone. *Nature* **312**, 271–275.

Havran, W. L., Di Giusto, D. L. and Cambier, J. C. (1984). mIgM:mIgD ratios on B cells: mean mIgD expression exceeds mIgM by 10-fold on most splenic B cells. *J. Immunol.* **132**, 1712–1716.

Herbert, W. J. (1973). Mineral-oil adjuvants and the immunization of laboratory animals. *In* "Handbook of Experimental Immunology" (D.M. Weir, ed), Vol. 3, pp. A2.1–2.14. Blackwell, Oxford.

Herrmann, S. H. and Mescher, M. F. (1979). Purification of the H-2K^k molecule of the murine major histocompatibility complex. *J. biol. Chem.* **254**, 8713–8716.

Herzenberg, L. A., Minna, J. D. and Herzenberg, L. A. (1967). The chromosome region for immunoglobulin heavy chains in the mouse: allelic electrophoretic mobility differences and allotype suppression. *Cold Spring Harbor Symp. quant. Biol.* **32**, 181–186.

Herzenberg, L. A. and Herzenberg, L. A. (1977). Mouse immunoglobulin allotypes: Description and special methodology. *In* "Handbook of Experimental Immunology" (D. M. Weir, ed), 3rd edition, Vol. 2, Chapter 12. Blackwell, Oxford.

Hirashima, M., Yodoi, J. and Ishizaka, K. (1981). Regulatory role of IgE-binding factors from rat T lymphocytes. V. Formation of IgE-potentiating factor by T lymphocytes from rats treated with *Bordellas pertussis* vaccine. *J. Immunol.* **126**, 838–842.

Hirayama, N., Hirano, T., Köhler, G., Kurata, A., Okumura, K. and Ovary, Z. (1982). Biological activities of antitrinitrophenyl and antidinitrophenyl mouse monoclonal antibodies. *Proc. natn. Acad. Sci. U.S.A.* **79**, 613–615.

Hitchcock, S. E. (1980). Actin-deoxyribonuclease I interaction. *J. biol. Chem.* **255**, 5668–5673.

Hood, L., Loh, E., Hubert, J., Barstard, P., Eaton, B., Early, P., Fuhrman, J., Johnson, N., Kronenberg, M. and Schilling, J. (1976). The structure and genetics of mouse immunoglobulins: an analysis of NZB myeloma proteins and sets of BALB/c myeloma proteins binding particular haptens. *Cold Spring Harb. Symp. quant. Biol.* **41**, 817–836.

Horibata, K. and Harris, A. W. (1970). Mouse myelomas and lymphomas in culture. *Exp. Cell Res.* **60**, 61–77.

Howard, J. C., Butcher, G. W., Galfré, G., Milstein, C. and Milstein, C. P. (1979). Monoclonal antibodies as tools to analyse the serological and genetic complexities of major transplantation antigens. *Immunol. Rev.* **47**, 139–174.

Huang, C-H., Huang, H-J. S., and Lee, S-C. (1984). Detection of immunoglobulin heavy chain IgG3 polymorphism in wild mice with xenogeneic monoclonal antibodies. *Immunogenetics* **20**, 565–575.

Huber, R., Deisenhofer, J., Colman. P. M., Matsushima, M. and Palm, W. (1976). Crystallographic structure studies of an IgG molecule and an Fc fragment. *Nature* **264**, 415–420.

Inbar, D., Hochman, J. and Givol, D. (1972). Localization of antibody-combining sites within the variable portions of light and heavy chains. *Proc. natn. Acad. Sci. U.S.A.* **69**, 2659–2662.

Ishida, N., Ueda, S., Hayashida, H., Miyata, T. and Honjo, T. (1982). The nucleotide sequence of the mouse immunoglobulin epsilon gene: comparison with the human epsilon gene sequence. *EMBO J.* **1**, 1117–1123.

Jeppsson, J-O., Laurell, C-B., and Franzen, B. (1979). Agarose gel electrophoresis. *Clin. Chem.* **25**, 629–638.

Kakimoto, K. and Onoue, K. (1974). Characterization of the Fv fragment isolated from a human immunoglobulin M. *J. Immunol.* **112**, 1373–1382.

Karpas, A., Fischer, P. and Swirsky, D. (1982). Human plasmacytoma with an unusual karyotype growing *in vitro* and producing light chain immunoglobulin. *Lancet* **i**, 931–933.

Kearney, J. F., Radbruch, A., Liesegang, B. and Rajewsky, K. (1979). A new mouse myeloma cell line which has lost immunoglobulin expression but permits the construction of antibody in secreting hybrid cell lines. *J. Immunol.* **123**, 1548–1550.

Kehry, M., Sibley, C., Fuhrman, J., Schilling, J. and Hood, L. E. (1979). Amino acid sequence of a mouse immunoglobulin μ chain. *Proc. natn. Acad. Sci. U.S.A.* **76**, 2932–2936.

Kehry, M. R., Fuhrman, J. S., Schilling, J. W., Rogers, J., Sibley, C. H. and Hood, L. E. (1982). Complete amino acid sequence of a mouse μ chain: homology among heavy chain constant region domains. *Biochemistry* **21**, 5415–5424.

Kemp, D. J., Tyler, B., Bernard, O., Gough, N., Gerondakis, S., Adams, J. M. and Cory, S. (1981). Organization of genes and spacers within the mouse immunoglobulin V_H locus. *J. molec. appl. Genet.* **1**, 245–261.

Kilmartin, J. V., Wright, B. and Milstein, C. (1982). Rat monoclonal antibodies derived by using a new non-secreting rat cell line. *J. Cell Biol.* **93**, 576–582.

Klein, J., Juretic, A., Baxevanis, C. N. and Nagy, Z. A. (1981). The traditional and a new version of the mouse H-2 complex. *Nature* **291**, 455–460.

Köhler, G. (1980). Immunoglobulin chain loss in hybridoma lines. *Proc. natn. Acad. Sci. U.S.A.* **77**, 2197–2199.

Köhler, G. and Milstein, C. (1975). Continuous cultures of fused cells secreting antibody of predefined specificity. *Nature* **256**, 495–497.

Köhler, G. and Milstein, C. (1976). Derivation of specific antibody-producing tissue culture and tumor lines by cell fusion. *Eur. J. Immunol.* **6**, 511–519.

Köhler, G., Howe, S. C. and Milstein, C. (1976). Fusion between immunoglobulin-secreting and non-secreting myeloma cell lines. *Eur. J. Immunol.* **6**, 292–295.

Köhler, G., Pearson, T. and Milstein, C. (1977). Fusion of T and B cells. *Somat. Cell. Genet.* **3**, 303–312.

Köhler, G., Hengartner, H. and Shulman, M. J. (1978). Immunoglobulin production by lymphocyte hybridomas. *Eur. J. Immunol.* **8**, 82–88.

Koshland, M. E. (1975). Structure and function of the J chain. *Adv. Immunol.* **20** 41–69.

Kozbor, D., Triputti, P., Roder, J. C. and Croce, C. M. (1984). A human hybrid myeloma for production of human monoclonal antibodies. *J. Immunol.* **133**, 3001–3005.

Krause, R. M. (1970). The search for antibodies with molecular uniformity. *Adv. Immunol.* **12**, 1–56.

Kühn, L. C. and Kraehenbuhl, J-P. (1981). The membrane receptor for polymeric immunoglobulin is structurally related to secretory component. *J. biol. Chem.* **256**, 12490–12495.

Lamm, M. E. (1976). Cellular aspects of immunoglobulin A. *Adv. Immunol.* **22**, 223–290.

Lancet, D., Isenman, D., Sjödahl, J., Sjöquist, J. and Pecht, I. (1978). Interaction between staphylococcal protein A and immunoglobulin domains. *Biochem. biophys. Res. Commun.* **85**, 608–614.

Lane, D. and Koprowski, H. (1982). Molecular recognition and the future of monoclonal antibodies. *Nature* **296**, 200–202.

Langone, J. J. (1982). Protein A of *Staphylococcus aureus* and related immunoglobulin receptors produced by streptococci and pneumococci. *Adv. Immunol.* **32**, 157–252.

Ledbetter, J. A. and Herzenberg, L. A. (1979). Xenogeneic monoclonal antibodies to mouse lymphoid differentiation antigens. *Immunol. Rev.* **47**, 63–90.

Lefkovits, I. and Waldmann, H. (1979). "Limiting Dilution Analysis of Cells in the Immune System." Cambridge University Press, Cambridge.

Lerner, R. A. (1982). Tapping the immunological repertoire to produce antibodies of predetermined specificity. *Nature* **299**, 592–596.

Lieberman, R. (1978). Genetics of the IgCH (Allotype) locus in the mouse. *Springer Seminars Immunopath.* **1**, 7–30.

Littlefield, J. W. (1964). Selection of hybrids from matings of fibroblasts *in vitro* and their presumed recombinants. *Science* **145**, 709–710.

Liu, F-T., Bohn, J. W, Ferry, E. L., Yamamoto, H., Molinaro, C. A., Sherman, L. A., Kliman, N. R. and Katz, D. H. (1980). Monoclonal dinitrophenyl-specific murine IgE antibody: preparation, isolation and characterization. *J. Immunol.* **124**, 2728–2737.

Lo, M. M. S., Tsong, T. Y., Conrad, M. K., Strittmatter, S. M., Hester, L. D. and Snyder, S. H. (1984). Monoclonal antibody production by receptor-mediated electrically induced cell fusion. *Nature* **310**, 792–794.

Lyon, M. F. (1961). Gene action in the X chromosome of the mouse. (Mus. musculus L.). *Nature* **190**, 372–373.

Mason, D. W. and Williams, A F. (1980). The kinetics of antibody binding to membrane antigens in solution and at the cell surface. *Biochem. J.* **187**, 1–20.

Medgyesi, G. A., Füst, G., Gergely, J. and Bazin, H. (1978). Classes and subclasses of rat immunoglobulins: interaction with the complement system and staphylococcal protein A. *Immunochemistry* **15**, 125–129.

Merwin, R. M. and Redmon, L. W. (1963). Induction of plasma cell tumors and sarcomas in mice by diffusion chambers placed in the peritoneal cavity. *J. natn. Cancer Inst.* **31**, 997–1017.

Metzger, H. (1978). The IgE-mast cell system as a paradigm for the study of antibody mechanisms. *Immunol. Rev.* **41**, 186–199.

Michaelides, M., Sandrin, M., Morgan, G., McKenzie, I. F. C., Ashman, R. and Melvold, R. (1981). Ir function in an I-A subregion mutant B6.C-H-2[bm12]. *J. exp. Med.* **153**, 464–469.

Miller, C. H., Carbonell, A., Peng, R., Paglieroni, T. and Mackenzie, M. R. (1982). A human plasma cell line. Induction and characterization. *Cancer* **49**, 2091–2096.

Milstein, C. and Cuello, A. C. (1983). Hybrid hybridomas and their use in immunocytochemistry. *Nature* **305**, 537–540.

Milstein, C., Brownlee, G. G., Harrison, T. M. and Mathews, M. B. (1972). A possible precursor of immunoglobulin light chains. *Nature (New Biol.).* **239**, 117–120.

Milstein, C. P., Richardson, N. E., Deverson, E. V. and Feinstein, A. (1975). Interchain disulphide bonds of mouse immunoglobulin M. *Biochem. J.* **151**, 615–624.

Mitchell, G. F. (1979). Responses to infection with metazoan and protozoan parasites in mice. *Adv. Immunol.* **28**, 451–511.

Morrison, S. L., Johnson, M. J., Herzenberg, L. A. and Oi, V. T. (1984). Chimeric human antibody molecules: Mouse antigen-binding domains with human constant region domains. *Proc. natn. Acad. Sci. USA* **81**, 6851–6855.

Mostov, K. E., Friedlander, M. and Blobel, G. (1984). The receptor for trans-epithelial transport of IgA and IgM contains multiple immunoglobulin-like domains. *Nature,* **308**, 37–43.

Mullock, B. M. and Hinton, R. H. (1981). Transport of proteins from blood to bile. *Trends. biochem. Sci.* **6**, 188–191.

Munoz, J. (1964). Effect of bacteria and bacterial products on antibody response. *Adv. Immunol.* **4**, 397–440.

Munoz, J. J. and Bergman, R. K. (1977). "*Bordetella pertussis.* Immunological and Other Biological Activities." Marcel Dekker, New York.

Munoz, J. J. and Sewell, W. A. (1984). Effect of pertussigen on inflammation caused by Freund's adjuvant. *Infect. Immun.* **44**, 637–641.

Nahm, M., Der-Balian, G. P., Venturini, D., Bazin, H. and Davie, J. M. (1980). Antigenic similarities of rat and mouse IgG subclasses associated with anti-carbohydrate specificities. *Immunogenetics* **7**, 199–203.

Neuberger, M. S. and Rajewsky, K. (1981). Activation of mouse complement by monoclonal mouse antibodies. *Eur. J. Immunol.* **11**, 1012–1016.

Niman, H. L., Houghten, R. A., Walker, L. E., Reisfeld, R. A., Wilson, I. A., Hogle, J. M. and Lerner, R. A. (1983). Generation of protein-reactive antibodies by short peptides is an event of high frequency: Implications for the structural basis of immune recognition. *Proc. natn. Acad. Sci. U.S.A.* **80**, 4949–4953.

Nisonoff, A., Hopper, J. E. and Spring, S. B. (1975). "The Antibody Molecule." Academic Press, New York.

Nose, M. and Wigzell, H. (1983). Biological significance of carbohydrate chains on monoclonal antibodies. *Proc. natn. Acad. Sci. U.S.A.* **80**, 6632–6636.

Nossal, G. J. V. and Lederberg, J. (1958). Antibody production by single cells. *Nature* **181**, 1419–1420.

Nussenzweig, M. C., Steinman, R. M., Witmer, M. D. and Gutchinov, B. (1982). A monoclonal antibody specific for mouse dendritic cells. *Proc. natn. Acad. Sci. U.S.A.* **79**, 161–165.

Ohno, S., Babonits, M., Wiener, F., Spira, J., Klein, G. and Potter, M. (1979). Nonrandom chromosome changes involving the Ig gene-carrying chromosomes 12 and 6 in pristane-induced mouse plasmacytomas. *Cell* **18**, 1001–1007.

Oi, V. T., Vuong, M., Hardy, R., Reidler, J., Dangl, J., Herzenberg, L. A. and Stryer, L. (1984). Correlation between segmental flexibility and effector function of anti-bodies. *Nature* **307**, 136–140.

Olden, K., Bernard, B. A., White, S. L. and Parent, J. B. (1982). Function of the carbohydrate moieties of glycoproteins. *J. Cell Biochem.* **18**, 313–335.

Ollo, R. and Rougeon, F. (1983). Gene conversion and polymorphism: Generation of mouse immunoglobulin γ2a chain alleles by differential gene conversion by γ2b chain gene. *Cell* **32**, 515–523.

Olsson, L. and Kaplan, H. S. (1980). Human–human hybridomas producing mono-clonal antibodies of predefined antigenic specificity. *Proc. natn. Acad. Sci. U.S.A.* **77**, 5429–5431.

Parham, P. (1983). On the fragmentation of monoclonal IgG1, IgG2a, and IgG2b from BALB/c mice. *J. Immunol.* **131**, 2895–2902.

Parkhouse, R. M. E. (1971). Immunoglobulin M biosynthesis: Production of inter-mediates and excess of light chain in mouse myeloma MOPC-104E. *Biochem. J.* **123**, 635–641.

Paul, W. E. and Bencerraf, B. (1977). Functional specificity of thymus-dependent lymphocytes. *Science* **195**, 1293–1300.

Peppard, J., Orlans, E., Payne, A. W. R. and Andrew, E. (1981). The elimination of circulating complexes containing polymeric IgA by excretion in the bile. *Immunology* **42**, 83–89.

Perlmutter, R. M., Crews, S. T., Douglas, R., Sorensen, G., Johnson, N., Nivera, N., Gearhart, P. J. and Hood, L. (1984). Generation of diversity in phosphoryl-choline-binding antibodies. *Adv. Immunol.* **35**, 1–37.

Pillemer, E. and Weissman, I. L. (1981). A monoclonal antibody that detects a V_K-TEPC-15 idiotypic determinant cross-reactive with a Thy-1 determinant. *J. exp. Med.* **153**, 1068–1079.

Poljak, R. J., Amzel, L. M., Avey, H. P., Becka, L. N. and Nisonoff, A. (1972). Structure of Fab' New at 6 Å resolution. *Nature (New. Biol.)* **235**, 137–140.

Pollock, R. R., Dorf, M. E. and Mescher, M. F. (1980). Genetic control of murine IgD structural heterogeneity. *Proc. natn. Acad. Sci. USA.* **77**, 4256–4259.

Pontecorvo, G. (1976). Production of indefinitely multiplying mammalian somatic cell hybrids by polyethylene glycol (PEG) treatment. *Somatic. Cell Genet.* **1**, 397–400.

Potter, M. (1972). Immunoglobulin-producing tumors and myeloma proteins of mice. *Physiol. Rev.* **52**, 631–719.

Potter, M. (1977). Antigen-binding myeloma proteins of mice. *Adv. Immunol.* **25**, 141–211.

Potter, M. and Boyce, C. R. (1962). Induction of plasma cell neoplasms in strain BALB/c mice with mineral oil adjuvants. *Nature* **193**, 1086–1087.

Potter, M. and Lieberman, R. (1967). Genetics of immunoglobulin in the mouse. *Adv. Immunol.* **7**, 92–145.

Richards, F. F., Konigsberg, W. H., Rosenstern, R. W. and Varga, J. M. (1975). On the specificity of antibodies. *Science* **187**, 130–137.

Ringertz, N. R. and Savage, R. E. (1976). "Cell Hybrids." Academic Press, New York.

Ritchie, K. A., Brinster, R. L. and Storb, U. (1984). Allelic exclusion and control of endogenous immunoglobulin gene rearrangement in κ transgenic mice. *Nature* **312**, 517–520.

Rogers, J. and Wall, R. (1984). Immunoglobulin RNA rearrangements in B lymphocyte differentiation. *Adv. Immunol.* **35**, 39–59.

Rogers, J., Early, P., Carter, C., Calame, K., Bond, M., Hood, L. and Wall, R. (1980). Two mRNAs with different 3' ends encode membrane-bound and secreted forms of immunoglobulin μ chain. *Cell* **20**, 303–312.

Roth, R. and Koshland, M. (1981a). Role of disulfide interchange enzyme in immunoglobulin synthesis. *Biochemistry* **20**, 6594–6599.

Roth, R. and Koshland, M. (1981b). Identification of a lymphocyte enzyme that catalyzes pentamer immunoglobulin M assembly. *J. biol. Chem.* **256**, 4633–4639.

Rousset, B. and Wolff, J. (1980). Lactoperoxidase-tubulin interactions. *J. biol. Chem.* **255**, 2514–2523.

Ruddle, F. H. (1981). A new era in mammalian gene mapping: somatic cell genetics and recombinant DNA methodologies. *Nature* **294**, 115–120.

Russell, M. W., Brown, T. A. and Mestecky, J. (1981). Role of serum IgA. Hepatobiliary transport of circulating antigen. *J. exp. Med.* **153**, 968–976.

Sakano, H., Kurosawa, Y., Weigert, M. and Tonegawa, S. (1981). Identification and nucleotide sequence of a diversity DNA segment (D) of immunoglobulin heavy-chain genes. *Nature* **290**, 562–565.

Sanger, F. and Thompson, E. O. P. (1953). The amino acid sequence in the glycyl chain of insulin. *Biochem. J.* **53**, 353–374.

Schulz, G. E. and Schirmer, R. H. (1978). "Principles of Protein Structure." Springer-Verlag, New York and Heidelberg.

Seppälä, I., Sarvas, H., Péterfy, F. and Mäkelä, O. (1981). The four subclasses of IgG can be isolated from mouse serum by using protein A-Sepharose. *Scand. J. Immunol.* **14**, 335–342.

Sewell, W. A., Munoz, J. J., Scollay, R. and Vadas, M. A. (1984). Studies on the mechanism of the enhancement of delayed-type hypersensitivity by pertussigen. *J. Immunol.* **133**, 1716–1722.

Sheppard, H. W. and Gutman, G. A. (1981a). Complex allotype of rat kappa chains are coded for by structural alleles. *Nature* **293**, 669–671.

Sheppard, H. W, and Gutman, G. A. (1981b). Allelic forms of rat kappa chain genes: Evidence for strong selection at the level of nucleotide sequence. *Proc. natn. Acad. Sci. U.S.A.* **78**, 7064–7068.

Shimizu, A., Watanabe, S., Yamamura, Y. and Putnam, F. W. (1974). Tryptic digestion of immunoglobulin M in urea: conformational lability of the middle part of the molecule. *Immunochemistry* **11**, 719–727.

Shulman, M., Wilde, C. D. and Köhler, G. (1978). A better cell line for making hybridomas secreting specific antibodies. *Nature* **276**, 269–270.

Sikorav, J-L., Auffray, C. and Rougeon, F. (1980). Structure of the constant and 3′ untranslated regions of the murine Balb/c γ2a heavy chain messenger RNA. *Nucleic Acids Res.* **8**, 3143–3155.

Spiegelberg, H. L. (1974). Biological activities of immunoglobulins of different classes and subclasses. *Adv. Immunol.* **19**, 259–294.

Stanisz, A. M., Lieberman, R., Kaplan, A. and Davie, J. M. (1983). IgA polymorphism in mice: NZB and BALB/c mice produce two forms of IgA. *Molec. Immunol.* **20**, 983–988.

Surolia, A., Pain, D. and Khan, M. I. (1982). Protein A:: nature's universal anti-antibody. *Trends biochem. Sci.* **7**, 74–76.

Tainer, J. A., Getzoff, E. G., Alexander, H., Houghten, R. A., Olson, A. J., Lerner, R. A. and Hendrickson, W. A. (1984). The reactivity of anti-peptide antibodies is a function of the atomic mobility of sites in a protein. *Nature* **312**, 127–134.

Takahashi, N., Tataert, D., Debuire, B., Lin, L-C. and Putnam, F. W. (1982). Complete amino acid sequence of the δ heavy chain of human immunoglobulin D. *Proc. natn. Acad. Sci. U.S.A.* **79**, 2850–2854.

Tartakoff, A. and Vassali, P. (1979). Plasma cell immunoglobulin M molecules. Their biosynthesis, assembly and intracellular transport. *J. Cell. Biol.* **83**, 284–299.

Tomasi, T. B. and Grey, H. M. (1972). Structure and function of immunoglobulin A. *Prog. Allergy* **16**, 81–185.

Tonegawa, S. (1983). Somatic generation of antibody diversity. *Nature* **302**, 575–581.

Tucker, P. W., Slighton, J. L. and Blattner, F. R. (1981). Mouse IgA heavy chain gene sequence: Implications for evolution of immunoglobulin hinge exons. *Proc. natn. Acad. Sci. U.S.A.* **78**, 7684–7688.

Tyler, B. M., Cowman, S. D., Gerondakis, S. D., Adams, J. M. and Bernard, O. (1982). Messenger RNA for surface immunoglobulin γ chains encodes a highly conserved transmembrane sequence and a 28-residue intracellular domain. *Proc. natn. Acad. Sci. U.S.A.* **79**, 2008–2012.

Uhr, J. W., Capra, J. D., Vitetta, E. S. and Cook, R. G. (1979). Organization of the immune response genes. *Science* **206**, 292–297.

Underdown, B. J. and Dorrington, K. J. (1974). Studies on the structural and conformational basis for the relative resistance of serum and secretory immunoglobulin A to proteolysis. *J. Immunol.* **112**, 949–959.

Unkeless, J. C. (1979). Characterization of a monoclonal antibody directed against mouse macrophage and lymphocyte Fc receptors. *J. exp. Med.* **150**, 580–596.

Vaerman, J. P., Heremans, J. F. and Laurell, C. B. (1968). Distribution of alpha chain subclasses in normal and pathological IgA globulins. *Immunology* **14**, 425–432.

Vassalli, P., Tartakoff, A., Pink, J. R. L. and Jaton, J-C. (1980). Biosynthesis of two forms of IgM heavy chains by normal mouse B lymphocytes. Membrane and secretory IgM. *J. biol. Chem.* **25**, 11822–11827.

Vitetta, E. S. and Uhr, J. .W. (1975). Immunoglobulin-receptors revisited. *Science* **189**, 964–969.

Wall, R. and Kuehl, M. (1983). Biosynthesis and regulation of immunoglobulins. *Ann. Rev. Immunol.* **1**, 393–422.

Walter, P. and Blobel, G. (1982). Signal recognition particle contains a 7S RNA essential for protein translocation across the endoplasmic reticulum. *Nature* **299**, 691–698.

Walter, G., Scheidmann, K. H., Carbone, A., Laudano, A. P. and Doolittle, R. F. (1980). Antibodies specific for the carboxy- and amino-terminal regions of simian virus 40 large tumor antigen. *Proc. natn. Acad. Sci. U.S.A.* **77**, 5197–5200.

Warner, N. L. (1975). Autoimmunity and the pathogenesis of plasma cell tumor induction in NZB inbred and hybrid mice. *Immunogenetics* **2**, 1–20.

Warner, N. L. and Marchalonis, J. J. (1972). Structural differences in mouse IgA myeloma proteins of different allotypes. *J. Immunol.*, **109**, 657–661.

Watanabe, M., Ishii, T. and Nariuchi, H. (1981). Fractionation of IgG1, IgG2a, IgG2b and IgG3 immunoglobulins from mouse serum by protein A-Sepharose column chromatography. *Japan J. exp. Med.* **51**, 65–70.

Westhof, E., Altschuh, D., Moras, D., Bloomer, A. C., Mondragon, A., Klug, A. and van Regenmortel, M. H. V, (1984). Correlation between segmental mobility and the location of antigenic determinants in proteins. *Nature*, **311**, 123–127.

Wiley, D. C., Wilson, I. A. and Skehel, J. J. (1981). Structural identification of the antibody binding sites of Hong Kong influenza haemagglutinin and their involvement in antigenic variation. *Nature* **289**, 373–378.

Winchester, R. J., Fu, S. M., Hoffman, T. and Kunkel, H. G. (1975). IgG on lymphocyte surfaces: technical problems and significance of a third cell population. *J. Immunol.* **114**, 1210–1212.

Wojciezsyn, J. W., Schlegel, R. A., Limley-Sapanski, K. and Jacobson, K. A. (1983). Studies on the mechanism of polyethylene glycol-mediated cell fusion using fluorescent membrane and cytoplasmic probes. *J. Cell. Biol.* **96**, 151–159.

Word, C. J. and Keuhl, W. M. (1981). Expression of surface and secreted IgG2a by a murine B-lymphoma before and after hybridization to myeloma cells. *Mol. Immunol.* **18**, 311–322.

3   Production of Monoclonal Antibodies

Although the technology of hybridoma production is now firmly established, there are a large number of steps involved, and each of these may be carried out in many different ways. The diversity of published approaches reflects both individual biological problems and previous experience. The methods also vary in convenience, speed, reliability and expense, but there is no one "right" approach, and ultimately each investigator must choose and adapt the published strategies to individual needs. An appreciation of the variables and compromises will help minimize the effort required.

Much useful information on general aspects of tissue culture will be found in the volume edited by Jakoby and Pastan (1979) and a monograph by Adams (1980).

3.1 Choice of Normal Lymphocyte Donor

In 1900, Ehrlich recognized that it is difficult to generate antibodies against "self" antigens, a phenomenon that he termed "horror autotoxicus". While the broad truth of this generalization still holds today, an excessively dogmatic adherence to Ehrlich's rule was probably the main reason for the initial rejection of the classic paper of Berson and colleagues (1956) demonstrating the presence of anti-insulin antibodies in certain patients with diabetes (see Yalow, 1978).

Notwithstanding the above, strong antibody responses are most easily obtained when the immunizing antigen differs structurally from components of the body of the recipient. This is usually achieved by immunizing across a species barrier. For example, mice will make large amounts of antibody to

IgG from chicken, human, rabbit or rat, but will not normally make antibody against mouse IgG unless the donor IgG structural genes differ from those of the recipient (Chapter 2). Such genetic differences need not be extensive. Chorney *et al.* (1982) have recently shown that a single amino acid substitution in mouse β_2 microglobulin is sufficient to induce allele-specific antibodies.

In most situations, the choice of species to be immunized will be limited to the mouse and rat. Some success has been obtained in generating hybridomas from human lymphocytes (Olsson and Kaplan, 1980; Schlom *et al.*, 1980; Nowinski *et al.*, 1980; Lane *et al.*, 1982), but the procedure is still difficult and not yet of general usefulness (see Chapter 2 for additional discussion and references).

The mouse is usually preferred as recipient, because of its convenience, the availability of suitable myeloma lines, and its rapid breeding (gestation time 21 days; first mating at 6–8 weeks). However, if it is desired to make antibodies against a *mouse* protein for which there are no known genetic variants, immunization of mice is unlikely to be successful. In such cases, rats may be used as recipients. The other advantage of rats is their larger size, resulting in higher volumes of serum per animal. Moreover, the breeding time of rats is not much longer than that of mice (Galfrè *et al.*, 1979; Galfrè and Milstein, 1981).

All the currently available mouse myeloma cell lines used for hybridoma production are of BALB/c origin, and unless there are compelling reasons to the contrary (e.g. inability of BALB/c to respond to the antigen), BALB/c mice should be used as recipients for the initial immunization. The resulting hybridomas may then be grown in BALB/c mice.

On the other hand, if C57Bl mice are used as recipients, the resulting hybridomas will be rejected by C57Bl mice because of the BALB/c histocompatibility antigens of the myeloma cells. Such hybridomas could only be grown in C57Bl $\times$ BALB/c F_1 mice. Hybridomas from outbred animals will usually fail to grow as tumours in any recipient, because they are unlikely to be histocompatible. Occasionally the need for histocompatibility can be overcome by injecting relatively large numbers (10^7) of hybridoma cells into BALB/c mice that have been sublethally irradiated (400–500R).

All available rat myelomas suitable for fuision are of LOU/C origin. These tumour lines will also grow in LOU/M rats, which are better breeders, but which do not have a high incidence of spontaneous myeloma (Bazin *et al.*, 1973). If, on the other hand, DA rats are used as recipients for antigen, the resulting hybridomas could only be grown in LOU $\times$ DA F_1 rats (see Kilmartin *et al.*, 1982).

Several investigators have successfully made hybridomas by fusing spleen cells from rats with myeloma cells from mice (e.g. Ledbetter and Herzenberg, 1979; McKearn *et al.*, 1980; Springer, 1980; Kincade *et al.*, 1981). These hybrids seem to be as stable as mouse–mouse hybrids, but in general they can only be grown in tissue culture. Occasionally, such hybrids will grow in "nude" (athymic) mice, but nude mice are difficult to breed and maintain in good health. Rat–mouse hydrids will sometimes grow in mice or rats which have been sublethally irradiated (400–500R).

3.2 Immunization Protocol

Protocols for immunization of animals vary widely. The first injection of antigen should be given in a highly aggregated form, because soluble monomeric proteins in their native state are poorly immunogenic and tend to induce tolerance (Dresser, 1962). Subsequent injections may be either soluble or aggregated.

When the antigen is a water-soluble protein, the use of an adjuvant is usually essential (see Chapter 2). By far the most widely used adjuvant is Freund's complete adjuvant. A detailed account of Freund's adjuvant is given by Herbert (1973). Alternatively, the antigen may be precipitated on alum, with or without the addition of killed *Bordetella pertussis* organisms.

The use of adjuvant may influence the class of antibody produced. Handman and Remington (1980) have shown that mice which are chronically infected with *Toxoplasma gondii* make substantial quantities of IgG2 and IgG3 antibodies, but virtually no IgG1. Hybridomas made from the spleens of these mice had a similar class distribution to the serum antibody. In contrast, Johnson *et al.* (1981) immunized mice with the same parasite in Freund's adjuvant, and obtained a substantial IgG1 response and many IgG1 hybridomas. The antigens recognized in these two cases appeared to be the same proteins, but it is not known whether the same determinants were involved.

If the antigen is of very low molecular weight, or is poorly immunogenic for any other reason, strong responses may be elicited by coupling it to an immunogenic carrier molecule (see Chapter 8).

3.2.1 Preparation of Antigen in Freund's Adjuvant

Vials of Freund's complete adjuvant are available from Difco. It is important that the vial be shaken to resuspend the mycobacteria prior to use. It is traditional to use equal volumes of antigen (in aqueous solution) and adjuvant, although it has been suggested that the formation of *water-in-oil* emulsion (rather than oil-in-water, which has little adjuvant effect) is more reliable ("infallible") if 2–4 volumes of oil are used for each volume of aqueous immunogen (Hurn and Chantler, 1980).

The antigen solution, in buffered saline or water, is sucked into a 5 ml *glass* syringe with a Luer lock attachment. A second glass syringe is filled with Freund's complete adjuvant. Any excess air is expelled, and the syringes connected together via a double-hub needle (Herbert, 1973) or a disposable plastic three-way stopcock (Top Surgical, Japan). The *aqueous phase is injected into the oil*, and then the mixture is passed rapidly back and forth between the syringes a few dozen times.

The emulsion should be tested by allowing a drop to fall onto the surface of a beaker of water. The first drop will often spread (Herbert, 1973), but subsequent drops should remain as discrete globules. The emulsion should be thick and creamy. Rapid dispersion of the drops is indicative of an oil-in-water emulsion. The presence of detergents such as sodium dodecyl sulphate, Triton X-100 or Nonidet P-40 in the antigen solution may prevent proper emulsification. Detergents may be removed by acetone precipitation of the antigen (Hager and Burgess, 1980).

Freund's adjuvant should be prepared with care. Accidental injection into the hand may result in permanently stiff or useless fingers, and hyper-sensitivity reactions can be very severe (Chapel and August, 1976). Glass syringes are recommended, because the plunger of plastic disposable syringes tends to swell and stiffen in oil. Failure to use Luer-lock fittings will usually result in the couplings coming undone, and the resultant widespread spraying of adjuvant may cause permanent eye damage.

The site of injection into the recipient is probably not of crucial import-ance. Intradermal injections often cause large painful ulcers, and the popular intra foot-pad route is also inhumane and probably unnecessary. Adequate priming can usually be achieved by subcutaneous, intraperitoneal or intra-muscular routes. A typical volume of emulsion is $50-200\,\mu l$ per mouse, and $1-2\,ml$ per rat. Although the older literature suggests that antigen doses of $1-50\,mg$ are necessary, more recent experience suggestst that $1-50\,\mu g$ are often adquate (see Chapter 8).

It is customary to give "booster" immunizations in *incomplete* Freund's adjuvant (i.e. without the tubercle bacilli) to prevent possible hypersensitivity reactions to the bacteria. Typically, 1–3 boosters may be given at intervals of 2–8 weeks. The final boost is best given 2–4 days prior to fusion, and is often given in aqueous form rather than in adjuvant. Some authors recommend that the final boost be given intravenously (e.g. Stähli *et al.*, 1980), but in my experience this often results in the animal dying of anaphylaxis within min-utes. Intraperitoneal boosting is safer, and probably nearly as effective.

In summary, a reasonable schedule would involve priming with $10\,\mu g$ antigen emulsified in $200\,\mu l$ complete Freund's adjuvant given intra-peritoneally, and boosting twice with the same dose in Freund's incomplete adjuvant at 3–4 weekly intervals. A final intraperitoneal boost of the same or somewhat higher dose in aqueous solution may be given (see Stähli *et al.*, 1980), and the fusion performed 3–4 days later. Both the spleen and the regional draining lymph nodes may be used for fusion (Kearney *et al.*, 1979). Lymph nodes are somewhat deficient in macrophages, and should usually be cultured together with feeder cells (see Section 3.9.3).

The syringes should be thoroughly washed in several changes of acetone, followed by standard wash procedure in detergent. It is difficult to clean metal adapters for joining the syringes, and disposable plastic three-way stopcocks are therefore preferable.

3.2.2 Preparation of Antigen Adsorbed to Alum

An alternative adjuvant system involves precipitation of protein antigen adsorbed to alum (Chase, 1967). The following protocol is adapted from that described by Hudson and Hay (1976):

(1) Make up the antigen solution in 10 ml 0.2 M aluminium potassium sulphate (alum; $AlK(SO_4)_2 \cdot 12H_2O$) in water. The pH will be about 3.0.

(2) Add 4.5 ml of 1.0 M $NaHCO_3$ (pH $\cong$ 8.0). Mix. A white precipitate should form. Leave for 15 min at room temperature.

(3) Centrifuge (300 g, 15 min). Discard supernate, and wash the precipitate three times in phosphate-buffered saline, pH 7.4.

(4) Resuspend the insolubilized protein to the desired concentration.

(5) Some authors add killed *Bordetella pertussis* vaccine ($1–2 \times 10^{10}$ organisms/ml; see Bradley and Shiigi, 1980). (Note that the adjuvanticity of *B. pertussis* may vary markedly between batches.)

(6) Inject the suspension 20–200 µg antigen, subcutaneously or intraperitoneally, and boost at 3–4 week intervals in the same way, until the antibody titre is strong. A final boost should be given 3–4 days prior to fusion, and is probably best given in water-soluble form intraperitoneally.

3.2.3 Immunization with Intact Cells

Intact living cells are highly immunogenic, and do not usually require the use of adjuvants. Cells should be washed 3–4 times in phosphate-buffered saline to remove serum components, and injected intraperitoneally. A typical dose is 10^7 cells, although any dose from 2×10^6 to 5×10^7 will probably be just as good. Recipients may be boosted at intervals of 3–8 weeks, and fusion performed 2–4 days after the last boost. There is some evidence that better yields of active hybridomas are obtained if the recipients are "rested" for 4–8 weeks between the penultimate and final boost (Oi and Herzenberg, 1980).

Long immunization schedules are probably unnecessary, and may even be counter-productive. Trucco *et al.* (1978) obtained many interesting hybrids by fusing 4 days after a single injection of human lymphoblastoid cells.

3.2.4 In Vitro *Immunization*

It has been shown that it is possible to immunize mouse lymphocytes *in vitro* prior to fusion (Luben and Mohler, 1980; Luben *et al.*, 1982). The main advantage of *in vitro* immunization is that extremely small amounts of antigen appear to be sufficient. Luben *et al.* immunized $\sim 2 \times 10^8$ spleen cells in 20 ml with only 60 μg of a partially purified preparation containing less than 1% growth hormone-releasing factor (GRF), and fused with a subline of the myeloma MPC-11 four days later. They obtained a number of hybridomas secreting antibodies to GRF. All were of the IgM class.

The spleen cells were cultured with antigen in a mixture of 10 ml of medium conditioned by 48 h of culture with mouse thymus cells. The authors stressed the importance of adhering strictly to the conditions for generation of conditioned medium as given below.

Thymuses from 10 day old mice were teased into a single cell suspension, and cultured at 10^7 per ml in MEM plus 20% FCS, 20 mM L-glutamine, I mM pyruvate and 50 μM mercaptoethanol. After removal of cells by centrifugation, the conditioned medium was filtered and stored at 4°C for up to 2 weeks prior to use. The medium for culture of spleen cells contained the same additives as the conditioned medium, added freshly just before culture. The antigen (purified by HPLC) was taken to dryness in the presence of 400 μg human serum albumin, dissolved in culture medium for immunization and sterilized by filtration. No antibiotics were used at any stage.

The use of *in vitro* immunization has not been widely adopted, but it is worth considering in cases where the supply of antigen is very limited. There is some controversy about its effectiveness, and some doubt about whether the presence of antigen in the cultures makes any difference. For further details, the primary literature should be consulted.

3.3 Choice of Myeloma Cell Line for Fusion

There are now numerous myeloma cells which have been used successfully for the generation of hybridomas. However, not all cultured myelomas are capable of forming hybridomas, and occasionally a subline of a previously satisfactory line may fail to work. If this is suspected, a new subline should be obtained from a laboratory where it is being used successfully. The advantages of "nonproducer" myelomas as fusion partners have been discussed in the previous chapter (Section 2.9.3). Such lines are now widely available.

3.3.1 Mouse Myelomas

By far the most widely used cell lines for hybridoma production are descendants of MOPC-21 which have been selected for HAT sensitivity and loss of endogenous immunoglobulin heavy chains (e.g. P3-NS1-Ag 4-1; abbreviated NS-1) or loss of both heavy and light chains (e.g. X63-Ag 8.653 or NSO/1). Of these, NS-1 has been the most popular, but the current line of choice is probably X63-Ag 8.653 (see Chapter 2).

Another widely used line is Sp2/O-Ag-14 (abbreviated Sp2), which is a total nonproducer variant selected from a hybridoma involving fusion of MOPC-21 and BALB/c spleen cells. Rightly or wrongly, Sp2 has a reputation for being somewhat more fastidious in its growth characteristics (especially intolerance to alkaline medium) and for giving a low fusion frequency. A variant of Sp2 termed "FO" has been produced by Fazekas and Scheidegger (1980). FO cells are claimed to have particularly rapid growth, high fusion frequency and good cloning efficiency, but they have not yet been widely used.

Other mouse lines that have been used by small numbers of workers include variants of the BALB/c myelomas MPC-11 (Yelton *et al.*, 1978) and S-194 (Trowbridge, 1978) but they do not appear to offer any significant advantages over NS-1, X63-Ag 8.653 or NSO/1.

3.3.2 Rat Myelomas

All of the currently available rat myelomas which have been used for hybridoma production are derived from the LOU/C strain of rats (Bazin *et al.*, 1973; Bazin, 1982). These include Y3-Ag 1.2.3 (abbreviated Y3) which is an azaguanine-resistant derivative of the myeloma R210.RCY3, and secretes κ chains (Burtonboy *et al.*, 1973; Galfrè *et al.* 1979). A second line that is suitable is IR983F (Bazin, 1982). The total nonproducer line YB2/O (Kilmartin *et al.*, 1982; Galfrè and Milstein, 1981) was derived from a fusion between Y3 myeloma cells and spleen cells from an AO rat. It must be grown in LOU/C × AO or LOU/M × AO F_1 rats.

At the time of writing, successful production of rat–rat hybridomas has been limited to a small number of laboratories. Several experienced investigators have had difficulty in keeping rat–rat hybrids alive for more than 2–3 weeks. The reason for such problems is not yet clear. The hybrids seem to grow initially, and then die. Perhaps rat cells are unduly susceptible to "natural killer" cells, or some rat colonies have unusually high numbers of natural killer cells in the spleen.

3.3.3 Human Myeloma Cell Lines

In contrast to mouse and rat myelomas, it has been extraordinarily difficult to adapt human myelomas to continuous growth as tissue culture lines. Over the years, several reports have claimed success, but in almost all cases the lines so produced have turned out to be lymphoblastoid lines derived from Epstein–Barr virus (EBV) transformed normal B cells (Karpas *et al.*, 1982 a, b).

Lines such as RPMI-8226 (Nilsson, 1971), H My-2 (Edwards *et al.*, 1982), IM9 (Everson *et al.*, 1973) and GM-1500 (Croce *et al.*, 1980) are all probably EBV-transformed lymphoblastoid lines, even though most of them arose from patients with myeloma. For a line to be acceptable as a true myeloma, it should secrete *large amounts* of immunoglobulin of the same idiotype and heavy and light chain isotope as the paraprotein in the patient's serum. EBV-transformed lymphoblastoid lines have low levels of sectretion, grow in large clumps, and possess the EBV nuclear antigen (Reedman and Klein, 1973). In a few cases, EBV-transformed cell lines have been found suitable for hybridoma production (Croce *et al.*, 1980; Edwards *et al.*, 1982), although many unpublished failures have occurred.

At present, there are only one or two human cell lines that appear to be true myelomas. The U-266 line was grown from a patient with an IgE(K) myeloma (Nilsson *et al.*, 1970), and continued to secrete IgE after adaption to continuous tissue culture growth. Many later sublines of U-266 have lost production of the ε heavy chain. A HAT-sensitive variant of U-266 (SK-007) has been produced by Olssen and Kaplan (1980) and has been shown to be suitable for fusion with normal human B cells, resulting in antibody-secreting hybridomas. A second human myeloma line (Karpas 707) has been described (Karpas *et al.*, 1982 a, b), but so far has not been widely used.

In view of the potential importance of human–human hybridomas, a massive effort to develop new human myeloma cell lines has been mounted. It is to be hoped that this search will soon be successful, and that such lines will be freely distributed. In the meantime, some success has been obtained by fusing human lymphocytes with mouse myeloma cells (Schlom *et al.*, 1980; Nowinski *et al.*, 1980; Lane *et al.*, 1982). (See Chapter 2 for additional discussion and references on human hybridomas).

3.4 Equipment Required for Fusion and Growth of Hybridomas

The production of hybridomas requires the following equipment:
   (1) *Laminar flow hood.* This is not absolutely essential, and a "still air" box to protect from airborne organisms will suffice.
   (2) *CO_2 incubator.* It is standard practice to buffer the cultures with CO_2

(7–10%) and sodium bicarbonate (2.0–3.7 g/l). The CO_2 regulation must be reliable, but need not be complex or expensive. Simple ball-type metering devices are inexpensive and trouble-free, while the more complex and expensive electronic CO_2 regulators break down frequently. In my opinion, it is best to avoid incubators with inbuilt fans, because they are impossible to clean, and if they become contaminated with moulds, the spores are blown into the cultures. Incubators with smooth unobstructed interiors are preferable. Temperature regulation and uniformity are important. The temperature gauge on most incubators cannot be trusted, and the internal temperature should be measured frequently with a thermometer in a beaker of water. It should be $37° \pm 0.2°$. It is important that the incubator be adequately humidified to prevent drying of cultures.

(3) *Liquid nitrogen facility.* This is absolutely essential for storage of cells, and must be organized so that there is no possibility of the nitrogen running out.

(4) *Inverted microscope*, preferably with phase optics. Absolutely essential for monitoring growth of cells.

(5) *37° water bath.*

(6) *Centrifuge.*

(7) *Sterile pipettes.* Disposable plastic pipettes are convenient, but very expensive. Alternatively, if glass pipettes are used, a hot air sterilizing oven will be required.

(8) *Gamma counter.* (Desirable for screening assays, but not absolutely essential, because it can be replaced by autoradiography or non-isotopic assays such as enzyme-linked immunoassay).

(9) *Others.* Animal holding facilities, small forceps, scissors, tissue culture ware, standard microscope, haemocytometers.

3.5 Preparation of Spleen Cells

Instruments needed are medium-sized scissors, fine scissors and fine forceps. They may be adequately sterilized by boiling in water for 5 min.

The animal may be killed by cervical dislocation or asphyxiation in CO_2. (The former is instantaneous, and therefore preferable). The animal should then be swabbed with 70% ethanol, the superficial skin pinched up over the left side of the abdomen, and a small cut made over the spleen. The skin is then torn back, revealing the abdominal muscles, through which the spleen will be visible. From this point on, sterile technique must be used.

The abdominal wall over the spleen is pinched up with fine forceps, and a small incision made with fine scissors, taking care to avoid the gut. The spleen is gently delivered through the incision, released by cutting its mesentery and placed into a sterile Petri dish.

A single-cell suspension is then made by gently teasing the spleen through a sterile sieve into culture medium, using fine forceps. The medium should be at room temperature. Alternatively, the spleen may be cut into a few pieces with scissors, and the cells gently released into medium by pressure between the frosted ends of two sterile glass microscope slides.

The cells are then harvested by centrifugation ($400\,g$ for 5 min), washed twice in medium, and counted. Erythrocytes may be removed from an aliquot of cells for counting by using 3% acetic acid as diluent. Typically, a mouse spleen will yield $\sim 10^8$ nucleated cells, and a rat spleen about 5–10 times as much.

3.6 Preparation of Myeloma Cells

3.6.1 Culture Medium

The two most popular media are Dulbecco's modified Eagle's medium (DME) or RPMI-1640, which is very similar. The main differences are that RPMI-1640 has no pyruvate, and DME has no asparagine. Neither of these ingredients is essential for hybridomas.

Most culture media are buffered with HCO_3^-/CO_2. Typically, one might use $3.4\,g\,NaHCO_3$/litre, in equilibrium with 10% CO_2 in air to give the desired pH. Supplementary buffering, especially with very small volume cultures, can be obtained by addition of HEPES up to 20 mM final concentration.

Glutamine is somewhat unstable, and some investigators add extra glutamine (2 mM final concentration), although it is doubtful whether this is necessary. Glutamine is stored as a concentrated solution at $-20°$. It is customary to add $100\,\mu g$/ml of streptomycin and pencillin. The addition of pyruvate (1.0 mM) and 2-mercaptoethanol (5×10^{-5} M) is optional; there is no evidence that they make any difference to hybridoma production.

It is strongly recommended that the tissue culture medium be stored protected from direct sunlight or room fluorescent light, because light generates highly toxic photoproducts (Stoien and Wang, 1974; Wang, 1976; Griffin *et al.*, 1981).

3.6.2 Fetal Calf Serum

As a general rule, fetal calf serum (10–15%) must be added to the medium. The quality of fetal calf serum has greatly improved in recent years, and extensive testing of many different batches is now usually unnecessary. Nonetheless, the serum chosen should be capable of supporting the growth of the myeloma cells at 1 cell per well, and this test should be carried out on each new batch. When a good batch is found, a bulk order (5–20 litres) should be placed. Serum is stable at $-20°$ for at least 1–2 years.

Occasional investigators have used horse serum or newborn calf serum, but in general the best results are obtained with fetal calf serum. The precise ingredients in serum which make cells grow are still poorly understood (reviewed by Barnes and Sato, 1980). Of particular importance are the iron transport protein transferrin, hormones (e.g. insulin, thyroxine) and possibly trace elements such as selenium. Some limited success has been obtained in growing hybridomas in serum-free medium (Chang et al., 1980; Murakami et al, 1982), but a general solution to the problem has still not been found.

3.6.3 Growth of Myeloma Cells

It is important to maintain a number of vials of myeloma cells in liquid nitrogen, as insurance against infection, genetic drift, and a host of other disasters which occur in the laboratory. When vials are removed from this stock, the cells should be grown in bulk, and fresh vials replaced as soon as possible.

The myeloma cells are maintained in the laboratory in exponential growth in medium with 10% fetal calf serum. A convenient way to do this is to have a series of small Petri dishes, each holding 5 ml medium. Cells are seeded at serial tenfold dilutions (six dishes are ample). Once a week they are passaged from a dish in which the cells are fairly dense but not overgrown. Typical doubling times are 14–16 h.

If the cells are in exponential growth, the doubling time (t_D) may be calculated from the expression

$$t_D = \frac{0.693\,t}{\log_e \dfrac{N}{N_0}}$$

where t = elapsed time
N_0 = starting number of cells
N = final number of cells
e = 2.7183.

Similarly, if the doubling time is known, and a certain number of cells are required, one may arrange the initial number of cells and the culture time according to the formula

$$\frac{N}{N_0} = e^{\frac{0.693\,t}{t_D}}$$

Understanding exponential growth is crucial for success in tissue culture. Healthy growing cells divide every 8–48 h, but notwithstanding claims to the contrary, the doubling times of mammalian cells in culture are virtually never less than 10 h. Exponential growth means that the cells will appear to be growing extremely slowly when dilute, but rapidly when concentrated.

3.6.4 Maximum Cell Density

As the cells become very dense, they start to look unhealthy, and viability drops. This happens quite suddenly; if the cultures are too dense on one day, by the next day most of the cells will be dead.

Most mouse myeloma cells will grow to approximately 10^6/ml in roller bottles (rotate at 3 revolutions/min), and somewhat lower density ($\cong 3 \times 10^5$/ml) in stationary culture. [Rat myeloma cells and hybrids involving rat cells tend to adhere loosely to the walls of tissue culture vessels. They do not usually grow well in roller bottles.] Cells may also be grown in "spinner" flasks (Galfrè and Milstein, 1981).

It is not necessary to use special "tissue culture" grade plastic dishes for myeloma cells. Standard bacteriological Petri dishes are adequate, and much less expensive.

3.7 Preparation of HAT and HT Medium

HAT and HT medium are prepared by addition of concentrated stock solutions to standard medium.

3.7.1 100X HT Stock Solution
(10 mM hypoxanthine,
1.6 mM thymidine)

Dissolve 136 mg hypoxanthine and 39 mg thymidine in 100 ml deionized distilled water warmed to 70–80°. Sterilize by filtration, and store in 1.0 ml aliquots at − 20°.

3.7.2 100X HAT Stock Solution
(10 mM hypoxanthine,
4×10^{-5} M aminopterin;
1.6 mM thymidine)

Prepare 100 ml of 100X HT medium as above. Add 1.8 mg aminopterin. If the aminopterin does not dissolve readily, add a few drops of 1.0 M NaOH. Sterilize by filtration, and store as for HT. Note that aminopterin is light sensitive, and may deteriorate, resulting in failure of HAT selection and growth of unfused myeloma cells. It is a good idea to test the HT and HAT concentrates for toxicity and effectiveness prior to use. The myeloma cells should grow normally in HT medium, but should all die within 1–3 days in HAT medium. As a final test, the HAT medium should allow the growth of established hybridoma lines. (It is conceivable that an established hybrid line grown in normal medium could regain HAT sensitivity by loss of the X chromosome derived from the spleen cell fusion partner.)

3.8 Fusion Protocol

The first hybridomas were made using Sendai virus as the fusing agent, but virtually all hybridomas are now produced with polyethylene glycol (PEG). PEG is commercially available and inexpensive, and its use results in a higher fusion frequency and greater reproducibility. PEG-induced fusion of myeloma cells was first described by Galfrè *et al.* (1977). Although there have been a number of minor modifications described since then, the procedure has not been changed in its essentials. The most important variables are:

(1) *The concentration of PEG.* Below about 30% PEG, very few hybrids are formed. Above 50% PEG, toxicity becomes overwhelming. If 40–50% PEG is used, dilution of PEG after fusion must be slow.

(2) *The purity of the PEG.* It seems likely that a contaminant in the PEG is essential for cell fusion (Chapter 2). Nonetheless, some batches of PEG are excessively toxic to cells, and cannot be used. If in doubt, try a new batch of PEG from a different source.

(3) *The pH of the PEG mixture.* Sharon *et al.* (1980) have shown that the fusion frequency is highly dependent on pH. Maximal numbers of hybridomas were obtained at pH 8.0–8.2.

(4) *The duration of exposure to PEG.* The fusion frequency, but also toxicity, increases with the time of exposure to PEG. Lower concentrations of PEG (30–35%) can be tolerated for longer times (e.g. 7 min) than higher concentrations (50% for no more than 1–2 min, see Gefter *et al.*, 1977).

Factors which seem to be of minor importance include temperature (20°–37°), cell numbers, the molecular weight of the PEG, the ratio of spleen cells to myeloma cells, and the presence or absence of serum or erythrocytes during fusion (Zola and Brooks, 1982). Fusions of mouse spleen cells to Y3 rat cells seem to work best if the ratio of spleen cells:Y3 cells is less than 2:1 (I. van Driel, personal communication). Norwood *et al.* (1976) have suggested that the addition of 15% (v/v) dimethyl sulphoxide to 42% (w/v) PEG results in better fusion, but the difference is probably small (Fazekas and Scheidegger, 1980).

It should be noted that there is always a certain percentage of experiments in which the fusions do not work, and a degree of variability in the yield of hybrids. *It is therefore essential to perform a number of fusions.* Sometimes, success will result from the first fusion. In other cases, it may be necessary to perform as many as 5–10 fusions before the desired hybrid is obtained.

3.8.1 Protocol of Galfrè and Milstein (1981)

Polythylene glycol (10 g), molecular weight 1500 (BDH cat. no. 29575) is autoclaved in a glass bottle. After allowing to cool somewhat, but while the PEG is still liquid, 10 ml of sterile Dulbecco's modified Eagle's medium (without serum) is added and thoroughly mixed. The pH should be slightly alkaline (pink; not orange or purple).

(1) Mix approximately 10^8 mouse spleen cells (i.e. 1 spleen) and 10^7 (mouse) or 6×10^7 (rat) myeloma cells in a sterile 50 ml conical-bottom tube; add serum-free medium to 50 ml.

(2) Spin at 400 g for 5 min.

(3) Remove *all* the medium by suction; tilt the tube to ensure its complete removal. The final concentration of PEG is critical, and any residual medium will result in dilution.

(4) Break the pellet by gently tapping the tube; place in a 200 ml beaker of water at 40°, inside a laminar flow hood.

(5) Add 0.8 ml 50% (w/v) PEG prewarmed to 40°, using a 1 ml pipette, over 1 min, continuously stirring with the tip.

(6) Continue stirring for 1–2 min.

(7) With the same pipette, add 1 ml serum-free medium at 37°, stirring for a further 1 min.

(8) Repeat 7.

(9) Repeat 7 twice, but adding over 30 s.

(10) Add 7 ml warm medium over about 2 min, stirring continuously.

(11) Add a further 12–13 ml warm medium.

(12) Spin at 400 g for 5 min.

(13) Discard the supernate; break the pellet by gently tapping the tube; resuspend in 49 ml medium containing 20% fetal calf serum (FCS).

(14) Distribute into 48 × 1 ml tissue culture wells (flat bottom).

(15) Add 1 ml medium with FCS, and 10^5 normal spleen cells per ml ("feeder cells").

(16) Incubate overnight at 37° in a CO_2 incubator.

(17) Remove half the supernate, taking care not to disturb the cells. Add 1 ml HAT medium to each well.

(18) Repeat 17 daily for next 2–3 days, then once a week until there is evidence of vigorous growth of hybrids.

3.8.2 The Protocol of Gefter et al. (1977)

Gefter *et al.* (1977) have shown that good fusion frequencies are obtained with less variation if the PEG concentration is lowered to 30–35%, and the cells exposed for 7–9 min at room temperature. The mixture of spleen and myeloma cells is centrifuged in serum-free medium, and the supernate removed. The cell pellet is then loosened by tapping the tube, and a solution of 30–35% PEG (molecular weight 1000; 1–5 ml) is added at room temperature. The cells are then centrifuged at 200 g for 2 min, and left for an additional 5–7 min at room temperature. They are then diluted in a large volume of medium without serum, harvested by centrifugation and cultured. The dilution step may be rapid.

3.8.3 Electrically Induced Fusion

Induction of fusion with polyethylene glycol is essentially random, and the fraction of hybrids of the desired specificity is therefore generally low. Recently, a new technique has been described in which a much higher percentage of hybrids secrete antibody of the desired specificity. The technique depends on bringing the antigen-binding B cell into contact with the myeloma cell via an antigen "bridge", and subsequent induction of fusion by a transient electrical field (Lo *et al.*, 1984).

The bridge between myeloma and antigen-binding cell involves the biotin–avidin system (see Section 7.4). Washed myeloma cells in PBS are derivatized with biotin using the succinimide ester dissolved in dimethyl formamide (10^7–10^8 cells in 5 ml PBS plus 50 μl dimethyl formamide containing 5×10^{-7} M biotin succinimide ester for 1 h at 4°C). They are then washed extensively with culture medium to remove unbound biotin. The wash medium should contain 50 μg/ml DNAse I to digest DNA released from cells killed by procedure.

The antigen is coupled with avidin as follows. Avidin (0.5 mg) is bound to 100 μl iminobiotin-agarose (Sigma Chemical Company), which binds avidin at alkaline pH but releases it at pH 4 (Heney *et al.*, 1981). After 2 h at 20°C, the beads are washed with 10 ml 0.1 M borate buffer at pH 8.5 and reacted with 1 μM 1,5-difluoro-2,4-dinitrobenzene (DFDNB) in 10μl methanol for 10 min at 20°C. Pure antigen (1 μg) is then reacted with the activated immobilized avidin for 12 h at 4°C, followed by washing and quenching unreacted sites with 0.1 μmole glycine. The antigen–avidin conjugate is eluted off the beads with 200 μl citrate-phosphate buffer, pH 4.

Spleen cells from immunized mice are held with the avidin-conjugated antigen in 5 ml medium for 4 h on ice, and then washed with medium containing DNAse I to remove excess conjugate, mixed with biotinylated myeloma cells, and centrifuged at 200 g for 5 min. The pellet is held for 3 h at 4°C, then washed in medium containing 10^{-6} M biotin. Finally, cells are resuspended in isosmotic (290 mosmol) sucrose containing 2 mM phosphate, pH 7.2.

Fusion is performed using $\sim 10^7$ myeloma cells and 10^7 B cells, by exposing them to four $5 \mu S$ pulses at 4 Kv/cm in an apparatus described by Kinosita and Tsong (1977) and Tsong (1983).

The advantages of electrofusion include economy in terms of amount of antigen, the routine production of high affinity antibodies, and a great reduction in the amount of cell farming and screening. The disadvantages include increased complexity and the need for special and expensive equipment. The procedure could probably be greatly simplified. For example, antigen could be coupled with biotin (Section 7.4), and the tetrameric structure of avidin used to form a bridge between cells (Wojchowski and Sytkowski, 1986).

3.9 Early Growth

Some investigators plate the cells into normal medium (containing 10–15% FCS) for 1 day prior to adding HAT (e.g. Galfrè and Milstein, 1981; Oi and Herzenberg, 1980), while many others plate directly into HAT (e.g. Hämmerling *et al.*, 1981; Zola and Brooks, 1982). There seems to be no clear reason for delaying the introduction of HAT selection, and direct plating into HAT is now becoming common practice.

3.9.1 Large or Small Cultures?

The other main area in which there is a good deal of variation concerns the size of the initial cultures. Galfrè and Milstein (1981) recommend plating a total of 10^8 spleen cells plus the myeloma cells into 48×1.0 ml Linbro plates, together with 10^5 normal spleen cells per ml (feeder cells). The latter are probably unnecessary, as each well already contains 2×10^6 spleen cells. Oi and Herzenberg (1980) have used a slightly different protocol, starting with a total of 3×10^8 cells and plating into $300 \times 100 \mu l$ wells (i.e. 10^6 cells per 100 ml). Depending on the frequency of hybridoma formation (typically 1 clone per 10^5–10^7 input cells), each well may have none, one or several clones. Plating at relatively low numbers of cells per well has the advantage that "positive" wells will probably contain monoclonal antibodies from the start. Thus, screening assays which are searching for antibody of a *particular specificity* (e.g. detecting a subpopulation of cells) will not be confused by the presence of more than one clonal product. On the other hand, some workers feel that the overall yield of hybrids is higher in large cultures. The matter is not yet resolved, but good results may be obtained using either strategy (see Fazekas and Scheidegger, 1980).

If 96-well plates are used, it is a good idea to leave the outermost row of wells empty. These wells are most prone to infection by airborne microorganisms.

3.9.2 Feeding the Cultures

Another area where some variation exists concerns the feeding of cultures after fusion. Feeding is carried out by removal of about half the culture medium by suction, followed by its replacement with fresh medium. Two purposes are served. The first is that feeding gradually dilutes out any antibody made by normal (unfused) antibody-secreting cells, which may remain alive for up to a week. The second reason for feeding is to remove waste products and to replenish nutrients. Some authors feed every 3–4 days (e.g. Oi and Herzenberg, 1980), but in this case the "feeding" also served the purpose of gradually phasing in the HAT selection. If the hybrids are plated immediately into HAT, it is usually sufficient to feed only after the first 7 days (Zola and Brooks, 1982). Subsequent feeding should be guided by the rate of cell growth. If the cultures become dense and the medium turns yellow, it may be necessary to feed more frequently.

3.9.3 Feeder Cells

Lymphoid cells often grow poorly or die when grown at low density. The reasons are not well understood, but may relate to toxic products from the tissue culture vessels and also to requirements for ill-defined "growth factors". Choice of the particular batch of FCS may make a big difference.

In some cases the growth of small numbers of cells is improved by incubating the tissue culture ware with medium overnight at 37°, and then replacing it with fresh medium before the cells are added. It is presumed that something toxic in the plastic is being washed out.

These problems can be overcome (at least partially) by culturing together with a slow-growing or non-growing population of cells. Although the mechanism is not understood, these cells are usually termed "feeders", implying that they make something needed for growth. If culture conditions are optimal, feeder cells may make little difference. They do no harm however, and may reduce variation between experiments (see Fazekas and Scheidegger, 1980).

Commonly needed feeder cells include thymocytes (typically $10^6/0.2$ ml well; Lernhardt *et al.*, 1978; Oi and Herzenberg, 1980), normal spleen cells (10^5/ml; Galfrè and Milstein, 1981) or peritoneal cells (Hengartner *et al.*, 1978; typically $2 \times 10^4/0.2$ ml). Peritoneal cells are harvested by washing out the peritoneal cavity with sterile saline, using a syringe and needle and taking care to avoid puncturing the gut. Roughly half are lymphocytes and half are macrophages. If the mice are from specific pathogen-free colonies, yields will be $3–5 \times 10^6$ cells per mouse. "Conventional" mice will yield up to ten times as many cells. The feeder cells do not have to be histocompatible with the hybrids. They do not even need to be from the same species. Rat thymocytes seem to function well for mouse–mouse hybrids.

3.9.4 Termination of HAT Selection

After a week in HAT medium, it is safe to assume that all the parental myeloma cells will be dead, and any growing cells will be hybrids. At this point, HAT selection may be terminated. It is generally recommended that the hybrids be cultured in HT medium for a few days prior to using normal medium. Theoretical considerations suggest that this step should be done carefully.

The inhibition constant (K_i) of aminopterin for dihydrofolate reductase is less than $10^{-9} M$ (Calabresi and Parks, 1975), and the concentration of aminopterin in HAT medium is $4 \times 10^{-7} M$. *The aminopterin concentration must therefore drop by more than 400-fold before the enzyme can regain activity.* Unlike hypoxanthine and thymidine, aminopterin is metabolized extremely slowly. [In man, the main route of elimination of the closely related drug methotrexate is via urinary excretion, and catabolism does not seem to occur to a significant degree (Calabresi and Parks, 1975).] *The main route of elimination of aminopterin from the cultures must therefore be by dilution.* Accordingly, it would seem prudent to remove as much of the HAT medium as possible prior to feeding with HT medium, and to repeat the process several times prior to using ordinary medium.

Zola and Brooks (1982) found that some hybrids died when taken out of HT medium, and suggested that the cells be grown in HT medium permanently. It may be that the very slow catabolism of aminopterin, together with its extremely high affinity for folate reductase, resulted in unexpectedly slow recovery of enzyme activity. The ingredients for HT medium are inexpensive, and the long-term growth in HT would provide little extra work, so their proposal should be considered.

3.10 Screening Assays

The choice of an appropriate screening assay is one of the most important parts of hybridoma production. In principle, any method which is capable of detecting antibody of the desired specificity may be used. The practical constraints on screening assays are reliability, speed, cost and labour. Many hundreds or thousands of assays will have to be performed during initial screening, cloning, expansion, recloning and bulk culture. Unless the assays can be done in large numbers, and at reasonable cost and effort, the production of hybridomas is likely to fail.

The screening assay should be set up and "de-bugged" well before the fusion is started, because there will not be enough time to eliminate problems later. A trial bleed from the immune spleen donor may be used as a source of antibody.

The required "dynamic range" of the assay (i.e. the ratio of the strongest signal to the weakest that can be detected above background) will depend on whether or not the test antigen is a pure substance. For example, if it is desired to make hybridomas against a purified protein, 100% of the test antigen will be relevant, and a plus/minus system will be adequate. On the other hand, if the desired antigen is a minor cell surface protein, the assay system may need to be capable of detecting very small signals, and should have a dynamic range of at least 10:1 (preferably 100:1).

Choice of screening assays is also influenced by the type of antibody required. Classes of antibody which fix complement might be chosen by using an assay based on cytotoxicity. If protein A-binding antibodies are desired, this will be guaranteed by incorporating protein A in the screening assay.

3.10.1 Removal of Supernates

The first step in any assay will involve sterile removal of the supernates. This may be accomplished by using sterile Pasteur pipettes, but if hundreds of supernates must be tested, it will be found to be very slow. There are now a variety of alternative procedures which vary in ease, complexity and cost. In my experience, the more complex and sophisticated devices are usually unreliable and cumbersome.

One of the best and cheapest procedures is to use standard laboratory pipettes with disposable conical tips (e.g. Eppendorf, Gilson, Finnpipette, Oxford). The lower part of the pipette should be wiped with 70% ethanol prior to use. A convenient autoclavable re-usable box for sterilizing 96 tips at the one time is made by Treff (Treff AG, CH 9113, Degersheim, Switzerland; cat. no. 9606). Each tip may then be placed onto the pipette without contact with the fingers.

Another alternative is the use of multi-channel pipettes, such as those made by Flow Laboratories (8 channel 100 μl Titertek multi-channel pipette; cat. no. 77-844-00). However, it is difficult to arrange for the secure attachment of all tips without finger contact, even if the expensive bracketed tips are used.

Gefter (personal communication) has produced a simple and convenient device for sampling supernates. A 96-well plastic tissue culture tray is modified by attaching a small loop of Nichrome wire beneath each well. The plate is sterilized, and the loops are dipped into the culture wells, where they are then transferred by dipping the loops into buffer-fitted wells of the test plate. Thus, 96 wells may be sampled in a few seconds. A commercial sampler based on a similar principle is available (Titertek Replicator; Flow Laboratories). It is relatively inexpensive, simple and effective. Automated harvesting devices, such as those described by Lefkovits and Kamber (1972) are yet another alternative. However, they are complex and expensive, and have not found widespread use.

3.10.2 Labour-saving Devices for Screening Assays

Screening assays constitute one of the most time-consuming and labour-intensive parts of hybridoma production, so it is important to eliminate any unnecessary steps, and to automate those steps which cannot be eliminated. It is neither necessary nor desirable to spend thousands of dollars on complex and sophisticated machines, because they are usually unreliable and insufficiently flexible to meet changing needs. However, a couple of hundred dollars spent on a repetitive dispenser will greatly facilitate the assays. The Eppendorf Multipette 4780 is ideal for such purposes, because it is inexpensive, robust and reliable, and can be adjusted to deliver a large range of volumes. Sterile disposable tips are available for feeding cultures.

The simultaneous washing of 8 or 12 wells may be accomplished by the use of the "Nunc Immuno Wash" or the "Skatron Mini-Microwash". These devices simultaneously deliver and aspirate wash fluid, and are reasonably priced. The Drummond Model 590 Microdispenser with microtest manifold and repeating dispenser, is also relatively inexpensive. It does not allow simltaneous delivery and aspiration.

3.10.3 Solid-phase Radioimmunoassay — Soluble Protein Antigen

The solid-phase radioimmunoassay (Catt and Tregear, 1967; Fig. 3.1) is a very simple, sensitive and precise assay for hybridoma antibodies. It is usually easy to set up, and is capable of a very low background and a large dynamic range. A detailed account is given by Tsu and Herzenberg (1980).

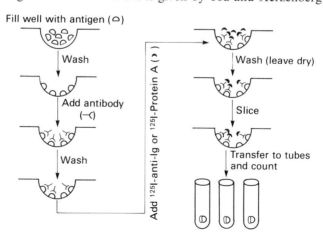

Fig. 3.1. Solid-phase radioimmunoassay for hybridoma screening.

The assay is based on the fact that polyvinyl surfaces will tightly adsorb nanogram amounts of most proteins. The antigen-containing solution is simply pipetted into the tube, left there for a few hours, and the unbound material washed out. Any remaining protein-binding sites are saturated by a large excess of irrelevant protein, which is usually bovine serum albumin (BSA). The antibody-containing solution is then added, left to react with the antigen, and any unbound material washed out. Finally, a "revealing" reagent is added. This is usually ^{125}I-labelled affinity-purified anti-immunoglobulin or ^{125}I-labelled staphylococcal protein A, which binds specifically to IgG (Goding, 1978). After 30–60 min, excess revealing reagent is removed, and the wells are washed and counted in a gamma scintillation counter. If a scintillation counter is not available, detection may be by autoradiography with intensifying screens (Parkhouse and Guarnotta, 1978; Nowinski *et al.*, 1979).

The assay most commonly used today is based on that described by Pierce and Klinman (1976). All steps may be carried out at room temperature. Ninety-six well polyvinyl plates (Cooke cat. no. 1-220-24; Dynatech Laboratories) are coated with 20–50 μl of antigen (10–50 μg/ml) in phosphate-buffered saline, pH 7.4 (PBS) for at least 30–60 min. (Although the optimal pH for coating may vary for each protein, in most cases adequate results are obtained at neutral pH.) The antigen should have no added carrier protein, and detergent will inhibit adsorption. The supernate is removed, but it may be re-used several times, as only a small fraction binds. The plate is then washed three times in "RIA buffer" (PBS plus 0.1% BSA and 0.1% NaN$_3$). Plates are then incubated with culture supernate (20–100 μl) for an hour. After a further three washes, ^{125}I-anti-immunoglobulin (10 μCi/μg) or ^{125}I-protein A (40 μCi/μg) is added (10 000 cpm per well are sufficient). After a further hour, plates are washed three more times and the wells removed for counting by cutting with scissors or slicing with a hot wire (see Tsu and Herzenberg, 1980, for details). The fumes are toxic, and slicing must be carried out in a fume cupboard. The assay is very flexible, and all concentrations and times given above may be varied by at least twofold with only minor changes in results.

It has recently been shown that non-fat powdered milk may be substituted for BSA in buffers and to block plates (Johnson *et al.*, 1984). These authors used 5% (w/v) milk in PBS plus 0.01% Antifoam A (Sigma), but similar results may be obtained with as little as 0.5% milk, and the Antifoam is not essential. The substitution of non-fat powdered milk for BSA results in a major saving in cost, and the results are at least as good, and often better.

If the antigen is pure, a typical positive well might have 3000 cpm, while negative wells should have less than 100 cpm. Even if the antigen is impure, the background should not rise significantly, but positive signals will be smaller. Providing the background is low and reproducible, wells with 2–3 times background may be considered positive.

Some thought should be given to the choice of revealing reagent. The use of ^{125}I-protein A has certain advantages, and also some disadvantages (Goding 1978, 1980). In the mouse, IgG2a, IgG2b and IgG3 bind at neutral pH, while IgG1 will bind only weakly at pH > 8 (Ey *et al.*, 1978). In general, mouse IgM, IgA, IgD and IgE do not bind. Very few rat IgG molecules bind protein A (Ledbetter and Herzenberg, 1979).

One often obtains ample numbers of positive wells from mouse fusions using protein A as the revealing reagent. Its use also guarantees that the antibodies may be subsequently purified by affinity chromatography on protein A-agarose. IgG antibodies are more stable and easier to handle than other classes. Some mouse IgM antibodies bind nonspecifically to the plates, causing false positive reactions (Goding, 1980). The use of protein A eliminates this problem by failing to detect IgM. Unless there are special reasons for wanting classes other than IgG2 or IgG3, protein A is often the reagent of choice for mouse antibodies. Sometimes, however, it may be found that the predominant response is IgG1, IgM or IgA. This is particularly likely for IgG1. In these cases, anti-immunoglobulin antibodies must be used instead.

If anti-immunoglobulin antibodies are used, they should be affinity-purified to ensure that the majority of counts can bind. Non-affinity purified antibodies will usually have less than 10% bindable counts, with consequent poor signal:noise ratio. Many anti-immunoglobulin antisera have substantial anti-light chain activity, and will therefore detect all antibody classes and subclasses. However, some display a marked preference for individual classes, and it is unwise to assume that a randomly chosen antiserum will detect all classes with equal efficiency. If all classes must be detected, the reagent of choice is an antiserum against the Fab fragments of normal polyclonal IgG. Such antisera usually detect all classes with approximately equal efficiency.

3.10.4 Solid-phase Radioimmunoassay
— Cell Surface and Viral
Antigens

The assay described in Section 3.10.3 is easily adapted to cell surface antigens (Oi *et al.*, 1978) or viruses (Nowinski *et al.*, 1979). One important difference is that if living cells are used, they should be kept cold to prevent antibody-induced "capping", endocytosis and shedding of antigen–antibody complexes (Taylor *et al.*, 1971). The polyvinyl 96-well plates must be kept on a bed of ice during the assay, and the centrifuge must be refrigerated.

Cell suspensions are prepared by standard techniques, and washed twice to remove soluble or loosely adsorbed material. In certain cases, adherent cells such as fibroblasts may actually be grown in the assay dish. Typically 10^4–10^6 cells are used per well. All steps are performed in RIA buffer (Section

3.10.3). It is advisable to pre-coat the trays to saturate protein-binding sites on the plastic.

The cells are held at 4° for 30–90 min with 20–100 μl hybridoma supernatant. The trays are then centrifuged in tray carriers (200–400 g, 2–5 min), and the supernatants removed by gentle vacuum aspiration from the edges of the wells. Cells are then washed 2–3 times by the addition of RIA buffer and centrifugation. (Resuspension is achieved by simply pipetting onto the cell pellet.) The cells are then resuspended in 50–100 μl ^{125}I-anti-immunoglobulin or ^{125}I-protein A (Section 3.10.3). After a further 30–90 min, cells are washed again (x2-3), and the wells cut and counted (Section 3.10.3). The "background" should be no more than 100–200 cpm, and positive wells may contain ~ 500–3000 cpm.

More recently, the cellular binding assay has been modified to avoid the tedious and time-consuming centrifugations. Viruses (Nowinski *et al.*, 1979) and crude cellular membrane preparations (Howard *et al.*, 1980) may be firmly coated onto polyvinyl plates by simple adsorption, and washes may be performed without centrifugation.

Sometimes, intact cells in serum-free medium will adhere to the plastic with sufficient tenacity to allow washing without centrifugation. In most cases, however, it is necessary to attach them by chemical means. Stocker and Heusser (1979) have described an assay in which cells are attached to the plate with glutaraldehyde. The chemistry of this reaction is somewhat obscure, and it was not demonstrated that the glutaraldehyde was necessary. Nonetheless, the method works well in the form in which it was published (see also Kincade *et al.*, 1981).

Cells are added to the plates (10^6/well) in protein-free PBS. The plates are then centrifuged at 50–100 g for 5 min and, without disturbing the cell layer, immersed in a 1 litre glass beaker containing freshly prepared 0.25% glutaraldehyde in PBS at 4°C. After 5 min, the plates are washed in RIA buffer. The remainder of the assay is essentially as described above, but omitting the centrifugations.

If glutaraldehyde treatment alone is not sufficient to bind the cells firmly to the plates, adequate adhesion is usually obtained by pre-coating the plates with poly-L-lysine (10–50 μg/ml in distilled water) prior to adding the cells in protein-free PBS. Kennett (1980) recommends treating the plates with 0.5% glutaraldehyde for 15 min after the cells have been added, but this is probably only necessary for certain cell types. Regardless of how the cells are attached to the plate, all subsequent steps must include carrier protein (0.1% BSA) to saturate any remaining protein-binding sites.

If the cells are fixed with glutaraldehyde, the plates may be stored for several months at 4°C without apparent deterioration. However, some antigenic determinants may be destroyed by glutaraldehyde treatment (Gatti *et al.*, 1974; Kincade *et al.*, 1981).

The solid-phase assay has also been adapted for glycolipid antigens

(Smolarsky, 1980). The glycolipids are dissolved in ethanol and added to the wells of polyvinyl plates. The ethanol is then evaporated by a stream of nitrogen followed by high vacuum for 5 min, and the plates washed three times in PBS containing 0.3% gelatin and 1 mM ethylenediamine tetra-acetic acid (EDTA). The remainder of the assays is similar to those previously described. Other assays for antibodies to glycolipids have been described by Gray (1979), Young *et al.* (1979), and Handman and Jarvis (1985). Glycolipids are also discussed in Section 5.1.1.

3.10.5 Enzyme-linked Immunosorbent Assays (ELISA)

The assays described in the previous sections are easily adapted to ELISA readout (Engvall and Pesce, 1978; Voller *et al.*, 1979; Maggio, 1980; Engvall, 1980). The revealing agent is simply conjugated with an enzyme (peroxidase, alkaline phosphatase or β-galactosidase) rather than [125]I. After washing away any unbound material, the bound enzyme is revealed by addition of substrate which undergoes a colour change (Fig. 3.2).

The advantages of ELISA readout are many. No isotopes or scintillation counters are required, and the readout may be by eye. The tedious cutting up of trays, loading into tubes, and loading and unloading the counter are all avoided. If a quantitative readout is needed (unnecessary for hybridoma screening) automated reading devices are available which will scan 96 wells in a minute or so, compared to 1–2 h for scintillation counting. Finally, the reagents for ELISA are inexpensive, and have a long shelf line. Enzyme-conjugated anti-immunoglobulin or protein A are available commercially from many suppliers.

The most commonly used enzymes are horseradish peroxidase and alkaline phosphatase. Horseradish peroxidase is much less expensive. Both are capable of giving good results, providing that no endogenous enzyme is present. This may be a serious problem in cell-binding assays. Macrophages and myeloid cells possess high levels of endogenous peroxidase (Williams *et*

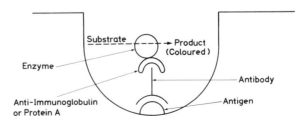

Fig. 3.2. The enzyme-linked immunosorbent assay (ELISA).

al., 1977) and B lymphocytes have high levels of alkaline phosphatase (Culvenor *et al.*, 1981; Garcia-Rozas *et al.*, 1982). Thus, these enzymes cannot be used if screening is performed on cells from spleen or lymph node; even thymus cell suspensions will have an unacceptable background. Attempts to destroy endogenous peroxidase require harsh chemical treatment (see Farr and Nakane, 1981) which may destroy antigenic determinants. However, peroxidase has been used very effectively (Douillard *et al.*, 1980), especially when cultured tumour lines were used as targets. Only one of 23 lines tested had significant endogenous peroxidase activity (Posner *et al.*, 1982). One ingenious way to overcome endogenous peroxidases is to use antibodies coupled with glucose oxidase to generate hydrogen peroxide from. glucose. A set amount of peroxidase and colour reagent is then added to detect the H_2O_2. Thus, endogenous peroxidases will not alter the background (D. Fayle, personal communication).

Alternatively, β-galactosidase (O'Sullivan *et al.*, 1979; Kincade *et al.*, 1981) or urease (Chandler *et al.*, 1982) may be used. These enzymes are not present in most mammalian cells. The urease assay depends on the pH change resulting from conversion of urea to ammonia. Ammonia is volatile, and the urease procedure is rather prone to false positives and other problems. In my experience, the sensitivity of β-galactosidase assays is considerably lower than peroxidase assays using O-phenylenediamine, and is inadequate for cell surface antigens (but see Kincade *et al.*, 1981) The use of fluorogenic substrates for β-galactosidase (O'Sullivan *et al.*, 1979) requires expensive equipment, and only increases the sensitivity slightly.

However, when enzymes with high turnover numbers, such as horseradish peroxidase, are combined with carefully chosen substrates (Al-Kaissi and Mostratos, 1983), the sensitivity of ELISA may equal that of RIA. ELISA is ideal for assays in which the antigen is relatively pure, but has not yet been widely accepted for cell surface antigen. Apart from the problem of endogenous enzymes, cell-binding ELISA assays suffer from a limited dynamic range. The strongest signals are seldom more than ten times background, and the background is not as low or as uniform as in RIA. When antibodies against low-abundance membrane proteins are sought, RIA will give much clearer discrimination between positives and negatives.

3.10.6 A Simple Method for Conjugating Horseradish Peroxidase to Antibodies or Staphylococcal Protein A

The method to be described is based on that of Wilson and Nakane (1978), but has been greatly simplified. It produces excellent conjugates for ELISA assays, but probably results in considerable polymerization, and has not been assessed for use in immunohistochemistry. A somewhat more refined but slightly more complex procedure is described by Tijssen and Kurstak (1984).

The method is based on the oxidation of the carbohydrate moieties of horseradish peroxidase (HRPO) by periodate ions, and the subsequent reaction of the resulting aldehyde groups with amino groups of proteins to form Schiff bases. The Schiff bases are stabilized by reduction with sodium borohydride.

pH 4.0 Acetate Buffer: 0.3 g sodium acetate (anhydrous) to 100 ml H_2O. Add 960 µl glacial acetic acid. Mix, and check pH. Adjust if necessary by adding acetic acid or NaOH ($\pm$ 0.2 pH units is satisfactory).

pH 9.5 Carbonate Buffer: 17.2 g $NaHCO_3$ plus 8.6 g Na_2CO_3 to 1 litre H_2O. Make up fresh on day of use. The pH should be close enough without adjustment ($\pm$ 0.2 pH units).

Practical procedure

(1) Dialyze affinity-purified IgG (1.0 ml of 5.0 mg/ml) against 1 litre pH 9.5 buffer overnight at 4°C.

(2) Weigh out 10 mg horseradish peroxidase (Sigma type VI, cat. no. P8375); dissolve in 1.0 ml H_2O.

(3) Add 200 µl pH 4 buffer. Mix.

(4) Add 200 µl 0.2 M $NaIO_4$ (freshly made up). Solution will turn green. Leave at room temperature for 15 min, protected from light.

(5) Equilibrate a Pharmacia PD-10 column of Sephadex G-25 with 20–30 ml pH 9.5 buffer.

(6) Let column run dry, then load sample and allow to run in.

(7) Add 1.0 ml pH 9.5 buffer. Discard effluent.

(8) Elute "activated HRPO" with 3.5 ml pH 9.5 buffer.

(9) Add activated HRPO to dialysed IgG.

(10) Leave at room temperature for 60 min.

(11) Add 100 µl $NaBH_4$ (4.0 mg/ml in H_2O). *(N.B. $NaBH_4$ is extremely unstable in water. Store powder in a dessicator, and make up solution immediately before use)*.

(12) Leave conjugate at room temperature for 1 h, then dialyze against PBS overnight at 4°C.

(13) Add glycerol to conjugate to 50% (v.v) and store at $-20°C$. The glycerol prevents freezing. The conjugate should be usable at a dilution of more than 1:1000.

[For conjugates of HRPO with staphylococcal protein A, use same procedure but use 4 mg HRPO and 1.0 mg protein A.]

3.10.7 Peroxidase ELISA Assays

The coating of the trays, binding of antibody and washing may be performed as for solid-phase RIA. The "carrier" protein in the buffers must be free of peroxidase activity (a common contaminant in BSA and milk). Note that azide ions must not be present, as they inhibit peroxidases. Water for buffers should be distilled but not de-ionized, as the hydrocarbons from de-ionizing resins often inhibit peroxidase. The conjugate is used at the maximum dilution that gives satisfactory results.

The substrate is made immediately before use as follows:

Distilled water	100 ml
Citric acid	0.47 g
Na_2HPO_4 (anhydrous)	0.73 g
o-phenylenediamine	40 mg
30% H_2O_2	30 μl

Positive wells should turn yellow after 5–60 min at room temperature. The tray should be read at a fixed time (e.g. 30 min), because the colour is not very stable. Note that the peroxide concentration is chosen to give rapid development of colour, but at this concentration there is a time-dependent inactivation of the enzyme. If difficulties are encountered, try varying the peroxide concentration. A test for H_2O_2 is given in Section 5.3.3.

3.10.8 Screening by Immunofluorescence

Screening of hybridomas by immunofluorescence has also been widely used (e.g. Ledbetter and Herzenberg, 1979). The sensitivity of immunofluorescence appears to be similar to RIA and ELISA. Immunofluorescence has the definite advantage that one may detect antibodies against subpopulations of cells or subcellular structures. A detailed account of immunofluorescence is given in Chapter 7.

The cellular antigen targets are held on ice with the hybridoma supernates for 30–90 min, washed, and then held for a similar period with fluorescein-conjugated anti-immunoglobulin antibodies. After a final wash, the cells are examined using a microscope with appropriate illumination and filters, or by the fluorescence-activated cell sorter (Ledbetter and Herzenberg, 1979; Loken and Stall, 1982). Screening by immunofluorescence may be quite rapid. A simple visual assessment takes only a few seconds. In the same time, the fluorescence-activated sorter can generate a histogram of the staining of 10 000 cells.

An interesting variation of screening by immunofluorescence was described by Parks *et al.* (1979), who used antigen-coated fluorescent latex microspheres to identify and simultaneously clone antigen-binding hybridoma cells by flow cytometry (see Chapter 7). Modification of the fluorescence-activated cell sorter to allow cloning of individual antigen-binding cells is now commercially available (Becton-Dickinson, Mountain View, California).

3.10.9 Cytoxicity Assays

Hybridoma supernates containing complement-fixing antibodies against cell surface antigens may be detected by cytotoxicity assays. It is customary to use two-step assays in which antibody is bound to the cells, unbound antibody is washed away, complement is added, and the cells are examined for lysis. The two-step assay was originally developed to circumvent "anti-complementary" activity in mouse serum. It is possible that a one-step assay (i.e. addition of complement together with the antibody) would be adequate for hybridoma screening.

Cells bearing the target antigen (10^5–10^6) are held with the supernate (10–100 μl) at 4°C for 30–60 min to allow antibody binding. They are then washed once or twice, and a source of complement added (usually guinea pig or rabbit serum). The cells are held at 37° for 30 min to allow lysis to occur, and then placed on ice until they are scored for lysis.

The source of complement is critical. Complement-containing serum must be processed rapidly, and stored in small aliquots at $-70°C$. Once thawed, aliquots should be used immediately and any excess discarded. Repeated freeze-thaw cycles will rapidly inactivate complement.

The optimal dilution of the complement must be determined for each individual batch. A certain degree of "background" lysis (5–10%) is unavoidable, and is largely due to the presence in the complement of naturally occurring antibodies against cells. These may be minimized by selection of serum from individual animals. Serum from baby rabbits is said to be less toxic. Absorption of natural antibodies on cells at 4°C in the presence of EDTA may be performed (Boyse *et al.*, 1970), but usually a dilution of unabsorbed complement can be found at which the background is acceptable and complement activity adequate. Typical dilutions of complement are 1:10–1:20.

Assessment of lysis may be performed using 0.2% trypan blue, or by staining with acridine orange and ethidium bromide (Lee *et al.*, 1975; Parks *et al.*, 1979). The acridine orange/ethidium bromide method is vastly superior in accuracy to the older methods. A stock solution of 1 part per million of acridine orange and ethidium bromide is made in PBS, and stored in a foil-wrapped bottle at 4°C. (Both acridine orange and ethidium bromide are potentially carcinogenic, and should be handled with care.) To assess viability, one drop of cells is placed on a glass slide, and one drop of stain solution added, followed by a cover slip. The slide is examined by fluorescence microscopy, using filters for fluorescein. Living cells stain bright green, while dead cells are bright orange.

The complement-mediated cytoxicity assay has many variants. It may be miniaturized by the use of Terasaki microcytotoxicity plates (Falcon 3034) and Hamilton syringes with repeating dispensers for aliquoting 1 μl and 5 μl volumes. The use of ^{51}Cr-release as a marker of cell death may be used instead of vital stains, but is not very satisfactory with resting lymphocytes, and works best with mitogen-stimulated blasts as targets (McKearn, 1980).

Screening by cytotoxicity is somewhat cumbersome, and has fallen from favour in recent years. Nonetheless, if only cytotoxic antibodies are of interest, the use of the assay will guarantee that they are selected.

3.10.10 Rosetting Assays

When an excess of anti-immunoglobulin or protein A-coated sheep erythrocytes are centrifuged with immunoglobulin-coated lymphocytes, the erythrocytes will adhere to the surface of the lymphocytes, forming rosettes. Rosetting is a very sensitive and simple method of detection of cell-bound antibody (Parish and McKenzie, 1978; Sandrin *et al.*, 1978) and the only equipment required is a centrifuge and a microscope. The assay may be divided into four parts. These are (i) coating of the red cells with antibody, (ii) removal of endogenous membrane immunoglobulins from B cells in the lymphocyte poulation, (iii) coating the lymphocytes with antibody and (iv) formation of rosettes.

Anti-mouse IgG antibodies (sheep, goat or rabbit) are precipitated by ammonium sulphate (final concentration 40% of saturation) and washed twice in 40% saturated ammonium sulphate, and dialysed extensively against 0.9% NaCl *without phosphate* (normal saline). The protein concentration is estimated from the optical density (1.0 mg/ml has an O.D. of 1.4 at 280 nm).

The red cells are coated with anti-immunoglobulin or protein A by the chromic chloride method (Goding, 1976; Parish and McKenzie, 1978). A 1% (w/v) stock solution of $CrCl_3 \cdot 6H_2O$ is prepared in normal saline and the pH adjusted to 5.0 with 1 M NaOH at weekly intervals for three weeks, after which it is stable indefinitely. The cells are washed $\times$ 4 in normal saline. To 2 ml normal saline is added 125 μl packed red cells and 800 μg of the globulin fraction of anti-mouse immunoglobulin serum or 50 μg protein A. The appropriate amount of $CrCl_3$ which has been predetermined to give the optimal coupling is added (typically 200 μl of 0.1% $CrCl_3$ in normal saline) with constant shaking. The cells are then held at room temperature for 10 min, the reaction stopped by addition of 4 ml PBS, and the cells washed twice in 6 ml PBS plus 10% FCS to make a final 2% suspension. Coated cells may be stored at 4° for 1–2 days, provided they are rewashed just prior to use.

If the red cells are coated with anti-immunoglobulin, endogenous membrane immunoglobulin (which is mostly IgM and IgD) on B cells in the lymphocyte preparation must be removed by "capping" (Parish and McKenzie, 1978). Lymphocytes (10^7/ml) are cultured at 37° for 75 min in Eagle's medium with 10% fetal calf serum and 50 μg/ml immunoadsorbent-purified anti-immunoglobulin antibodies. They are then washed twice in PBS plus 10% FCS, and diluted to a concentration of 5 × 10^6/ml in the same medium. Very few normal B cells possess membrane IgG, and it is not usually necessary to "cap off" membrane IgM and IgD if protein A rather than anti-immunoglobulin is used for coating the red cells.)

The lymphocytes (50 μl of 5 × 10^6/ml) are then held with hybridoma supernatant (10–100 μl) for 30–60 min at 4°C, washed twice, and resuspended in 50 μl PBS/FCS. Fifty microlitres of coated erythrocytes (2%) are added. Rosette formation occurs after 10 min at unit gravity on ice (Sandrin *et al.*, 1978) or by centrifugation at 200 g for 5 min at 4°C (Parish and McKenzie, 1978). The cell pellets are gently resuspended in their own supernatants, and kept on ice prior to examination. Once formed, the rosettes are stable for many hours at 4°C. True rosettes may be distinguished from aggregates of red cells by staining the central lymphocytes with 0.1% methyl violet (Parish and McKenzie, 1978).

Rosette assays have the advantage of requiring little equipment, and are capable of recognizing antibodies which detect subpopulations of cells. However, they have not achieved widespread poplarity.

3.10.11 Screening by Immunoprecipitation and Polyacrylamide Gel Electrophoresis

It is customary to identify positive hybridoma wells by simple binding assays, to clone the cells, grow bulk cultures, and finally to identify the antigen biochemically. However, Brown *et al.* (1980) have shown that it is feasible to reverse this order and identify the antigen as part of the screening procedure. The method is unlikely to be the first choice in most circumstances, but when antibodies against a particular polypeptide in a complex mixture are sought, it should be considered.

In order to minimize the number of supernates to be tested, two strategies were adopted. First, all supernates were screened for IgG production by testing their ability to compete with ^{125}I-IgG for binding to protein A-containing staphylococci. About 25% of wells with growth contained IgG. The second strategy involved pooling a series of horizontal rows (1–12), and pooling a series of vertical columns (A–H), with each primary well contributing $10 \mu l$ supernatant. The pools were held for 1 h at $0°C$ with $100–200 \mu l$ ^{125}I-labelled lysate of the immunizing cell type ($\sim 10^8$ cpm), and then 1 mg of heat-killed and formalin-fixed protein A-bearing *Staphyloccus aureus* was added. The staphylococci, to which the immune complexes were bound, were harvested and washed twice. Bound antigen was released by heating the bacteria to $100°C$ in SDS-sample buffer, and identified by SDS-polyacrylamide electrophoresis and autoradiography. If, for example, an M_r 50 000 polypeptide was present only in row pool C and column pool 11, the relevant antibody would be found in primary well C11. The cells in this well could then be cloned and grown in large numbers. A more detailed account of immunoprecipitation analysis will be found in Chapter 5.

3.10.12 Other Assays

A great many other assays are possible. Indeed, any way in which antibodies have been used may be considered. For example, antibodies against hormones could be identified by standard radioimmunoassay techniques in which ^{125}I- or ^3H-labelled hormone is precipitated. In many cases, biological assays might be used. For example, antibodies to an enzyme or hormone might be identified by inhibition of its activity (Frackelton and Rotman, 1980; Secher and Burke, 1980). Antibodies which cause passive cutaneous anaphylaxis (PCA) may be identified by subcutaneous injection into rats (Böttcher *et al.*, 1978; Eshhar *et al.*, 1980).

3.11 Cloning

As soon as positive wells are identified, the hybrid cells should be cloned. Cloning is important to reduce the risk of overgrowth by nonproducer cells, and to ensure that the antibodies are truly monoclonal.

Cells may be cloned by growth in soft agar (Coffino *et al.*, 1972; reviewed by Metcalf, 1977). Typically, two layers are used. A firm underlayer, consisting of 0.5% (w/v) agar in culture medium, is allowed to gel. A second "soft" agar layer (0.3% agar) which contains the cells to be cloned, is added. If feeder cells are used, they may be grown in the dishes beforehand, and the culture medium removed just prior to addition of the lower agar layer. Further details are given elsewhere (Köhler, 1979; Goding, 1980; Galfrè and Milstein, 1981).

Cloning in soft agar usually requires the additional step of reculturing in liquid medium before antibody production can be assessed. In contrast, cloning by limit dilution (see below) allows direct testing of supernatants. In a few limited cases, however, actively secreting colonies can be identified by haemolytic overlay techniques (Köhler and Milstein, 1975; Köhler, 1979) or formation of immune precipitates surrounding the colonies (Cook and Scharff, 1977).

The advantages of cloning by limiting dilution are so great that detailed protocols for agar cloning will not be given here.

3.11.1 Cloning by Limit Dilution

The theory of cloning by limiting dilution has been described in Section 2.9.1. Since the cloning efficiency will seldom be 100% (especially for newly isolated hybrids), cells should be plated at 10,3 and 0.5 cells per 200 μl well in 96-well plates (30 wells per group). Cloning efficiency will often be improved by the presence of feeder cells (Section 3.9.3). Probably the simplest and most convenient source of feeder cells is mouse or rat thymocytes (10^6 per 200 μl well).

Macroscopic colonies, visible by looking at the under surface of the plate, should become visible 1–2 weeks after cloning is commenced. The group where about half the wells show growth may be assumed to contain single clones. Clones should be assayed as soon as they become visible, but will survive and grow for several days afterwards. In the first cloning, only a minority of wells with growth may be active. Recloning should always be carried out, because cloning by limit dilution does not guarantee clonality.

It is also possible to "clone" by limiting dilution *without* performing cell counts. The hybrids are simply plated out in serial twofold dilutions in 200 μl cultures, and the well with the highest dilution in which growth occurs is considered to contain the progeny of a single cell. As previously noted, recloning is highly desirable, because the method does not guarantee clonality.

3.11.2 Cloning Using the Fluorescence-activated Cell Sorter (FACS)

Parks *et al.* (1979) have described a modification of the FACS which allows individual hybridoma cells to be cloned. Intact, healthy cells are identified by their low-angle forward light scatter characteristics, and the cell-containing droplet is electrostatically deflected into the appropriate culture well. The electronics are arranged to inhibit subsequent deflections until reset, and to "abort" any situation in which two cells may end up in one well.

The main advantage of cloning by the FACS is that it allows the selection of cells of desired antigen-binding specificity. Some antibody-secreting cells possess small amounts of membrane immunoglobulin (Goding, 1982), but often insufficient to allow detection of bound soluble antigen by fluorescence. This problem is solved by the use of highly fluorescent hydrophilic microspheres (Covaspheres; Covalent Technology, Ann Arbor, Michigan) to which antigen may be bound (Parks *et al.*, 1979). Even single spheres bound to cells are detectable (see also Chapter 7).

So far, the FACS has not been used for cloning hybridomas against cell surface antigens, but the possibility of exploiting rosette formation with target cells might be considered (see Section 3.10.8; Tong *et al.*, 1983).

3.12 Large-scale Cultures

Once the active hybrids have been identified and cloned, they must be grown in larger numbers for freezing and antibody production. These steps seldom cause any problems. The cells are gradually moved to larger and larger cultures, taking care to maintain exponential growth. As soon as there are around 10^7 cells, it is wise to set some aside for freezing in liquid nitrogen (Section 3.13).

It is important to realize that the risk of overgrowth by nonproducer variants never completely ceases, and any stress on the cells (e.g. overgrowth) increases this probability. Adequate frozen stocks are an important insurance against disaster. In addition, it is wise to test the supernatants for antibody at frequent intervals. A falling antibody level is a sign of overgrowth by nonproducers, and is a warning of the need for recloning before it is too late.

Typical antibody levels in the culture supernatant range from 5–50 μg/ml, depending on the individual clone and on cell density. When large amounts of antibody are required, 1-litre cultures (e.g. roller bottles) may be set up and allowed to grow until the cells begin dying. This will maximize antibody levels.

If very large amounts of antibody are needed, it is generally easier to grow the cells as tumours in animals. The serum or ascites will usually contain around 1000 times the antibody concentration in culture (Section 3.14).

3.13 Storage of Hybrids in Liquid Nitrogen

Hybridoma cells may be frozen in liquid nitrogen and stored for several years with good recovery. Aliquots of cells ($\sim 10^7$ per vial) are resuspended in 1–2 ml of a mixture of 90% (v/v) fetal calf serum and 10% dimethyl sulphoxide. They should then be placed immediately into a cooling chamber where the rate of cooling is approximately 1°C per minute, particularly in the critical range of 0°C to − 30°C. Once the cells reach a temperature of below − 60°C, they may be transferred directly into the liquid nitrogen (− 196°C) or stored in the vapour phase ($-$ 120°C or colder, depending on position and insulation).

Makers of liquid nitrogen containers (e.g. Union Carbide) supply suitable equipment for controlled freezing. The narrow-neck containers may be fitted with "freezing cones" which possess a rubber ring which can be set to allow the correct rate of freezing. Other types of liquid nitrogen containers have cardboard drawers for storage of the vials in the vapour phase, and simply inserting the vial into a drawer will result in an adequate rate of cooling. Finally, it is possible to place a vial in a foam-insulated box inside a $-$ 70°C freezer, and transfer the vial to liquid nitrogen a few hours later. Cells will not usually survive for more than a few weeks at $-$ 70°C.

Cells may be frozen in sealed glass ampoules, or preferably in "NUNC" Cryotubes (32 $\times$ 12.5, with screw cap; 1077-1A/3-66656; A/S NUNC, Kamstrup-DK-4000, Ruskilde, Denmark), which are far more convenient in terms of labelling, recovery of cells and safety.

Regardless of how the cells are frozen, it is essential to "test-thaw" a vial to make sure that the cells may be recovered in a viable and sterile state. The vials should be thawed rapidly in a 37°C water bath, taking care to avoid contact of the water with the seal area of the vial. The vial should then be swabbed with 70% ethanol, dried, and opened. The cells are immediately recovered by centrifugation, placed in normal medium (RPMI-1640 or Eagle's with 10–15% FCS) and placed in culture. It is a good idea to plate the cells at several different dilutions (serial 10-fold dilutions) after thawing.

Even if the cells from the test vial look very healthy under the microscope upon thawing, they should be cultured for a day or two and re-examined, because sometimes a poor freezing will not reveal itself until 1–2 days after thawing. It is not unknown for apparently healthy cells to be all dead the day after thawing.

3.14 Growth of Hybridomas in Animals

The need for histocompatibility for hybridoma growth has already been mentioned (Section 3.1). In most instances, injection of 10^6–10^7 histocompatible hybrid cells into mice or rats will result in tumour formation after 2–4 weeks. Intraperitoneal injection is the preferred route, because it will often result in the development of ascites in some individuals. The antibody levels in ascites are not greatly different to those in serum, and range from 5–15 mg/ml. However, it is not uncommon to obtain 2–5 ml or more ascites from a single mouse, compared with 0.5–1 ml serum.

The success rate in tumour development, and the probability of ascites formation, are increased by injecting 0.5 ml pristane (2,6,10,14-tetramethyl pentadecane; Aldrich Chemical Company, Milwaukee, WI) intraperitoneally a few days prior to injecting the cells. If tumours fail to appear, sublethal irradiation (350–500 R) prior to injection of the cells may help.

Mice may be bled from the retrobulbar sinus (the widely used term "retro-orbital sinus" is incorrect) or the tail. The blood is allowed to clot, and the tube should be "rimmed" with a wooden stick to detach the clot and allow maximal retraction to occur over a period of several hours. The blood is then centrifuged (5000 g for 5–10 min) and the serum collected. Ascites does not usually clot, but it is essential to remove the cells by centrifugation prior to freezing.

Serum or ascites should be examined by electrophoresis on agarose or cellulose acetate strips for the presence of a "spike" of monoclonal antibody in the gamma globulin region (Fig. 2.3). It is then stored in small aliquots, preferably at $-70°C$. It should not be subjected to multiple freeze–thaw cycles, because these may cause denaturation of the antibody, especially IgM. Stability and storage of monoclonal antibodies will be discussed in Chapter 4.

3.15 Mix-ups of Cells

It is extremely easy to contaminate one cell line with another, although most investigators do not believe it until it happens to them personally. The notorious contamination of cell lines with HeLa cells (Nelson-Rees and Flandermeyer, 1976) should serve as a warning. Only one cell is enough to take over a culture if it grows rapidly.

The risk of contamination is minimized if a few simple precautions are taken. It is preferable to passage only one cell line at a time, keeping the remainder in the incubator. Care should be taken to avoid aerosols. A pipette that has contacted cells must obviously never be put into a bottle of medium.

Contamination of cell lines can also occur during passaging of tumours in animals. Instruments should be boiled before use, and cleaned and boiled again after use. Adequate frozen stocks of cells from early passages will help if a mix-up is suspected. Wherever possible, controls should be built into experiments to allow mix-ups to be detected. Serum electrophoresis (Fig. 2.3) is also useful for detecting mix-ups.

3.16 Mycoplasma Contamination

3.16.1 Nature of the Problem

Most laboratories around the world working with continuous cell lines have either chronically or periodically suffered from the problem of mycoplasma contamination (Chen, 1977; McGarrity *et al.*, 1978; Birke *et al.*, 1981). Any of a large number of species of mycoplasma or the related genus *Acholeplasma* can become chronic contaminants of cell lines without necessarily causing any grossly observable effect on cell growth or morphology. Some random surveys show incidences of infection of greater than 50% in U.S. laboratories.

Since such contamination was first recognised some 25 years ago, it has gradually come to be recognized as a significant source of misleading and invalid observations on cultured cells. For example, Vennegoor *et al.*, (1982) unintentionally produced monoclonal antibodies to *Mycoplasma hyorhinis* by immunizing with cultured cells that had been contaminated.

There is now a long list of ways in which the organisms interfere with research on cells. The most obvious are biochemical studies, and a number of reported differences between different types of cell lines proved subsequently to be due to differences between contaminated and noncontaminated cells. Infection has been shown to affect the ability of cells to form hybrids, and it may cause complete failure of hybridoma production. Mycoplasma infection may also affect the cloning efficiency in culture and the ability to form tumours *in vivo*.

The current belief of most workers who specialize in mycoplasma–cell relationships is that the common primary source of contamination are bovine (fetal calf serum), porcine (possibly from trypsin) and human, but not the tissue of origin of the cells. Many mycoplasmas are small and pliable enough to pass through even 0.22 μm filters. Better quality control by the commercial suppliers of fetal calf serum and routine heating of serum (56°C for 1 h) before use seems to be progressively reducing the incidence of fresh contaminations of bovine origin.

It is likely that the main sources at present are laboratory workers handling the cultures and existing chronically contaminated cell lines. Mouth pipetting should never be used for cultured cell lines. Some epidemiological studies of individual tissue culture laboratories suggest that existing lines are by far the major source of new contaminations. Contaminated lines have not been recognized as a biohazard either to laboratory personnel or to mice. They do, however, represent a threat to cell lines that are presumed to be clean, and will earn the laboratory no gratitude if they are sent to other laboratories.

Thus, for a laboratory which has a clean set of lines it is important to identify any newly contaminated lines or imported contaminated lines and to eliminate them promptly. A programme of regular testing of existing lines and immediate testing of imports is highly desirable. Complete cure of infections is usually difficult to achieve, and therefore not worth the effort unless there is no alternative.

3.16.2 Detection of Mycoplasma Contamination

Monitoring by microbiological culture techniques has been somewhat unreliable, particularly in non-specialist hands, because some mycoplasma species are extremely fastidious (Hessling *et al.*, 1980). In the last few years, however, some tests have developed that are not so dependent on specialist expertise (Chen, 1977; Razin, 1985). Kaplan *et al.* (1984) have published a procedure for mycoplasma detection based on incorporation of tritiated thymidine, but this test has been criticized by McGarrity (1984). Gobel and Stanbridge (1984) have developed a test for mycoplasma based on hybridization with a 23S ribosomal RNA gene probe. The probe hybridized to all mycoplasma species, but not to eucaryotic DNA. The approach using DNA hybridization will probably prove to be the most satisfactory (see also Razin *et al.*, 1984; Razin, 1985; Taylor *et al.*, 1985; McGarrity and Kotani, 1986).

The following is an adaptation of Chen's procedure:

(1) Remove and discard most of the supernatant from an exponentially growing 6 ml culture, and add 5 ml of fixative (3:1 methanol:glacial acetic acid) to the cells remaining in the dish. Leave for 5 min at room temperature.

(2) Transfer cells to a centrifuge tube, spin at 1500 rpm for 5 min.

(3) Discard supernatant. Resuspend in fixative, spin as in 2.

(4) Discard supernatant. Resuspend in 1 ml fixative.

(5) Place 1–2 drops on a clean slide. Allow liquid to evaporate by standing at room temperature or with a gentle stream of warm air from a hair dryer.

(6) Make up stock solution of 1.0 mg/ml Hoechst 33258 (Calbiochem cat. no. 382061) in distilled water. (May be kept for two weeks at 4°C, protected from light).

(7) Stain with 0.05 μg/ml Hoechst 33258 in PBS for 20 min at room temperature. (Dilute from stock solution immediately before use.)

(8) Rinse in distilled water.

(9) Examine under high power oil immersion, using a fluorescence microscope. The filter combination is 48 77 02 (UV) (Zeiss), which consists of an excitation filter G365, an FT 420 dichroic mirror and an LP 418 barrier filter.

The nuclear DNA of the cells will stain brightly. There should be no discrete fluorescence in the cytoplasm, although some uncontaminated cell lines may show a very pale cloudy fluorescence. The presence of mycoplasma will be seen as tiny fluorescent dots that appear to lie in the cytoplasm or in clusters around or between cells (see Chen, 1977; Hessling *et al.*, 1980).

3.16.3 Elimination of Mycoplasma

Elimination of mycoplasma is not easy, and should only be attempted if the cell line is particularly valuable. The organisms rapidly acquire resistance to antibiotics. Staehelin *et al.* (1981) treated cells with chlortetracycline (50 μg/ml) and passaged the cells through mice. The resulting tumour cells were mycoplasma-free. Kaplan and Olsson (1981) exposed cells to 41°C for approximately 40 h, followed by subcloning and/or treatment with kanamycin and clindamycin followed by recloning. Other possibilities include passage through mice, or culture for 72 h with 100 μg/ml of lincomycin and tylosin on top of a monolayer of mouse peritoneal macrophages (Schimmelpfeng *et al.*, 1980; Birke *et al.*, 1981; see also Marcus *et al.*, 1980).

References

Adams, R. L. P. (1980). "Cell Culture for Biochemists." Elsevier/North Holland, Amsterdam, New York and Oxford.

Al-Kaissi, E. and Mostratos, A. (1983). Assessment of substrates for horseradish peroxidase in enzyme immunoassay. *J. immunol. Methods* **58**, 127–132.

Barnes, D. and Sato, G. (1980). Methods for growth of cultured cells in serum-free medium. *Anal. Biochem.* **102**, 255–270.

Bazin, H. (1982). Production of rat monoclonal antibodies with the LOU rat non-secreting IR983F myeloma cell line. *In* "Protides of the Biological Fluids" (H. Peeters, ed), 29th Colloquium, pp. 615–618. Pergamon Press, Oxford and New York.

Bazin, H., Beckers, A., Deckers, C. and Moriamé, M. (1973). Transplantable immunoglobulin-secreting tumours in rats. V. Monoclonal immunoglobulins secreted by 250 ileocecal immunocytomas in LOU/WsI rats. *J. natn. Cancer. Inst.* **51**, 1359–1361.

Berson, S. A., Yalow, R. S., Bauman, A., Rothschild, M. A. and Newerly, K. (1956). Insulin-^{131}I metabolism in human subjects: demonstration of insulin-binding globulin in the circulation of insulin treated subjects. *J. clin. Invest.* **35**, 170–190.

Birke, C., Peter, H H., Langenberg, U., Müller-Hermes, W. J. P., Peters, J. H., Heitmann, J., Leibold, W., Dallügge, H., Krapf, E. and Kirchner, H. (1981). Mycoplasma contamination in human tumor cell lines: effect on interferon induction and susceptibility to natural killing. *J. Immunol.* **127**, 94–98.

Böttcher, I., Hammerling, G. and Kapp, J.-F. (1978). Continuous production of monoclonal mouse IgE antibodies with known allergenic specificity by a hybrid cell line. *Nature* **275**, 761–762.

Boyse, E. A., Hubbar, L., Stockert, E. and Lamm, M. E. (1970). Improved complementation in the cytotoxic test. *Transplantation* **10**, 446–449.

Bradley, L. M. and Shiigi, S. M. (1980). Secondary immunization to nitrophenyl haptens, *In* "Selected Methods in Cellular Immunology" (B. B. Mishell and S. M. Shiigi, eds.), pp. 45–47. Freeman, San Francisco.

Brown, J. P., Wright, P. W., Hart, C. E., Woodbury, R. G., Hellström, K. E. and Hellström, I. (1980). Protein antigens of normal and malignant human cells identified by immunoprecipitation with monoclonal antibodies. *J. biol. Chem.* **255**, 4980–4983.

Burtonboy, G., Bazin, H., Deckers, C., Beckers, A., Lamy, M. and Heremans, J. F. (1973). Transplantable immunoglobulin-secreting tumors in rats. 3. Establishment of immunoglobulin-secreting cell lines from LOU-Ws1 strain rats. *Eur. J. Cancer* **9**, 259–262.

Calabresi, P. and Parks, R. E. (1975). Alkylating agents, antimetabolites, hormones and other antiproliferative agents. *In* "The Pharmacological Basis of Therapeutics" (L. S. Goodman and A. Gilman, eds), 5th ed., pp. 1254–1307. MacMillan, New York.

Catt, K. J. and Tregear, G. (1967). Solid-phase radioimmunoassay in antibody-coated tubes. *Science* **158**, 1570–1572.

Chandler, H. M., Cox, J. C., Healey, K., MacGregor, A., Premier, R. R. and Hurrell, J. G. R. (1982). An investigation of the use of urease-antibody conjugates in enzyme immunoassays. *J. immunol. Methods* **53**, 187–194.

Chang, T. H., Steplewski, Z. and Koprowski, H. (1980). Production of monoclonal antibodies in serum free medium. *J. immunol. Methods* **39**, 369–375.

Chapel, H. M. and August, P. J. (1976). Report of nine cases of accidental injury to man with Freund's complete adjuvant. *Clin. exp. Immunol.* **24**, 538–541.

Chase, M. W. (1967). Preparation of immunogens. *In* "Methods in Immunology and Immunochemistry. Vol. 1. Preparation of Antigens and Antibodies" (C. A. Williams and M. W. Chase, eds), pp. 197–200. Academic Press, London.

Chen, T. R. (1977). *In situ* detection of mycoplasma contamination in cell cultures by fluorescent Hoechst 33258 stain. *Exp. Cell. Res.* **104**, 255–262.

Chorney, M., Shen, F. W., Michaelson, J., Taylor, B. and Boyse, E. A. (1982). Monoclonal antibody to an alloantigenic determinant on beta 2 microglobulin (B2M). *Immunogenetics* **16**, 91–93.

Coffino, P., Baumal, R., Laskov, R. and Scharff, M. (1972). Cloning of mouse myeloma cells and detection of rare variants. *J. Cell Physiol.* **79**, 429–440.

Cook, W. D. and Scharff, M. D. (1977). Antigen-binding mutants of mouse myeloma cells. *Proc. natn. Acad. Sci. U.S.A.* **74**, 5687–5691.

Croce, C. M., Linnenbach, A., Hall, A., Steplewski, Z. and Koprowski, H. (1980). Production of human hybridomas secreting antibodies to measles virus. *Nature* **288**, 488–489.

Culvenor, J. G., Harris, A. W., Mandel, T. E., Whitelaw, A. and Ferber, E. (1981). Alkaline phosphatase in hematopoietic tumor cell lines of the mouse: high activity in cells of the B lymphoid lineage. *J. Immunol.* **126**, 1974–1977.

Douillard, J. Y., Hoffman, T. and Herberman, R. B. (1980). Enzyme-linked immunosorbent assay for screening monoclonal antibody production: use of intact cells as antigen. *J. immunol. Methods* **39**, 309–316.

Dresser, D. W. (1962) Specific inhibition of antibody production. II. Paralysis induced in adult mice by small quantities of antigen. *Immunology* **5**, 378–388.

Edwards, P. A. W., Smith, C. M., Neville, A. M. and O'Hare, M. J. (1982). A human–human hybridoma system based on a fast-growing mutant of the ARH-77 plasma cell leukemia-derived line. *Eur. J. Immunol.* **12**, 641–647.

Ehrlich, P. (1900). On immunity with special reference to cell life. (Croonian lecture.) *Proc. R. Soc. Lond. B.* **66**, 424–448.

Engvall, E. (1980). Enzyme immunoassay ELISA and EMIT. *Meth. Enzymol.* **70**, 419–438.

Engvall, E. and Pesce, A. J. (1978). "Quantitative Enzyme Immunoassay." *Scand. J. Immunol.* **8**, Suppl. 7.

Eshhar, Z., Ofarim, M. and Waks, T. (1980). Generation of hybridomas secreting murine reaginic antibodies at anti-DNP specificity. *J. Immunol.* **124**, 775–780.

Everson, L. K., Buell, B. N. and Rogentine, G. N. (1973). Separation of human lymphoid cells into G_1, S and G_2 cell cycle populations by use of a velocity sedimendation technique. *J. exp. Med.* **137**, 343–358.

Ey, P. L., Prowse, S. J. and Jenkin, C. R. (1978). Isolation of pure IgG1, IgG2a and IgG2b immunoglobulins from mouse serum using protein A-Sepharose. *Immunochemistry* **15**, 429–436.

Farr, A. G. and Nakane, P. K. (1981). Immunohistochemistry with enzyme labeled antibodies: a brief review. *J. immunol. Methods* **47**, 129–144.

Fazekas de St. Groth, S. and Scheidegger, D. (1980). Production of monoclonal antibodies: strategy and tactics. *J. immunol. Methods* **35**, 1–21.

Frackelton, A. R. and Rotman, B. (1980). Functional diversity of antibodies elicited by bacterial β-D-galactosidase. *J. biol. Chem.* **255**, 5286–5290.

Galfrè, G. and Milstein, C. (1981). Preparation of monoclonal antibodies: strategies and procedures. *Meth. Enzymol.* **73**, 1–46.

Galfrè, G., Howe, S. C., Milstein, C., Butcher, G. W. and Howard, J. C. (1977). Antibodies to major histocompatibility antigens produced by hybrid cell lines. *Nature* **266**, 550–552.

Galfrè, G., Milstein, C. and Wright, B. (1979). Rat × rat hybrid myelomas and a monoclonal anti-Fd portion of mouse IgG. *Nature* **277**, 131–133.

Garcia-Rozas, C., Plaze, A., Diaz-Espada, F., Kreisler, M. and Martinez-Alonso, C. (1982). Alkaline phosphatase activity as a membrane marker for activated B cells. *J. Immunol.* **129**, 52–55.

Gatti, R. A., Östborn, A. and Fagraeus, A. (1974). Selective impairment of cell antigenicity by fixation. *J. Immunol.* **113**, 1361–1368.

Gefter, M. L., Margulies, D. H. and Scharff, M. D. (1977). A simple method for polyethylene glycol-promoted hybridization of mouse myeloma cells. *Somat. Cell. Genet.* **3**, 231–236.

Gobel, U. B. and Stanbridge, E. (1984). Cloned mycoplasma ribosomal RNA genes for the detection of mycoplasma contamination in tissue culture. *Science.* **226**, 1211–1213.

Goding, J. W. (1976). The chromic chloride method of coupling antigens to erythrocytes: definition of some important parameters. *J. immunol. Methods* **10**, 61–66.

Goding, J. W. (1978). Use of staphylococcal protein A as an immunological reagent. *J. immunol. Methods* **20**, 241–253.

Goding, J. W. (1980). Antibody production by hybridomas. *J. immunol. Methods* **39**, 285–308.

Goding, J. W. (1982). Asymmetrical surface IgG on MOPC-21 plasmacytoma cells contains one membrane heavy chain and one secretory heavy chain. *J. Immunol.* **128**, 2416–2421.

Gray, B. M. (1979). ELISA methodology for polysaccharide antigens: protein coupling of polysaccharides for adsorption to plastic tubes. *J. immunol. Methods* **28**, 187–192.

Griffin, F. M., Ashland, G. and Capizzi, R. L. (1981). Kinetics of photoxicity of Fischer's medium for L5178Y leukemic cells. *Cancer Res.* **41**, 2241–2248.

Hager, D. A. and Burgess, R. R. (1980). Elution of proteins from sodium dodecyl sulfate-polyacrylamide gels, removal of sodium dodecyl sulfate, and renaturation of enzymatic activity: results with sigma subunit of *Escherichia coli* RNA polymerase, wheat germ DNA topoisomerase, and other enzymes. *Anal. Biochem.* **109**, 76–86.

Hämmerling, G. J., Hämmerling, U. and Kearney, J. F. (1981). "Monoclonal Antibodies and T-Cell Hybridomas", p. 569. Elsevier/North-Holland, Amsterdam, p. 569.

Handman, E. and Jarvis, H. M. (1985). Nitrocellulose-based assays for the detection of glycolipids and other antigens: Mechanism of binding to nitrocellulose. *J. immunol. Methods* **83**, 113–123.

Handman, E. and Remington, J. (1980). Serological and immunochemical characterisation of monoclonal antibodies to *Toxoplasma gondii. Immunology*, **40**, 579–588.

Heney, G. and Orr, G. A. (1981). The purification of avidin and its derivatives on 2-Iminobiotin-6-aminohexyl-Sepharose 4B. *Anal. Biochem.* **114**, 92–96.

Hengartner, H., Luzzati, A. L. and Schreier, M. (1978). Fusion of *in vitro* immunized lymphoid cells with X63Ag8. *Current Topics Microbiol. Immunol.* **81**, 92–99.

Herbert, W. J. (1973). Mineral-oil adjuvants and the immunization of laboratory animals. *In* "Handbook of Experimental Immunology" (D. M. Weir, ed), Vol. 3, Chapter 2. Blackwell, Oxford.

Hessling, J. J., Miller, S. E. and Levy, N L. (1980). A direct comparison of procedures for the detection of mycoplasma in tissue culture. *J. immunol. Methods* **38**, 315–324.

Howard, F. D., Ledbetter, J. A., Mehdi, S. Q. and Herzenberg, L. A. (1980). A rapid method for the detection of antibodies to cell surface antigens: a solid phase radioimmunoassay using cell membranes. *J. immunol. Methods* **38**, 75–84.

Hudson, L. and Hay, F. C. (1976). "Practical Immunology." Blackwell, Oxford.

Hurn, B. A. L. and Chantler, S. M. (1980). Production of reagent antibodies. *Meth. Enzymol.* **70**, 104–142.

Jakoby, W. B. and Pastan, I. H. (1979). Cell culture. *Meth. Enzymol.* **LVIII**.

Johnson, A. M., McNamara, P. J., Neoh, S. H., McDonald, P. J. and Zola, H. (1981). Hybridomas secreting monoclonal antibody to *Toxoplasma gondii. Aust. J. exp. Biol. med. Sci.* **59**, 303–306.

Johnson, D. A., Gautsch, J. W., Sportsman, J. R. and Elder, J. H. (1984). Improved technique utilizing nonfat dry milk for analysis of proteins and nucleic acids transferred to nitrocellulose. *Gene Anal. Techn.* **1**, 3–8.

Kaplan, D. R., Henkel, T. J., Braciale, V. and Braciale, T. J. (1984). Mycoplasma infection of cell cultures: Thymidine incorporation of culture supernatants as a screening test. *J. Immunol.* **132**, 9–11.

Kaplan, H. S. and Olsson, L. (1981). Stanford hybridoma cured of mycoplasma. *Immunology Today* October, 1981, p. ii.

Karpas, A., Fischer, P. and Swirsky, D. (1982a). Human myeloma cell line carrying a Philadelphia chromosome. *Science* **216**, 997–999.

Karpas, A., Fischer, P. and Swirsky, D. (1982b). Human plasmacytoma with an unusual karyotype growing *in vitro* and producing light-chain immunoglobulin. *Lancet* **i**, 931–933.

Kearney, J. F., Radbruch, A., Liesengang, B. and Rajewsky, K. (1979). A new mouse myeloma cell line that has lost immunoglobulin expression but permits the construction of antibody-secreting hybrid cell lines. *J. Immunol.* **123**, 1548–1550.

Kennett, R. H. (1980). Enzyme-linked antibody assay with cells attached to polyvinyl chloride plates. *In* "Monoclonal Antibodies Hybridomas: a new dimension in biological analyses" (R. H. Kennett, T. J. McKearn and K. B. Bechtol, eds), pp. 376–377. Plenum Press, New York.

Kilmartin, J. V., Wright, B. and Milstein, C. (1982). Rat monoclonal antitubulin antibodies derived by using a new nonsecreting rat cell line. *J. Cell Biol.* **93**, 576–582.

Kincade, P. W., Lee, G., Sun, L. and Watanabe, T. (1981). Monoclonal rat antibodies to murine IgM determinants. *J. immunol. Methods* **42**, 17–26.

Kinosita, K. and Tsong, T. Y. (1977). Hemolysis of human erythrocytes by a transient electric field. *Proc. natn. Acad. Sci. U.S.A.* **74**, 1917–1927.

Köhler, G. (1979). Soft agar cloning of lymphoid tumor lines: detection of hybrid clones with anti-SRBC activity. *In* "Immunological Methods" (I. Lefkovits, and B. Pernis, eds), pp. 397–401. Academic Press, London and Orlando.

Köhler, G. and Milstein, C. (1975). Continuous cultures of fused cells secreting antibody of predefined specificity. *Nature* **256**, 495–497.

Lane, H. C., Shelhamer, J. H., Mostowski, H. S. and Fauci, A. S. (1982). Human monoclonal anti-keyhole limpet hemocyanin antibody-secreting hybridoma produced from peripheral blood B lymphocytes of a keyhole limpet hemocyanin-immune individual. *J. exp. Med.* **155**, 333–338.

Ledbetter, J. A. and Herzenberg, L. A. (1979). Xenogeneic monoclonal antibodies to mouse lymphoid differentiation antigens. *Immunol. Rev.* **47**, 63–90.

Lee, S-K., Singh, J. and Taylor, R. B. (1975). Subclasses of T cells with different sensitivities to cytotoxic antibody in the presence of anesthetics. *Eur. J. Immunol.* **5**, 259–262.

Lefkovits, I. and Kamber, O. (1972). A replicator for handling and sampling micro-cultures in tissue culture trays. *Eur. J. Immunol.* **2**, 365–366.

Lernhardt, W., Anderson, J., Coutinho, A. and Melchers, F. (1978). Cloning of murine transformed cell lines in suspension culture with efficiencies near 100%. *Exp. Cell. Res.* **111**, 309–316.

Lo, M. S., Tsong, T. Y., Contad, M. K., Strittmatter, S. M., Hester, L. D. and Snyder, S. H. (1984). Monoclonal antibody production by receptor-mediated electrically induced cell fusion. *Nature* **310**, 792–794.

Loken, M. R. and Stall, A. M. (1982). Flow cytometry as an analytical and preparative tool in immunology. *J. immunol. Methods* **50**, 85–112.

Luben, R. A. and Mohler, M. A. (1980). *In vitro* immunization as an adjunct to the production of hybridomas producing antibodies against the lymphokine osteoclast activating factor. *Molec. Immunol.* **17**, 635–639.

Luben, R. A., Brazeau, P., Böhlen, P. and Guillemin, R. (1982). Monoclonal antibodies to hypothalamic growth hormone-releasing factor with picomoles of antigen. *Science* **218**, 887–889.

Maggio, E. T. (1980). "Enzyme-immunoassay." CRC Press, Florida.

Marcus, M., Lari, U., Nattenberg, A., Rottem, S. and Markowitz, O. (1980). Selective killing of mycoplasmas from contaminated mammalian cells in cell cultures. *Nature* **285**, 659–661.

McGarrity, G. J. (1984). Letter to Editor. *J. Immunol.* **133**, 1683. (Reply by Kaplan *et al.* is on same page).

McGarrity, G. J., Murphy, D. G. and Nichols, W. W. (1978) "Mycoplasma Infection of Cell Cultures." Plenum Press, New York and London.

McGarrity, G. J. and Kotani, H. (1986). Detection of cell culture mycoplasmas by a genetic probe. *Exp. Cell Res.* **163**, 273–278.

McKearn, T. J. (1980). ^{51}Cr-release cytotoxicity assay. *In* "Monoclonal Antibodies. Hybridomas: a new dimension in biological analyses" (R. H. Kennett, T. J. McKearn and K. B. Bechtol, eds), pp. 393–394. Plenum Press, New York.

McKearn, T. J., Smilek, D. E. and Fitch, F. W. (1980). Rat–mouse hybridomas and their application to studies of the major histocompatibility complex. *In* "Monoclonal Antibodies" (R. H. Kennett, T. J. McKearn and K. B. Bechtol, eds), pp. 219–234. Plenum Press, New York.

Metcalf, D. (1977). "Hemopoietic Colonies. *In vitro* cloning of normal and leukemic cells." Recent Results in Cancer Research, Vol. 61. Springer-Verlag, Berlin.

Murakami, H., Masui, H., Sato, G. H., Sueoka, N., Chow, T. P. and Kano-Sueoka, T. (1982). Growth of hybrdoma cells in serum-free medium: Ethanolamine is an essential component. *Proc. natn. Acad. Sci. U.S.A.* **79**, 1158–1162.

Nelson-Rees, W. and Flandermeyer, N. R. (1976). HeLa cultures defined. *Science* **191**, 96–98.

Nilsson, K. (1971). Characteristics of established myeloma and lymphoblastoid cell lines derived from an E myeloma patient: a comparative study. *Int. J. Cancer* **7**, 380–396.

Nilsson, K., Bennich, H., Johansson, S. G. O. and Ponten, J. (1970). Established immunoglobulin producing myeloma (IgE). *Clin. exp. Immunol.* **7**, 477–489.

Norwood, T. H., Zeigler, C. J. and Martin, G. M. (1976). Dimethyl sulfoxide enhances polyethylene glycol-mediated cell fusion. *Somat. Cell Genet.* **2**, 263–270.

Nowinski, R. C., Lostrom, M. E., Tam, M. R., Stone, M. R. and Burnette, W. N. (1979). The isolation of hybrid cell lines producing monoclonal antibodies against the p15(E) protein of ecotropic murine leukemia viruses. *Virology*, **93**, 111–126.

Nowinski, R. C, Boglund, J., Lane, M., Lostrum, M., Bernstein, I., Young, W., Hakomori, S., Hill, L. and Cooney, M. (1980). Human monoclonal antibody against Forsmann's antigens. *Science* **210**, 537–539.

Oi, V. T., Jones, P. P., Goding, J. W., Herzenberg, L. A. and Herzenberg, L. A. (1978). Properties of monoclonal antibodies to mouse Ig allotypes, H-2 and Ia antigens. *Current Topics Microbiol. Immunol.* **81**, 115–129.

Oi, V. T. and Herzenberg, L. A. (1980). Immunoglobulin-producing hybrid cell lines. *In* "Selected Methods in Cellular Immunology", (B. B. Mishell and S. M. Shiigi, eds), pp. 351–372. Freeman, San Francisco.

Olsson, L. and Kaplan, H. S. (1980). Human–human hybridomas producing monoclonal antibodies of predefined antigenic specificity. *Proc. natn. Acad. Sci. U.S.A.* **77**, 5429–5434.

O'Sullivan, M. J., Gnemmi, E., Simmonds, A. D., Chieregatti, G., Heyderman, E., Bridges, J. W. and Marks, V. (1979). A comparison of the ability of β-galactosidase and horseradish peroxidase enzyme-antibody conjugates to detect specific antibodies. *J. immunol. Methods* **31**, 247–250.

Parish, C. R. and McKenzie, I. F. C. (1978). A sensitive rosetting method for detecting subpopulations of lymphocytes which react with alloantisera. *J. immunol. Methods* **20**, 173–183.

Parkhouse, R. M. E. and Guarnotta, G. (1978). Rapid binding test for detection of alloantibodies to lymphcoyte surface antigens. *Current Topics Microbiol. Immunol.* **81**, 142.

Parks, D. R., Bryan, V. M., Oi, V. T. and Herzenberg, L. A. (1979). Antigen-specific identification and cloning of hybridomas with a fluorescence-activated cell sorter. *Proc. natn. Acad. Sci. U.S.A.* **76**, 1962–1966.

Pierce, S. K. and Klinman, N. R. (1976). Allogeneic carrier-specific enhancement of hapten-specific secondary B-cell responses. *J. exp. Med.* **144**, 1254–1262.

Posner, M. R., Antoniou, D., Griffin, J., Schlossman, S. F. and Lazarus, H. (1982). An enzyme-linked immunosorbent assay (ELISA) for the detection of monoclonal antibodies to cell surface antigens on viable cells. *J. immunol. Methods* **48**, 23–31.

Razin, S., Gross, M., Wormser, M., Pollack, Y. and Glaser, G. (1984). Detection of mycoplasmas infecting cell cultures by DNA hybridization. *In Vitro.* **20**, 404–408.

Razin, S. (1985). Molecular biology and genetics of Mycoplasmas (Mollicutes). *Microbiol. Rev.* **49**, 419–455.

Reedman, B. M. and Klein, G. (1973). Cellular localization of an Epstein–Barr virus (EBV)-associated complement-fixing antigen in producer and non-producer lymphoblastoid cell lines. *Int. J. Cancer* **11**, 499–520.

Sandrin, M. S., Potter, T. A., Morgan, G. M. and McKenzie, I. F. C. (1978). Detection of mouse alloantibodies by rosetting with protein A-coated sheep red blood cells. *Transplantation* **26**, 126–130.

Schimmelpfeng, L., Langenberg, U. and Peters, J. H. (1980). Macrophages overcome mycoplasma infections of cells *in vitro*. *Nature* **285**, 661–662.

Schlom, J., Wonderlich, D. and Teramoto, Y. A. (1980). Generation of human monoclonal antibodies reactive with human mammary carcinoma cells. *Proc. natn. Acad. Sci. U.S.A.* **77**, 6841–6846.

Secher, D. S. and Burke, D. C. (1980). A monoclonal antibody for large-scale purification of human leucocyte interferon. *Nature* **285**, 446–450.

Sharon, J., Morrison, S. L. and Kabat, E. A. (1980). Formation of hybridoma clones in soft agarose: effect of pH and medium. *Somat. Cell. Genet.* **6**, 435–441.

Smolarsky, M. (1980). A simple radioimmunoassay to determine binding of antibodies to lipid antigens. *J. immunol. Methods* **38**, 85–93.

Springer, T. A. (1980). Cell-surface differentiation in the mouse. Characterization of "jumping" and "lineage" antigens using xenogeneic rat monoclonal antibodies. *In* "Monoclonal Antibodies" (R. H. Kennett, T. J. McKearn and K. D. Bechtol, eds), pp. 185–217. Plenum Press, New York.

Staehelin, T., Durrer, B., Schmidt, J., Takacs, B., Stocker, J., Miggiano, V., Stahli, C., Rubinstein, M., Levy, W. P., Hershberg, R. and Pestka, S. (1981). Production at hybridomas secreting monoclonal antibodies to the human leukocyte interferons. *Proc. natn. Acad. Sci. U.S.A.* **78**, 1848–1852.

Stähli, C., Staehelin, T., Miggiano, V., Schmidt, J. and Haring, P. (1980). High frequencies of antigen-specific hybridomas: dependence on immunization parameters and prediction by spleen cell analysis. *J. immunol. Methods* **32**, 297–304.

Stocker, J. W. and Heusser, C. H. (1979). Methods for binding cells to plastic: application to a solid-phase radioimmunoassay for cell-surface antigens. *J. immunol. Methods* **26**, 87–95.

Stoien, J. D. and Wang, R. J. (1974). Effect of near-ultraviolet and visible light on mammalian cells in culture. II. Formation of toxic photoproducts in tissue culture medium by blacklight. *Proc. natn. Acad. Sci. U.S.A.* **71**, 3961–3965.

Taylor, M. A., Wise, K. S. and McIntosh, M. A. (1985). Selective detection of Mycoplasma hyorhinis using cloned genomic DNA fragments. *Infect. Immun.* **47**, 827–830.

Taylor, R. B., Duffus, W. P. H., Raff, M. C. and de Petris, S. (1971). Redistribution and pinocytosis of lymphocyte surface immunoglobulin molecules by anti-immunoglobulin antibody. *Nature (New Biol.)* **233**, 225–229.

Tijssen, P. and Kurstak, E. (1984). Highly efficient and simple methods for the preparation of peroxidase and active peroxidase-antibody conjugates for enzyme immunoassays. *Anal. Biochem.* **136**, 451–457.

Tong, A. W., Vandenbark, A. A., Kraybill, W., Regan, D. and Burger, D. R. (1983). Detection of antigen specific rosette formation with the FACS. *J. immunol. Methods* **56**,63–74.

Trowbridge, I. S. (1978). Interspecies spleen-myeloma hybrid producing monoclonal antibodies against mouse lymphocyte surface glycoprotein T200. *J. exp. Med.* **148**, 313–323.

Trucco, M. M., Stocker, J. W. and Ceppellini, R. (1978). Monoclonal antibodies against human lymphocyte antigens. *Nature* **273**, 666–668.

Tsong, T. Y. (1983). Voltage modulation of membrane permeability and energy utilization in cells. *Biosci. Rep.* **3**, 487–505.

Tsu, T. T. and Herzenberg, L. A. (1980). Solid-phase radioimmunoassays. *In* "Selected Methods in Cellular Immunology" (B. B. Mishell and S. M. Shiigi, eds), pp. 373–397. Freeman, San Francisco.

Vennegoor, C., Polak-Vogelzang, A. A. and Hekman, A. (1982). Monoclonal antibodies against Mycoplasma hyorhinis. A secondary effect of immunization with cultured cells. *Exp. Cell. Res.* **137**, 89–94.

Voller, A., Bidwell, D. E. and Bartlett, A. (1979). "The Enzyme Linked Immunosorbent Assay (ELISA). A guide with abstracts of microplate applications." Published by Dynatech Europe, Burough House, Rue du Pre, Guernsey, G. B.

Wang, R. J. (1976). Effect of room fluorescent light on the deterioration of tissue culture medium. *In Vitro* **123**, 19–22.

Williams, W. J., Beutler, E., Erslev, A. J. and Rundles, R. W. (1977). "Hematology", 2nd ed. McGraw-Hill, New York.

Wilson, M. B. and Nakane, P. K. (1978). Recent developments in the periodate method of conjugating horseradish peroxidase (HRPO) to antibodies. *In* "Immunofluorescence and Related Staining Techniques" (W. Knapp, K. Holubar and G. Wick, eds.), pp 215–224. Elsevier/North-Holland, Amsterdam and New York.

Wojchowski, D. M. and Sytkowski, A. J. (1986). Hybridoma production by simplified avidin-mediated bridging. *J. immunol. Methods* (In press).

Yalow, R. (1978). Radioimmunoassay: a probe for the fine structure of biologic systems. *Science* **200**, 1236–1245.

Yelton, D. E., Diamond, B. A., Kwan, S-P. and Scharff, M. D. (1978). Fusion of mouse myeloma and spleen cells. *Curr. Topics Microbiol. Immunol.* **81**, 1–7.

Young, W. W., Regimbal, J. W. and Hakomori, S. (1979). Radioimmunoassay of glycosphingolipids: application for the detection of Forssman glycolipid in tissue extracts and cell membranes. *J. immunol. Methods* **28**, 59–69.

Zola, H. and Brooks, D. (1982). Techniques for the production and characterization of monoclonal hybridoma antibodies. *In* "Monoclonal Hybridoma Antibodies: Techniques and Applications", (J. G. Hurrell, ed), pp. 1–57. CRC Press, Florida.

4   Purification, Fragmentation and Isotopic Labelling of Monoclonal Antibodies

In many cases, purification of monoclonal antibodies is not necessary. For example, if fluorescein-conjugated anti-immunoglobulin is used as a second step in indirect immunofluorescence experiments (Chapter 7), there is little reason to purify the first antibody. Similarly, most analytical-scale experiments in which antigens are isolated by immunoprecipitation can be performed using unfractionated culture supernates or serum from hybridoma-bearing animals. On the other hand, if monoclonal antibodies are to be coupled to fluorochromes, biotin or solid-phase affinity matrices, or if it is desired to make proteolytic fragments, at least partial purification is essential.

Typical antibody concentrations in serum or ascites of hybridoma-bearing mice range from 2–20 mg/ml, and thus represent a significant fraction of all protein present. In contrast, the antibody levels in culture supernatants of hybridomas are of the order of 5–50 μg/ml. It is therefore obvious that purification of antibodies from serum or ascites will be much easier than from culture supernatants. If antibodies must be purified from culture supernatants, affinity chromatography is usually the method of choice.

The literature abounds with "recipes" for the purification and fragmentation of antibodies. Often, these procedures have been developed for a particular species (e.g. human, rabbit), and applied with little thought to other species. The result is poor reproducibility and recovery, especially when attempts are made to generate defined proteolytic fragments. Frequently, the procedures for purification of antibodies were designed for polyclonal antisera, and were optimized to make a reasonable compromise between yield and purity. The homogeneity of monoclonal antibodies makes them much easier to purify, but in order to obtain good results it is advisable to individualize the conditions for each antibody. The methods to be described in this chapter have proven reliable and usually involve minimal effort.

The descriptions of antibody purification will concentrate on IgG and IgM, because these are the classes most frequently encountered. Fortunately, IgG is both the most common antibody and the easiest to purify. The purification and fragmentation of mouse IgA, IgD and IgE are specialized subjects, and the primary literature should be consulted (Tomasi and Grey, 1972; Grey *et al.*, 1970; Goding, 1980; Perez-Montgort and Metzger, 1982).

Much useful practical information on protein purification is provided in the monograph by Scopes (1982).

4.1 Determination of Antibody Class

Knowledge of antibody class and subclass is a great help in determining the strategy of purification. Unless special immunization and screening procedures have been used, the most frequent antibodies will be IgM and IgG. Hybridomas secreting IgE are rare (Böttcher *et al.*, 1978; Eshhar *et al.*, 1980; Liu *et al.*, 1980), and hybridomas secreting IgA are usually only obtained when the lympocytes for fusion are from gut-associated lymphoid tissue (Komisar *et al.*, 1982). If the screening procedure uses staphylococcal protein A (Sections 3.10.3 and 4.3.2), it is unlikely that classes other than IgG will be detected.

4.1.1 Ouchterlony (Double Diffusion) Analysis

Perhaps the simplest means of determining antibody class is via Ouchterlony analysis (formation of precipitin lines in agar). A typical analysis is shown in Figure 4.1. Glass slides (50 × 75 mm) are coated with 6 ml molten agar (1% in phosphate-buffered saline, pH 7.4) and the agar is allowed to set. [Alternatively, the gel may be poured on the hydrophilic side of "Gelbond" flexible plastic sheets (Marine Colloids division of FMC Corporation). The use of Gelbond allows a permanent unbreakable record to be mounted in a notebook]. Then, holes of 1–2 mm in diameter are punched, usually in a circular pattern around a central hole. The distance between holes is typically 3–5 mm.

The best source of test immunoglobulin is probably culture supernatant from densely grown hybridoma cells obtained after cloning. This ensures that the only mouse immunoglobulin present in the desired antibody. The testing of antibody class from serum or ascites may cause ambiguous results due to

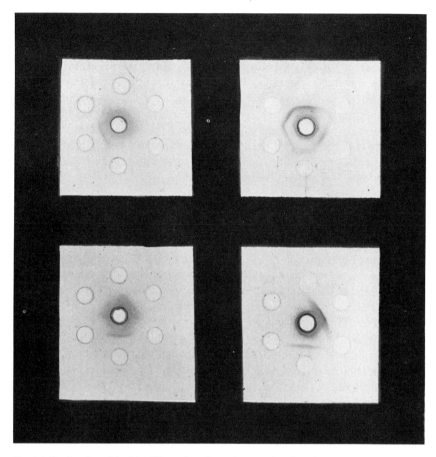

Fig. 4.1. Ouchterlony (double diffusion) analysis of monoclonal antibodies. The wells contain the following proteins (clockwise from top): IgG1κ, IgG2aλ, IgG2bκ, IgG3λ, IgAκ and IgG3κ. The central wells contain anti-K (upper two panels) and anti-λ (lower two panels). The two right-hand panels contain 3% polyethylene glycol, while the two left panels do not. It can be seen that the typing sera are specific, but the IgG3λ protein contains κ-bearing contaminants. Precipitation lines in the right hand panels are strengthened by the presence of polyethylene glycol.

the concurrent presence of normal immunoglobulins, although these can often be diluted out.

The optimal concentration of immunoglobulin for detection in Ouchterlony analysis is 100–1000 μg/ml, when strong anti-immunoglobulin sera are used. This concentration may be achieved by diluting hybridoma antibody-containing serum or ascites by about 20-fold. On the other hand, culture fluid will have to be concentrated by a similar factor. This is easily achieved by addition of an equal volume of saturated ammonium sulphate (Section 4.2.1) followed by centrifugation and resuspension of the pellet in an appropriate volume of phosphate-buffered saline, and dialysing against the same buffer overnight to remove ammonium sulphate.

The central well is filled with the immunoglobulin-containing solution (typically 2–3 μl), and the peripheral wells are filled with undiluted class-specific anti-immunoglobulin antisera (Meloy, Nordic, Litton Bionetics or numerous other suppliers). It is strongly recommended that any laboratory engaged in the production of monoclonal antibodies should possess a set of these antisera. Diffusion is allowed to proceed at room temperature for several hours.

Strong "home-made" class-specific anti-immunoglobulin antibodies will usually produce intense precipitin lines in 3–12 h, using antigen at 1.0 mg/ml. Commercial antibodies are usually much weaker, and appear to be "watered down" to the maximum acceptable dilution, and often beyond. They should generally be used undiluted, and the antigen should be at about 100 μg/ml. Under these conditions, faint precipitin lines should appear after 12–18 h.

If, as is often the case with commercial antisera, the reaction is too weak to be visible, the lines may become visible after staining with Coomassie blue. Before staining is carried out, unprecipitated protein must be removed. This may be accomplished by soaking the wet slide in PBS with agitation for 1–2 days, but in my experience the agar often lifts off the slide. A better method is to wrap the slide in Whatman No. 1 filter paper that has been wet with water, and allow it to dry overnight at 37°C. Most of the uncomplexed protein and buffer salts will diffuse into the filter paper. Once the slide is dry, the paper is wet again with water and removed. The slide is then soaked overnight in PBS to allow residual uncomplexed protein to diffuse out of the gel. The slide is then stained for 5 min in 0.1% Coomassie blue in 40% methanol/10% acetic acid, and destained in 12% ethanol/7% glacial acetic acid until the background is acceptable. It may then be dried at room temperature for a permanent record.

Sometimes the precipitin lines are poor, even after staining. Addition of 3% (w/v) polyethylene glycol (molecular weight 4000–6000) to the agar before pouring the plate will often enhance precipitation (Figure 4.1).

4.1.2 Other Methods

Alternatively, the antibody class might be determined by radioimmunoassay, enzyme-linked immunosorbent assay or indirect immunofluorescence with class-specific fluorescent antibodies. The method chosen will often be governed by the availability of reagents and techniques in the individual laboratory. It may be possible to adapt the screening assay to include class-specific antibodies.

4.2 Methods Used in Antibody Purification

4.2.1 Precipitation with Ammonium Sulphate

One of the oldest and most useful methods of purification of immuno-globulins is based on the observation that they are precipitated by lower concentrations of ammonium sulphate than most other serum proteins. Precipitation of immunoglobulins by ammonium sulphate is gentle, effective and simple. While it is not possible to purify immunoglobulins to homogeneity by this method, it provides a substantial enrichment, and reduces the protein load on subsequent purification steps.

Ammonium sulphate precipitation of immunoglobulins is simple to perform, but there are a few technical points which can greatly influence the degree of purification obtained. It is preferable to add ammonium sulphate slowly in the form of a saturated aqueous solution, rather than as solid crystals. High local concentrations of ammonium sulphate cause unwanted precipitation of proteins such as albumin, and thus degrade the degree of purification.

Saturated ammonium sulphate may be prepared by adding 1 kg of the crystals to 1 litre of distilled water, and stirring for 1–2 days. To be sure of saturation, there must always be undissolved crystals in the bottom of the vessel. The pH should be approximately 6–7. The solution may be stored at 4°C. It is customary to perform ammonium sulphate precipitations at 4°C, although most antibodies can be fractionated at room temperature without adverse effects. The percentage of saturation changes slightly with temperature, but for practical purposes the effect is negligible.

The serum to be fractionated should be placed in a beaker on a magnetic stirrer. Stirring should be slow, as frothing denatures protein. Saturated ammonium sulphate is added dropwise, allowing each drop to disperse before the next is added. When the concentration of ammonium sulphate reaches about 20% of saturation, the serum will begin to turn milky. Most immunoglobulins will be precipitated by 35–40% of saturation, although occasionally it may be necessary to use up to 50%. Higher concentrations do not increase the yield of immunoglobulins, but will cause increasing contamination by other proteins, especially transferrin and albumin.

The suspension should be stirred for 15–30 min, and then centrifuged at 2000 g or preferably 10 000 g. The supernate should be clear, but may contain a layer of lipoprotein on the top. The pellet should be washed 2–3 times in 50% saturated ammonium sulphate. Washing the pellet considerably reduces contamination with non-immunoglobulin proteins, and does not lower the yield significantly. The volume of the pellet should not change greatly after washing. [In the previous edition of this book, it was recommended to wash with 40% saturated ammonium sulphate, but I have since encountered occasional monoclonal antibodies that were soluble in 40% ammonium sulphate.]

It should be noted that ammonium sulphate solutions are dense and resist mixing. Care must be taken that the stock solutions are adequately mixed. A few end-over-end mixings are desirable, as the mixing by magnetic flea may fail to disperse a dense lower layer.

Solutions of saturated ammonium sulphate should not be stored in containers that were previously used for laboratory wash-up detergents. I have found that traces of these detergents can inhibit precipitation of immunoglobulins by ammonium sulphate.

Finally, the precipitate is dissolved in phosphate-buffered saline. It will virtually always redissolve easily. Ammonium ions will interfere with many subsequent procedures, especially conjugation of antibodies with fluorochromes, biotin or agarose. Ammonium sulphate may be removed by overnight dialysis against 500–1000 volumes of phosphate-buffered saline, or any buffer compatible with subsequent manipulations. The dialysis fluid should be changed several times at intervals of a few hours.

4.2.2 Precipitation at Low Ionic Strength

In the early days of serum fractionation, it was noted that some serum proteins were soluble in distilled water, while others were not. The soluble fraction was known as *albumin* and the insoluble fraction as *globulin*. Subsequently, it was found that many globulin-like proteins were soluble in distilled water. These proteins were termed "*pseudoglobulins*", to distinguish them from the water-insoluble "*euglobulins*". Subsequently, the definition of globulins was broadened to include proteins precipitated by 50% saturated ammonium sulphate. Later still, the globulins were redefined to include any protein whose anodic mobility on electrophoresis (Section 2.3.7) was less than that of albumin. The term "pseudoglobulin" is now obsolete, but the term "euglobulin" persists.

The euglobulin fractions of serum is mainly composed of a subpopulation of immunoglobulins, notably the majority of IgM molecules and a significant fraction of IgG and other classes. Precipitation of immunoglobulins at low ionic strength ("euglobulin precipitation") is still occasionally used as a preliminary purification method. Some monoclonal antibodies are insoluble at low ionic strength, while others are not. Euglobulin properties are common amongst mouse IgM, IgG2b and IgG3 proteins, but rare in IgG1.

Euglobulin precipitation is usually carried out by dialysing the protein against distilled water. The pH should be about 6, because like all proteins, immunoglobulins are least soluble near their isoelectric point. If necessary, low concentrations ($\sim 5\,mM$) of citrate-phosphate buffer, pH 5.8, may be used. Dialysis should proceed at 4° for 24–96 h, with several changes. The resulting precipitate is harvested by centrifugation, washed twice in the dialysis fluid, and resuspended in isotonic phosphate-buffered saline. One disadvantage of euglobulin precipitation is that it is sometimes difficult to redissolve the precipitate. Addition of NaCl to a final concentration of 0.3–0.5 M may help.

According to Garvey *et al.* (1977), euglobulins precipitate more readily when dialysed against 2% boric acid (pH ~ 6), and the boric acid precipitate is more readily solubilized than other precipitates. The effectiveness of the boric acid is said to derive from its low ionic strength (it ionizes only weakly) and the fact that its pH is close to the isoelectric point of many immuno-globulins, especially IgM. In addition, the complexing of borate with the carbohydrate moieties on glycoproteins may aid precipitation. The boric acid–glycoprotein complexes that are insoluble at low ionic strength are dissociable by higher salt concentrations.

4.2.3 Zone Electrophoresis

As discussed in Section 2.3.7, antibody molecules are contained in the gamma-globulin fraction of serum, and are the most cathodal serum com-ponent when analysed by electrophoresis at pH 8.6. While normal gamma globulins migrate as a broad smear, individual clonal products migrate as sharp bands (Fig. 2.3).

In addition to its analytical uses, zone electrophoresis may be scaled up for preparative applications (Kunkel, 1954). The support matrix may be starch (granular or gel), Pevikon C-870 beads (a copolymer of polyvinyl chloride and polyvinyl acetate),Sephadex or Sepharose or acrylamide beads, or agarose (Weiss, 1976; Garvey *et al.*, 1977; Radola, 1973).

Zone electrophoresis is now rarely used for immunoglobulin purification, because it is slow and cumbersome, and has limited capacity. However, it is capable of excellent separations, and is especially useful for monoclonal IgM and IgA.

Equipment

Typical apparatus is described by Weiss (1976) and by Garvey *et al.* (1977). For fractionation of 1–2 ml serum, a Perspex (Plexiglass) tray about 300 mm long × 70 mm wide and 10 mm deep is suitable. The tray is placed with each end resting on an electrode chamber (100 mm × 100 mm × 100 mm) con-taining 1–2 perforated baffles and platinum wire electrodes.

The most commonly used buffer system is barbital buffer (pH 8.6, $\mu = 0.1$), which gives excellent resolution of immunoglobulins. Barbital buffer is some-what tricky to get into solution, but the following procedure works well:
   (1) Dissolve 20.6 g sodium barbitone in 400 ml water.
   (2) Add 4.0 g barbitone to 500 ml water, and heat to dissolve.
   (3) Before the barbitone solution cools, add it to the sodium barbitone solution and mix well.
   (4) Add 1.0 g sodium azide and mix.
When used as drugs, barbiturates have addictive potential, and their distribution is restricted in some countries. An alternative buffer system is Tris-Tricine, pH 8.6 (Monthony *et al.*, 1978). To 1 litre of distilled water, add 9.8 g Tris, 4.3 g Tricine and 0.2 g sodium azide. Tris-Tricine has the added advantages of improved buffering, and that unlike barbitone it does not absorb light at 280 nm.

Preparation of the support matrix

Potato starch powder (1 kg; Mallinckrodt Chemical Works, St. Louis, MO) should be placed in a 10-litre plastic beaker and wet with several litres of distilled water. After allowing the starch to settle (several hours), the super-nate is discarded, and the process repeated several times. Finally, the starch is washed twice in barbital buffer and stored as a damp slurry at 4°C.

The tedious nature of the preparation of starch has encouraged a search for more convenient matrices. Pevikon C-870 (Calbiochem) is a suitable substitute, although it should also be washed prior to use. Other matrices include Sephadex G-100 superfine (Radola, 1973) or 1% agarose. If agarose is used, Seakem Seaprep 15/45 (gelling temperature 15°C; melting tem-perature 45°C) may be found convenient, as it may be possible to recover the sample by cutting and melting individual slices of the gel.

The wicks should be made of heavy filter paper, such as Whatman 3MM, soaked in buffer, and put in place prior to pouring the support matrix. Granulated matrices should be poured as thick slurries, and excess fluid removed by blotting until the surface has no visible sheen.

The sample may be neat serum or ascites fluid. If any prior fractionation (such as ammonium sulphate precipitation) has been used, the sample should be dialysed against barbitone buffer before loading. If this is not done, the separation may fail completely.

The sample may be loaded by scooping out a narrow trough about 100 mm from the cathode end, and not quite reaching the sides. Typical sample volumes are 1–2 ml. A few grains of bromphenol blue added to the sample will bind to albumin, and provide a convenient indication of separation. The block should be placed on the electrode chambers with the wicks dipping into the buffer. To prevent evaporation, the bed should be wrapped in kitchen plastic, and electrophoresis is best carried out in the cold room. Typical voltage gradients are 0.3–0.5 V/mm, and separation takes 8–36 h until the dye reaches the end of the trough.

After electrophoresis, the power is turned off, the bed cut into 10 mm segments and scooped into glass test tubes, and 10 ml phosphate-buffered saline added. The contents are mixed by vortexing, and the matrix allowed to settle. Owing to the strong absorbance of barbitone at 280 nm, it is necessary to measure the protein profile by the Lowry method (Lowry *et al.*, 1951). The Tris-Tricine buffer does not absorb at 280 nm. Alternatively, it is possible to make an imprint of the bed by blotting and staining with filter paper (Radola, 1973).

4.2.4 Ion Exchange Chromatography

Ion exchange chromatography is one of the simplest and most useful ways of purifying immunoglobulins, especially IgG. It is particularly suitable for the purification of monoclonal antibodies, because simple gradient elution allows the correct compromise between yield and purity to be made without

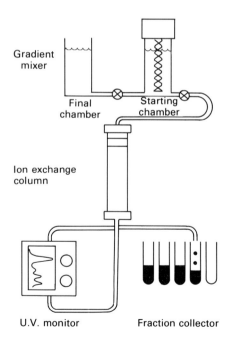

Fig. 4.2. Purification of monoclonal IgG antibodies by ion exchange chromatography. The antibody-containing solution is bound to the column at low ionic strength and pH 8.0, and eluted by a linear gradient of NaCl.

guesswork. The technique is gentle, and is capable of very high capacity. A 10 ml column will easily handle 100–200 mg protein, and the recovery should be virtually 100%. Modern ion exchange resins are inexpensive, easy to use and require a minimum of preparation. Ion exchange chromatography can be done with no special equipment, although work is greatly facilitated by the use of a gradient mixer, an ultraviolet absorbance monitor and a fraction collector (Fig. 4.2). These should be standard equipment in most biological laboratories.

The most commonly used matrix consists of cellulose or agarose to which is attached ionizable diethylaminoethyl-(DEAE) groups (Peterson, 1970). At pH 8, the matrix has a strong positive charge which must be balanced by negative ions (anions). The bound anions may be inorganic (e.g. chloride ions) or organic, such as the charged side chains of proteins, or a mixture of both. Hence, DEAE-cellulose is known as an anion exchanger. The cellulose matrix is sometimes referred to as a "resin", but strictly speaking this term should be confined to amorphous structures (Peterson, 1970).

The immunoglobulins are amongst the most basic of serum proteins, with isoelectric points in the range 6–8. At pH 8, almost all serum proteins will be negatively charged, and thus bind to DEAE-cellulose at low ionic strength. With increasing concentration of competing anions (e.g. Cl^-) or lowering of pH, the proteins will be eluted, approximately in order of their isoelectric points. Because the immunoglobulins are the most basic of the major serum proteins, they will be the first to be eluted.

Preparation of the ion exchanger

The most convenient matrices are those which are supplied pre-swollen. DEAE-Sepharose (agarose) or DEAE-Sephacel (beaded cellulose) are suitable, and there is little to choose between them for immunoglobulin purification. They are supplied in aqueous suspension, with Cl^- counterions.

The ion exchanger beads must be thoroughly equilibrated with the starting buffer prior to use. Unlike the older matrices, DEAE-Sephacel and DEAE-Sepharose do not require "precycling" prior to use. The slurry (50–100 ml) should be poured into a large conical flask, and 1 litre of starting buffer (10 mM Tris-HCl, pH 8) added. After the beads have settled, the supernatant may be decanted, and another litre of buffer added. The process should be repeated several times. The beads are then ready for use, and may be transferred to a smaller container. Alternatively, the beads may be equilibrated by washing with a few litres of buffer on a sintered glass funnel or a Büchner funnel.

The size of the gel bed will be determined by the mass of protein to be bound. The column shape is not very important; plastic disposable syringes are ideal. As a general rule, it is recommended that for optimal resolution, no more than 10% of the available capacity should be used. As a rough approximation, the bed volume should be at least 10 ml for each 100 mg of protein. Immunoglobulins are, in general, fairly resistant to the action of proteases, and ion exchange chromatography can usually be performed at room temperature.

Air is less soluble in water at room temperature than at 4°C. If it is desired to work at room temperature and the gel slurry and the buffers have been stored in the cold, they must be degassed by application of vacuum for a few seconds before pouring the column. Otherwise, the column will become filled with air bubbles, degrading its performance. The need to degas is eliminated if the gel and buffers are allowed to reach room temperature before pouring the column.

The pouring of the colomn is straightforward, and no special precautions are necessary. Gravity feed is adequate; a head of pressure of 100–200 mm of water will be sufficient. The pressure head is measured from the free end of the outlet tube to the free surface of the buffer reservoir.

Preparation of the sample

To ensure that all the protein in the sample will bind to the resin, the sample should be equilibrated with the starting buffer before application. If the salt concentration in the sample is physiological (i.e. ~ 150 mM for serum), simple dilution in 20–50 volumes of starting buffer may be adequate. Alternatively, the sample should be dialysed overnight against 500–1000 volumes of starting buffer.

Occasionally, immunoglobulins will precipitate in the low ionic strength starting buffer (see Section 4.2.2). For this reason, transfer into the starting buffer by desalting on small gel filtration columns (e.g. Sephadex) is only recommended if it is known that the protein will remain in solution. However, even immunoglobulins which precipitate in the starting buffer may be fractioned by ion exchange chromatography. The precipitate is simply loaded onto the column, where it will bind. As the salt concentration is raised during elution, the protein will go back into solution, and the recovery and resolution are indistinguishable from normal.

After the sample has been loaded, the column should be washed with 2–3 times its volume of starting buffer. Only occasional exceptionally basic immunoglobulins will emerge. Once the ultraviolet absorbance monitor tracing is steady, elution may be performed.

Step gradient elution

Bound proteins may be eluted by applying steps of increasing salt concentration (10 mM Tris-HCl, pH 8, plus NaCl 50 mM, 100 mM, 150 mM,

200 mM). Most IgG molecules will emerge by 200 mM. Step gradient elution has the attraction of extreme simplicity, but it also has many disadvantages. It is necessary to try a number of conditions before the appropriate ones are found, and the process must be repeated for each new monoclonal antibody. Step gradient elution results in sharp leading edges of peaks, but the trailing edges are often broad, leading to excessive dilution. Step gradients are also prone to artefacts. The successive application of two steps may result in the elution of two successive peaks of protein, yet when analysed these fractions may be found to consist of the same protein, even if the sample is perfectly homogeneous. These cases are probably manifestations of heterogeneity in the strength of binding sites of the beads.

Linear gradient elution

Elution of monoclonal antibodies by a linear gradient of NaCl in 10 mM Tris-HCl, pH 8, is simple to perform, and gives much better results than step gradients. There is no need for individualization of conditions for each monoclonal antibody, because the gradient can be constructed to cover all elution conditions. Gradient elution subjects the trailing edge of each protein to a higher salt concentration than the leading edge. The leading edge is therefore relatively retarded while the trailing edge is advanced, and the eluted peaks are sharp and symmetrical, with minimal dilution.

Simple gradient mixers are available commercially (e.g. Pharmacia). Alternatively, they may be made in any workshop, or improvised by connecting two beakers via a short length of capillary tubing. Mixing is achieved using a magnetic flea.

If the two chambers have the same shape and dimensions, it can be calculated that the gradient will be linear, with the starting conditions being those in the mixing chamber and the final conditions being those in the reservoir chamber. For purification of monoclonal IgG, one might typically start with 10 mM Tris-HCl, pH 8.0, and end with the same buffer containing 300–500 mM NaCl. The volume of the gradient is arbitrary; good results are obtained using 10–20 times the bed volume of the ion exchanger. Larger volumes will result in somewhat better separation at the expense of increased dilution. The gradient should be run slowly (over a period of 4–12 h) for best resolution. The speed may be adjusted by altering the head of pressure.

A typical fractionation might proceed as follows. Ten millilitres of mouse serum containing a monoclonal IgG antibody is made up to 50% saturated ammonium sulphate by slow addition of 10 ml saturated ammonium sulphate (Section 4.2.1). After two washes in 50% saturated ammonium sulphate, the precipitate is redissolved in phosphate-buffered saline, and the optical density at 280 nm measured. (Assuming that all the protein is IgG, 1 mg/ml will have an absorbance of 1.4 in a cell with 10 mm path length.) A yield of protein of 250 mg is obtained. The protein is dialysed against two changes of 1 litre of 10 mM Tris-HCl, pH 8, and applied to a 20 ml column of DEAE-Sephacel equilibrated with the same buffer. After washing with 50 ml starting buffer, no protein emerges. Then, a gradient mixer is set up with 100 ml of starting buffer in the mixing chamber and 100 ml of the same buffer plus 300 mM NaCl in the reservoir chamber. The gradient is allowed to run over 4 h, and 40 × 5 ml fractions collected. The monoclonal antibody is the first sharp peak to emerge (at approximately 50 ml), and is recovered in 3–4 tubes (yield 70 mg). The purity of individual fractions may be assessed by agarose gel electrophoresis (Section 2.3.7).

> *Isolation of ribonuclease and protease-free*
> *monoclonal antibodies on DEAE Affi-Gel Blue*

The use of ion exchange chromatography for purification of mouse mono-clonal antibodies has been extended by Bruck *et al.* (1982), who reported the use of DEAE Affi-gel blue (Bio-Rad) for the one-step purification of IgG. Ascitic fluid was centrifuged at 1000 g to remove cells, then 100 000 g for 30 min to remove debris and fibrin clots. The fluid was then dialysed over-night against 100 volumes of 20 mM Tris-HCl, pH 7.2, and centrifuged again at 100 000 g. The protein was then passed over a column of DEAE Affi-gel blue equilibrated with the same buffer. The column was washed with the same buffer containing added NaCl (25 mM) to elute transferrin. Finally, mono-clonal antibodies (IgG1 and IgG2) were eluted with 3 bed volumes of 20 mM Tris-HCl pH 7.2 plus 50 mM NaCl. Antibodies were found to be free of contamination by protease, nuclease or albumin. Recovery was said to be 77–80%.

4.2.5 Gel Filtration

Gel filtration separates proteins according to their size (Fischer, 1969). The procedure is simple to perform, and is capable of good recoveries. However, it usually results in greater dilution and a smaller factor of purification than ion exchange or affinity chromatography. The main role of gel filtration in purification of IgG is as an adjunct to other methods, if a higher degree of purification is needed. Gel filtration has a very important role in the purifi-cation of IgM.

Gel filtration is usually carried out in long, thin columns (typically 0.5–1 m in length and 15–30 mm in diameter). The gel itself occupies about 70% of the volume of the column, and the space between the beads the remaining 30%. Very small molecules are freely permeable into the beads, and hence emerge at a volume equal to the *total volume* (V_T) of the column ($\Pi r^2 h$). Very large molecules are totally excluded from the beads, and therefore emerge after a volume equal to about 30% of V_T. This is known as the *void volume* (V_0) of the column. Thus, all fractionation must occur between V_0 and V_T. The emergence of proteins after V_T is indicative of adsorption to the beads, an undesirable property.

The elution position of a protein is best described by the term K_{av}, where

$$K_{av} = (V_E - V_0) \div (V_T - V_0)$$

and V_E is the elution volume.

As a general rule, the best separations will result when the gel type is selected to give a K_{av} of about 0.3–0.6 for the protein of interest. It should be obvious that the selection of a gel which totally excludes the desired protein (e.g. Sephadex G-200 for IgM) will only result in chromatographic separation of the undesired impurities; the desired protein will not be chromatographed. It is surprising how often this combination is described in the literature.

Selection of a suitable gel

The range of gels available has increased enormously in recent years. The main types of gel are granulated dextran (Sephadex), acrylamide (Bio-gel P), agarose (Sepharose, Bio-gel A) and various combinations of these. Sephacryl is a mixture of dextran and acrylamide; Ultrogel is a mixture of agarose and acrylamide.

The main requirements are resolution of the desired molecular weight range, lack of nonspecific adsorption, and ease of use. The newer matrices (Sephacryl and Ultrogel) are much more resistant to compression and easier to pack. They may be run at higher pressures and faster flow rate than the classical gels such as Sephadex. Their resolution is at least as good, and often better. A list of suitable gels is given in Table 4.1.

Table 4.1 Suitable gels for separation of immunoglobulins and their fragments

Immunoglobulin	Molecular weight	Suitable gel
IgG	150 000	Sephacryl S-300 (Pharmacia)
IgM	900 000	Sepharose 6B (Pharmacia)
		Sephacryl S-500 (Pharmacia)
		Ultrogel AcA 22 (LKB)
Fab	50 000	Sephadex G-100 (Pharmacia)
F(ab')$_2$	100 000	Sephacryl S-200 or S-300

Pouring the column

Sephadex is supplied as dry powder, and must be swollen in water for 1–2 days prior to use. The more loosely cross-linked forms of Sephadex (e.g. G-100, G-200) swell by up to 40 ml per gram of dry powder, and must be swollen in a large excess of water. Sepharose, Sephacryl and Ultrogel beads are supplied pre-swollen.

Gel filtration of immunoglobulins can usually be carried out at room temperature. It is essential to degas the buffers and gel if they have been stored in the cold. Sometimes, it may be possible to omit degassing if buffers and gel are allowed to reach room temperature before pouring the column. In general it is wise to degas, because bubbles in the column will seriously degrade its performance.

Resolution in gel filtration is critically dependent on a well-poured column. The free booklets supplied by Pharmacia are highly recommended for details. The column should be poured as follows:

(1) Close the outlet valve. Pour in a small quantity of buffer (10% of bed volume). Arrange the outlet tubing such that the vertical distance between the free end of the tube and the top of the gel is equal to the desired packing pressure. [It is a good idea to include a "safety loop" of inlet tubing which dips below the free end of the outlet tubing. This will prevent the column from running dry and cracking if the buffer runs out.]

(2) Attach a reservoir cylinder to the top of the column.

(3) Mix a thick slurry of gel (~ 50% suspension) by inverting the bottle. Do not use a magnetic flea, as it will fragment the gel.

(4) Gently pour the gel into the column, preferably down the side of the column along a glass rod. It is important that enough gel is poured to fill the column in one operation.

(5) Immediately open the outlet valve and start flow. The column should be packed at a slightly greater pressure than the desired running pressure (typically 150–400 mm water). Pharmacia recommends that Sephacryl gels be poured with the aid of a peristaltic pump. Run through at least 2–3 bed volumes of buffer before using the column.

(6) It is a good idea to run a small amount (1–3% of bed volume) of 10 mg/ml blue dextran (Pharmacia) to check that the column is packed evenly. The leading edge of the dye should run as a horizontal straight line.

Running the column

The buffer should have a pH of 7–8 and a total salt concentration of at least 100 mM to prevent adsorption effects. It is also desirable to include a preservative such as 10 mM sodium azide to inhibit microbial growth. The sample should have a volume of 2–5% of the column volume, should not be too viscous (maximum 50 mg/ml). It must be free of any particulate or insoluble material.

The best resolution will be obtained if the flow rate is slow. The column should take 1–2 days to run, although the newer matrices with very fine particle sizes are capable of good resolution in shorter times. Band broadening due to diffusion is not significant at realistic flow rates.

4.2.6 Affinity Chromatography

Affinity chromatography is a method of separation which is based on the irreversible immobilization of one component of a system on a solid-phase matrix (usually agarose), and the subsequent binding and elution of a complementary *ligand* in free solution (Fig. 4.3). (The question of whether the solid or liquid phase component is designated the "ligand" is arbitrary.)

Fractionation of monoclonal antibodies by affinity chromatography offers excellent purification in a single step, even if the sample is very dilute. The volume of recovered protein is independent of the sample volume. Affinity chromatography is therefore ideally suited to purifying monoclonal antibodies from culture fluid. The main disadvantages of affinity chromatography are the relatively low capacity and high cost of immobilized ligands, and the need to subject the antibody to denaturing conditions for elution. Affinity columns may be used an unlimited number of times, so the cost per separation decreases with increasing use.

The principles involved in purification of antigen or antibodies by affinity chromatography are identical. The use of monoclonal antibodies in affinity chromatography will be discussed in detail in Chapter 6.

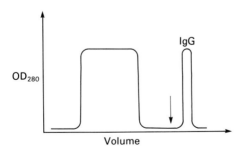

Fig. 4.3. Purification of IgG by affinity chromatography on protein A-Sepharose. The IgG-containing mixture is passed over a column of protein A-Sepharose, and the column washed until the ultraviolet absorption tracing is at baseline. Elution buffer is then applied (arrow; see text), releasing the bound IgG.

Affinity chromatography on immobilized antigen

If the antigen recognized by a monoclonal antibody is available in large (milligram) quantities, it may be coupled to agarose beads and used to isolate the antibody (see Chapter 6). The antibody should be bound at neutral pH and physiological salt concentrations. Depending on the individual antibody, elution may be accomplished by minor changes in pH or ionic strength (Herrman and Mescher, 1979), or by more drastic denaturing conditions such as 0.1 M glycine-HCl, pH 2.5 or 0.1 M diethylamine, pH 11. Other eluants include potassium thiocyanate (up to 3.5 M), urea (up to 8 M), guanidine-HCl (up to 6 M), or propionic acid (1 M). (See Chapter 6 for a detailed discussion of elution). The denaturing agent should be removed immediately by dialysis.

If the antigen is available in milligram quantities, there may be little reason for making monoclonal antibodies in the first place. In addition, purification of monoclonal antibodies by more gentle techniques such as ion exchange chromatography is less likely to cause denaturation and aggregation, and should result in a product of adequate purity.

Affinity chromatography on protein A or
anti-immunoglobulin antibodies

A more generally useful way to purify monoclonal antibodies, particularly from tissue culture supernatants, is to bind to and elute from immobilized anti-immunoglobulin antibodies or staphylococcal protein A (see Section 4.3.2). If the antibody is of a class and species that binds to protein A (Table 2.2), affinity chromatography on protein A-Sepharose (Section 4.3.2) is preferable because of its commercial availability, high capacity and gentle elution conditions. However, there are many situations in which monoclonal antibodies do not bind to protein A, notably the majority of rat immuno-globulins, mouse IgG1, and classes other than IgG. In these cases, anti-immunoglobulin may be substituted for protein A.

To take a concrete example, consider the purification of rat antibodies from culture fluid by affinity chromatography on goat anti-rat immuno-globulin antibodies coupled to agarose beads. A typical hyper-immune goat anti-rat immunoglobulin antiserum might contain 10 mg/ml total IgG and 1.0 mg/ml of specific antibody. In order to prepare a column of binding capacity of 100 mg (adequate for 1–2 litres of hybridoma supernatant), it would be necessary to use at least 100 ml of goat serum. If the IgG fraction were partially purified by precipitation with 40% ammonium sulphate and coupled to cyanogen bromide-activated Sepharose (protein binding capacity ∼ 10 mg/ml), a column of 100 ml of gel would be needed. (All the above assumes that no antibody activity is lost during the coupling.)

Once made, such a column should last virtually indefinitely, provided that care is taken to prevent drying or contamination with micro-organisms. Prior to first use, the column should be "pre-cycled" with normal rat serum followed by elution with glycine-HCl, pH 2.5, to saturate any irreversibly binding antibodies. The column should then be returned to neutral pH and stored in phosphate-buffered saline containing 0.005% merthiolate.

The column should also be pre-cycled prior to each use with glycine-HCl, pH 2.5, to remove any loosely bound material remaining from previous uses. Culture fluid should then be passed over the column and washed through with phosphate-buffered saline until no further protein emerges. (An ultraviolet absorbance monitor is useful). The bound material is then eluted with glycine-HCl, pH 2.5, and dialysed to restore neutral pH. Finally, the column is regenerated as in the previous paragraph.

Somewhat better results will be achieved if the affinity matrix is coupled with affinity-purified antibodies rather than an ammonium sulphate fraction. This will allow a much smaller column, and has the additional advantage that the antibodies have been selected to release their ligand under defined conditions.

Perhaps the ideal affinity matrix for purification of monoclonal antibodies would be a column of immobilized monoclonal anti-immunoglobulin antibodies. These might be selected for appropriate specificity and affinity, such that they release their ligand under defined gentle conditions. It seems likely that such matrices will eventually become commercially available.

4.3 Purification of Monoclonal IgG

4.3.1 Purification of Monoclonal IgG by Ammonium Sulphate Precipitation and Anion Exchange Chromatography

This procedure is the method of choice for monoclonal IgG-containing ascites fluid and serum. It is suitable for any species and IgG subclass. The main purification occurs during ion exchange chromatography; the ammonium sulphate fractionation serves mainly to reduce the protein load on the column.

(1) Slowly add saturated ammonium sulphate to the serum, with constant stirring at room temperature, to a final concentration of 50%. Stir for 30 min.

(2) Centrifuge at 2000–10 000 g for 5 min. Discard supernatant, which should be clear.

(3) Resuspend pellet in original volume of 50% saturated ammonium sulphate. Repeat centrifugation. The volume of the pellet should not diminish significantly.

(4) Repeat step 3.

(5) Resuspend pellet in phosphate-buffered saline.

(6) Dialyse against 2–3 changes of 1 litre 10 mM Tris-HCl, pH 8, at 4°C overnight.

(7) Take a small aliquot ($\sim$ 100 μl) of the dialysed protein; dilute 1:10 in phosphate-buffered saline. Measure optical density at 280 nm. A 1 mg/ml solution will have an optical density of $\sim$ 1.4 (1 cm cell). Calculate the total amount of protein.

(8) Set up DEAE-Sephacel column (Section 4.2.4; Fig. 4.2), with a bed volume of at least 10 ml for each 100 mg protein. The DEAE-Sephacel must be thoroughly equilibrated with starting buffer.

(9) Load sample. Wash column with starting buffer until chart recorder is stable.

(10) Elute with linear gradient of 0–300 mM NaCl in starting buffer (Section 4.2.4). Collect fractions.

(11) Pool the first peak. As a general rule, IgG2 antibodies will elute at a lower salt concentration than IgG1. The latter class may be slightly contaminated with transferrin (molecular weight 80 000). Most monoclonal antibodies will emerge in the first half of the gradient. The yield should be 3–10 mg IgG per ml serum or ascites, and the monoclonal antibody will often be more than 95% pure. Further purification may be achieved by gel filtration on Sephacryl S-300 (Section 4.2.5).

If the fusion was performed using a total nonproducer myeloma such as Sp2, NS/0 or X63-Ag 8.653, the monoclonal antibody should emerge as a single symmetrical peak. If mixed molecules are present (e.g. NS-1 hybrids), there may be more than one peak, reflecting the separation of the different species. If this occurs, each peak should be tested for antibody activity separately.

4.3.2 Purification of Monoclonal IgG by Affinity Chromatography on Protein A-Sepharose

Staphylococcal protein A is a protein made by most strains of *Staphylococcus aureus*, and has the remarkable property of binding IgG with high affinity and specificity (reviewed by Goding, 1978; Surolia *et al.*, 1982; Langone, 1982). There is considerable variation in the strength of binding among the different IgG subclasses in each species. In certain species, some IgG and IgA also binds. The binding of the various IgG subclasses of mouse and rat has been intensively studied (Ey *et al.*, 1978; Ledbetter and Herzenberg, 1979; Rousseaux *et al.*, 1981; Seppälä *et al.*, 1981; Watanabe *et al.*, 1981). Some of this information is summarized in Table 4.2.

Table 4.2 Conditions for binding to and elution from staphylococcal protein A

IgG Subclass	Species	Binds	Elutes	Reference	Comments
IgG1	Mouse	pH > 8.0	pH < 6.0	1–3	Some variability experienced; affinity chromatography on protein A is not recommended.[†]
IgG2a	Mouse	pH > 7.0	pH < 4.5	1–3	Allotype influences binding (2)
IgG2b	Mouse	pH > 7.0	pH < 3.5	1–3	May aggregate after elution.
IgG3	Mouse	pH > 7.0	pH < 4.5	1–3	
IgG1	Rat	Weak and variable binding at pH 8.0		4,5	Ocassional monoclonal antibodies bind (4)
IgG2a	Rat	No significant binding at pH 8.0		4,5	
IgG2b	Rat	Very weak binding at pH 8.0		4,5	Rat homologue of mouse IgG3 (6)
IgG2c	Rat	pH > 7.0	pH 4–5		Monoclonals which bind most strongly are most basic (5)

References: 1. Ey et al., 1978; 2. Sepällä et al., 1981; 3. Watanabe et al., 1981; 4. Ledbetter and Herzenberg, 1979; 5. Rousseaux et al., 1981; 6. Der Balian et al., 1980. [†]Monoclonal mouse IgG1 may be purified on Affi-Gel Protein A (Bio-Rad) using a special buffer (Monoclonal Antibody Purification Scheme; MAPS). Details of the composition of this buffer have not been released, but the kit is available from Bio-Rad.

Protein A, covalently attached to Sepharose beads, is now available commercially from Pharmacia. Five millilitres of wet gel (1.5 g dried beads) is capable of binding 100–125 mg IgG. The matrix will last virtually indefinitely, provided it is protected from drying and microbial contamination. The conditions for elution of IgG from protein A are fairly mild, depending on the IgG subclass, species and allotype (Table 4.2). Affinity chromatography on protein A-Sepharose is the method of choice for the purification of appropriate IgG subclasses from hybridoma supernatants.

As a general rule, purification of mouse IgG on protein A-agarose is most satisfactory for IgG2a, IgG2b and IgG3. Although there are reports that IgG1 binds to protein A-Sepharose at pH 8.0 (Ey *et al.*, 1978), the yield is often low and variable, and the technique is not recommended for mouse IgG1.

Recently, however, Bio-Rad have produced a new system which is said to allow purification of mouse IgG1 on protein A-agarose. The system consists of a special affinity matrix (Affi-gel Protein A) and a special buffer system, the details of which have not been disclosed. Recovery of IgG1 is claimed to be close to 100%. Since many monoclonal antibodies are IgG1, the system may become very popular.

As in all affinity chromatography, it is good practice to "precycle" the column with the eluting buffer just prior to each use. The tissue culture supernatant should be cleared of cells and debris by centrifugation, and sodium azide added (final concentration 10 mM) to discourage microbial growth. The concentration of monoclonal antibody in culture supernatants is unlikely to exceed 50–100 μg/ml, and batches of one litre may be processed on a 5 ml column. (The concentration of protein A-binding IgG in fetal calf serum is usually negligible.) The column is then washed with phosphate-buffered saline until the chart recorder reaches baseline (Fig. 4.3), and then the eluting buffer is applied. Although the information given in Table 4.2 may help in choosing the mildest conditions for elution, it is usually more convenient to elute all immunoglobulins using 0.1 M glycine-HCl, pH 2.5. If it is found that the acid conditions inactivate the antibody, a trial of elution at higher pH is indicated.

In general, acid-eluted antibodies should be rapidly neutralized with 1 M Tris-HCl, pH 8.0, as soon as they are eluted. Alternatively, the pH may be returned to neutrality by dialysis against a large volume of ice-cold phosphate-buffered saline. It is fairly unusual for antibodies to be inactivated by a brief encounter of an acidic environment. There have been a few instances, however, in which affinity chromatography on protein A has caused aggregation or loss of activity of monoclonal antibodies. The reasons are obscure; the problem may be more common with mouse IgG3.

Affinity chromatography on protein A-Sepharose may also be used to purify immunoglobulins from serum or ascites of hybridoma-bearing animals. However, the capacity of ion-exchange chromatography is greater, and ion-exchange also provides some separation of the monoclonal antibody from the normal immunoglobulins which are present in mouse serum. Occasionally, the columns may become blocked by fibrin deposition if ascites is applied directly. It is far cheaper to ruin a column of DEAE-cellulose than a column of protein A-Sepharose.

4.4 Purification of IgM

The purification of IgM is not as easy as that of IgG. IgM may be prepared in good yield and reasonable purity by precipitation with 40% saturated ammonium sulphate followed by gel filtration on Ultrogel AcA 22, Sepharose 6B or Sephacryl S-500. It is important to choose a gel filtration medium which includes IgM, so that it is chromatographed rather than simply dropped through the column (Section 4.2.5). The choice of an appropriate gel filtration medium allows separation of IgM from high molecular weight lipoproteins and protein aggregates, which would emerge with IgM in Sephadex G-200. Even on an appropriate gel, there is likely to be some contamination of IgM with α_2-macroglobulin (M_r 725 000). Contamination with α_2-macroglobulin may be reduced by substitution of euglobulin precipitation (Section 4.2.2) for ammonium sulphate in the first step. However, euglobulin precipitation causes some denaturation, as evidenced by the frequent difficulties in redissolving the precipitates. In addition, not all IgM proteins are euglobulins.

Zone electrophoresis (Section 4.2.3) is a very effective way of purifying IgM, especially when followed by a gel filtration step. Although the method is cumbersome and of low capacity, separation of IgM from α_2-macroglobulin is easily achieved.

Jehanli and Hough (1981) have recently shown that monoclonal human IgM may be purified to homogeneity by filtration on Ultrogel AcA 34 followed by ion exchange chromatography on DEAE-Sepharose CL6B with salt gradient elution. The IgM was bound to the ion exchanger in 0.05 M phosphate/citrate buffer at pH 6.8, and eluted with a linear gradient to 0.1 M phosphate/citrate, pH 5.0. Recovery was approximately 70%. This procedure may become the method of choice, and would probably be applicable to mouse IgM without modification. It would be preferable to use Ultrogel AcA 22, which chromatographs IgM, rather than AcA 34, which does not.

4.5 Fragmentation of Monoclonal Antibodies

In certain circumstances, it may be desirable to generate antigen-binding fragments of monoclonal antibodies. For example, when cells with receptors for the Fc portion of IgG are present (e.g. macrophages, monocytes), intact IgG molecules may bind nonspecifically via their Fc portions. Removal of the Fc will prevent this mode of binding. The production of small fragments of IgM (intact M_r 900 000) may aid penetration into the tissues for cytochemical studies.

The immunological literature is replete with accounts of the fragmentation of mouse antibodies, often using conditions that were established for other species such as rabbit or human. In many cases, it was assumed that the procedures worked, and no experimental verification was offered. In a few, it is now possible to state with hindsight that they could not possibly have worked. In others, the fragments were identified incorrectly.

It is therefore important to examine the claims in the literature on fragmentation of mouse immunoglobulins with a critical eye. One should not be too surprised if one is unable to reproduce them. In the succeeding paragraphs, I will summarize what I consider to be the most reliable procedures, and point out areas where uncertainty still exists.

4.5.1 Preparation of Fab Fragments of Mouse and Rat IgG

Cleavage of IgG at the hinge by the nonspecific protease papain (Stanworth and Turner, 1978) is one of the more straightforward ways of producing defined fragments of mouse and rat IgG. It is easy to find conditions for complete cleavage. However, it should be pointed out that even in this case, evaluation of the literature is not as straightforward as it would seem.

Part of the problem arises from the fact that papain is a thiol protease (i.e. it has a SH group in the active site, which must be in the reduced form for activity). The presence of reducing agents necessary for the activation of papain (cysteine, mercaptoethanol or dithiothreitol, in order of increasing potency) may also facilitate digestion by their effects on the substrate. Cysteine used to be a popular reducing agent in the older literature. However, it is very easily oxidized to cystine by air, and results of such experiments may be poorly reproducible unless oxygen is excluded during digestion. All these reducing agents have the potential of cleaving the labile inter-chain disulphide bonds of immunoglobulins, but the extent to which these effects occur depends on the individual reducing agent and its concentration. In some published work, it is difficult to decide whether apparent heterogeneity in digestion is due to proteolytic cleavage, partial reduction, or a mixture of the two.

Papain is inactivated by heavy metals, which complex with its sulphdryl group. It is often supplied as "mercuripapain" to prevent autodigestion. Regardless of whether mercury is present or not, it is good practice to chelate any divalent cations with EDTA to ensure maximal activity of the enzyme.

Papain should be "activated" by a brief incubation in 0.1 M Tris-HCl, pH 8.0, containing 2 mM EDTA and 1 mM dithiothreitol, just prior to use.

Digestion may be terminated by the irreversible alkylation of the thiol group of papain with iodoacetamide. A two-fold molar excess of iodo-acetamide over all thiol groups present is recommended. Reduction of iodo-acetamide by thiol groups causes the release of HI, so the reaction should be well buffered.

Iodoacetamide absorbs light significantly at 280 nm. In addition, iodo-acetamide is light-sensitive, and must be stored and used in the dark. The presence of any brown colour is an indication of decomposition, and such preparations should not be used.

Practical procedure

The extent of digestion of mouse and rat IgG is highly dependent on the concentration of reducing agent. The procedure given below (Oi and Herzenberg, 1979) should be monitored by SDS-polyacrylamide gel electrophoresis (reducing conditions). Digestion should result in complete disappearance of the γ heavy chain (M_r 55 000) and appearance of the Fd fragment of γ (M_r 27 000) and light chains (M_r 22 000–25 000). An example of a typical digestion is shown in Fig. 4.4.

(1) Activate papain (1–2 mg/ml) in 0.1 M Tris-HCl, pH 8.0, containing 2 mM EDTA and 1 mM dithiothreitol, for 15 min at 37°C.

(2) Digest IgG (1–10 mg/ml) in the same buffer at 37°C, using an enzyme: substrate ratio of 1:100, for 1 h.

(3) Terminate digestion by addition of iodoacetamide (final concentration 20 mM), and hold on ice for 1 h, protected from light.

(4) Dialyse overnight against phosphate-buffered saline, to remove iodoacetamide.

Comments: It is absolutely essential to monitor the completeness of digestion by SDS-polyacrylamide gel electrophoresis, as the individual IgG subclasses vary in their susceptibility to digestion. The rate of digestion is also influenced by the concentration of reducing agent. Mouse IgG2a and IgG2b are extremely susceptible to cleavage, even in 0.1 mM dithiothreitol, while IgG1 is more resistant, and requires at least 1 mM dithiothreitol, and sometimes more. At 1 mM, there will be considerable reduction of inter-chain disulphide bonds, but antibody activity will probably remain intact. If cleavage is incomplete, the problem will usually be solved by increasing the concentration of reducing agent. All rat IgG subclasses are easily cleaved by papain in the presence of reducing agent (Rousseaux *et al.*, 1980; 1983). It was found that Fab fragments could be produced from all rat IgG subclasses by treatment with 1% (w/w) papain at pH 7.0 in the presence of 10 mM cysteine for 2–4 h at 37°C. Fragments could be separated by ion exchange chromatography or protein A-Sepharose (IgG2c only).

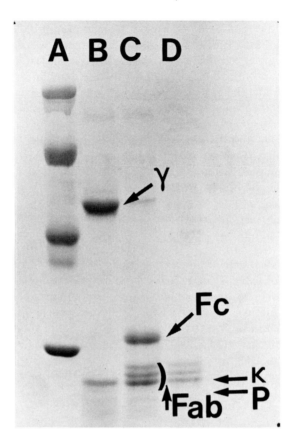

Fig. 4.4. SDS-polyacrylamide gel electrophoresis of mouse IgG1 and its fragments after digestion with papain. Digestion was terminated with iodoacetamide. The concentration of acrylamide was 10%, and all samples were reduced. A: Molecular weight standards (top to bottom); 95 000; 68 000; 43 000; 30 000. B: Undigested IgG. C: IgG after digestion with papain. D: Fab fragment after purification. The lowest band is κ chain. The upper bands are Fd fragments, although it is not clear why two bands are present. The mobility of papain ($M_r \simeq 20\,000$) is indicated (P) although there is not enough enzyme present to be visible. I thank Annette Blane for providing this gel.

Separation of Fab and Fc

Separation of Fab fragments from Fc and residual intact IgG may usually be accomplished with ease. In the case of IgG subclasses with strong affinity for staphylococcal protein A (mouse IgG2a, IgG2b and IgG3; rat IgG2c), the digest is passed over a column of protein A-Sepharose (Goding, 1976, 1978). (Failure to inactivate the papain with iodoacetamide may result in destruction of the column.) The Fab fragments pass through the column, while Fc and undigested IgG are bound (Fig. 4.5; upper panel). Note that the Fc

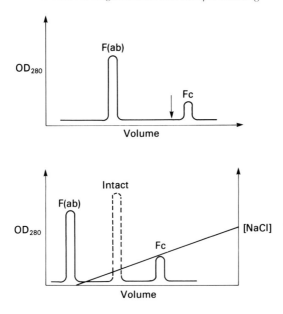

Fig. 4.5. Two methods for separation of Fab fragments of IgG from Fc fragments. Upper panel: Separation on protein A-Sepharose. The IgG digest is passed over protein A-Sepharose; the Fab fragment drops through the column. When the pen recorder reaches baseline, the elution buffer (arrow; see text) is applied, and the Fc fragment and any undigested IgG eluted. Lower panel: Separation by ion exchange chromatography. The digest is passed over a column of DEAE-cellulose. The Fab drops through the column or elutes early in the gradient, followed by undigested IgG, and finally Fc.

fragment of IgG3 is very insoluble in water, and may precipitate. The column may be regenerated and the bound material recovered by elution with 0.1 M glycine-HCl, pH 2.5.

Alternatively, the fragments may be separated by ion exchange chromatography (see Section 4.2.4), which is the method of choice for IgG subclasses which do not bind to protein A. The digest should be transferred to 0.01 M Tris-HCl, pH 8.0, by gel filtration on a small column or by dialysis or dilution. (The Fc fragment of IgG3 will precipitate in this buffer, and should be removed by centrifugation.) The Fab fragments are generally more basic than the Fc or the intact molecule; they will emerge in the "drop-through" or early in the salt gradient (Fig. 4.5; lower panel). The intact molecules and Fc fragments emerge at higher salt concentrations. [Occasionally, the Fab and Fc fragments may have similar charge, and may co-elute from DEAE-cellulose. This is mainly a problem for classes other than IgG1, and is an indication for use of protein A rather than DEAE to separate them.]

*A potential disadvantage of Fab fragments of
monoclonal antibodies*

If both antigen-combining sites of an intact IgG molecule have simultaneous and equal access to identical determinants on a multimeric antigen, the functional affinity ("avidity") may approach the product of the individual affinities, because if one site temporarily unbinds, the antibody remains bound via the other site. The strength of binding of monovalent Fab fragments might therefore be weaker than that of the intact molecule. Thus,if a monoclonal antibody were to have a low affinity for its antigen (as is often the case) the problem would be aggravated by the use of Fab fragments. Normally stable antigen–antibody complexes might dissociate during washing or prolonged incubations.

4.5.2 Preparation of $F(ab')_2$ Fragments of Mouse and Rat IgG

Pepsin is a nonspecific protease which is only active at acid pH, and is irreversibly denatured at neutral or alkaline pH. Treatment of human or rabbit immunoglobulin with pepsin (enzyme:substrate 1:100 at 37°C overnight at pH 4.5 in acetate buffer) usually results in cleavage at the C-terminal side of the inter-heavy chain disulphide bonds (Stanworth and Turner, 1978; Fig. 2.2). The resulting large fragment is named $F(ab')_2$, because it contains two antigen-combining sites. $F(ab')_2$ fragments do not bind to Fc receptors. The production of $F(ab')_2$ fragments of monoclonal antibodies would be very useful, because they would be expected to have considerably higher avidity than Fab.

Unfortunately, the rote application of these procedures to mouse and rat IgG does not always produce satisfactory results. While there have been many claims for production of $F(ab')_2$ fragments of mouse IgG (e.g. Svasti and Milstein, 1972; Dissanayake and Hay, 1975; Secher *et al.*, 1977), experience using rigorous techniques to assess the digestion products indicates that the recommended procedures do not always work (se Nisonoff *et al.*, 1975; Oi and Herzenberg, 1979).

Mouse IgG

Recently, the problem of production of $F(ab')_2$ fragments of mouse IgG has been re-investigated (Lamoyi and Nisonoff, 1983). Immunoglobulins were purified by conventional techniques, and digestion was carried out at pH 4.2 (IgG1 and IgG2a) or pH 4.5 (IgG3). The enzyme:substrate ratio was 1:33

(w/w) and the temperature was 37°C. Reducing agents were not used. F(ab')₂ fragments were obtained in good yield from IgG1, IgG2a and IgG3 proteins, with the relative rates of digestion being IgG3 > IgG2a > IgG 1. One IgG1 protein out of four tested was rapidly degraded, as were all of five different IgG2b proteins.

Optimal digestion times varied depending on the antibody class, and times which resulted in no undigested IgG generally resulted in somewhat lower yields, presumably due to further digestion into smaller fragments. Suitable times are 8 h for IgG1 (yield ∼ 70%), 4–8 h for IgG2a (yield 25–50%) and 15 min for IgG3 (yield ∼ 60%). It was not possible to find suitable conditions for production of F(ab')₂ fragments from mouse IgG2b. In general, it appears that the best yields are obtained by accepting a certain amount of undigested IgG, which may be removed by gel filtration (Table 4.1).

The production of F(ab')₂ fragments of mouse IgG has been analysed in detail by Parham (1983). It was found that IgG1 was resistant to cleavage with pepsin, but stable F(ab')₂ fragments could be produced by cleavage in 0.1 M citrate, pH 3.5 at 37°C, with an IgG concentration of 1–2 mg/ml and a pepsin concentration of 25 μg/ml. Cleavage was generally complete by 8 h, and yields varied from 25–90% for seven different proteins. The Fc portion was completely degraded.

In the case of mouse IgG2a, Parham found that a pH of 4.1 was optimal for the three proteins examined, but that it was not possible to find conditions that were general and ideal. Pepsin was capable of cleaving on both sides of the three inter-heavy chain disulphide bonds. At short times, F(ab')₂ predominated, but was contaminated by intact IgG. At longer times, a monomeric Fab' fragment became the major product, and a compromise between yield and purity was unavoidable.

Digestion of mouse IgG2b with pepsin was unsatisfactory, and resulted in asymmetrical cleavage. IgG3 was not examined.

Since there are often very large differences in amino acid sequences between mouse IgG subclasses of different allotypes (Section 2.3.6), it cannot be assumed that the results obtained with BALB/c immunoglobulins can be applied to IgG of other allotypes.

Rat IgG

Rousseaux *et al.* (1983) have studied the production of F(ab')₂ fragments of rat IgG in detail. Their results may be summarized as follows. Rat IgG1 and to a lesser extent IgG2a were resistant to pepsin, but complete cleavage to F(ab')₂ fragments occurred if the IgG (15 mg/ml) was dialyzed against 0.1 M formate buffer, pH 2.8 for 16 h at 4°C, followed by 0.1 M acetate buffer, pH 4.5 before peptic digestion. Cleavage into F(ab')₂ was complete after 4 h at

37°C with 1% (w/w) pepsin, and no other fragments were seen. It would appear that the pH 2.8 treatment caused irreversible change in the conformation of the Fc, probably the $C\gamma_2$ domain.

Cleavage of rat IgG2b with pepsin was less satisfactory, and gave results reminiscent of mouse IgG2a (see Parham, 1983 and above). However, it was possible to generate $F(ab')_2$-like fragments of rat IgG2b in good yield using staphylococcal V8 protease (3% w/w) in 0.1 M sodium phosphate pH 7.8, for 4 h at 37°C. Digestion was stopped by rapid freezing.

Rousseaux *et al.* (1983) found that IgG2c was the most susceptible of the rate IgG subclasses to peptic cleavage. Using an enzyme:substrate ratio of 1% (w/w) for 4 h at 37°C in 0.1 M citrate pH 4.5, rat IgG2c was completely cleaved into $F(ab')_2$, and the Fc subfragment pFc (Section 2.2.3) was also obtained. Longer times resulted in appearance of monomeric Fab' fragments.

The foregoing should serve to emphasize the importance of testing individual IgG proteins for peptic cleavage, and warn against the rote use of "recipes". Fragmentation must always be monitored by SDS-polyacrylamide gel electrophoresis, and failure to do so invites trouble.

4.5.3 Proteolytic Fragmentation of Mouse IgM

Information concerning the proteolytic fragmentation of mouse IgM is limited. Simply applying procedures developed for human IgM is unlikely to result in success. Bourgois *et al.* (1977) published a method for the fragmentation of mouse IgM into Fab and Fc fragments using tryptic digestion of the native proteins at 37°C, but the results have not been reproduced by others (e.g. Matthew and Reichardt, 1982). Shimizu *et al.* (1974) were able to digest human IgM with trypsin in the presence of 5 M urea, resulting in Fab and $(Fc)_5$. The Fc began at residue 326, and the majority of the $C_\mu 2$ domain was destroyed. Kehry *et al.* (1982) digested mouse IgM with trypsin in the presence of 5 M urea (enzyme:substrate 1:100; 25°C for 18 h). They apparently obtained a cleavage at residue 220 (near the end of C_H1 domain), cleaving the IgM into Fab and $(Fc)_5$ fragments. The Fab and $(Fc)_5$ fragments were separated by gel filtration on Ultrogel AcA 22. However, the yield was poor, and the procedure had to be modified for individual monoclonal IgM proteins (L. Hood, personal communication).

An interesting new cleavage was recently reported by Matthew and Reichardt (1982). Mouse IgM (1 mg/ml in 50 mM Tris-HCl, 150 mM NaCl, 20 mM $CaCl_2$, pH 8.0) was digested with 0.01 mg/ml TPCK trypsin for 5 h at 37°C. Mercaptoethanol was added to 10 mM. After 5 additional minutes at 37°C, the solution was adjusted to 60 mM iodoacetamide and left at room temperature for 10 min. The samples were then dialysed against four changes of 1 litre phosphate-buffered saline over 48 h.

The combination of tryptic digestion followed by reduction and alkylation produced active fragments of molecular weight 230 000 and 110 000. Both trypsinization and reduction were necessary. Analysis of the fragments indicated that the light chains were intact and the heavy chains intact or nearly intact. The M_r 230 000 fragments appeared to consist of two light chains and two heavy chains, while the M_r 110 000 fragments consisted of one light chain and one heavy chain.

The mechanism of this cleavage is not entirely clear. The authors postulated disulphide rearrangements and proteolytic attack on the J chain, reducing stability of the pentamer. It is interesting to note that the C-terminal 20 residues contain three potential tryptic cleavage sites (Kehry *et al.*, 1982). This region of the molecule is though to be crucial to the polymerization process, and cleavage at these residues might result in depolymerization with virtually no change in apparent size of the heavy chain. Contamination of IgM with the trypsin inhibitor α_2-macroglobulin (Travis and Salvesen, 1983) may prevent digestion.

4.6 Radiolabelling of Monoclonal Antibodies

Radiolabelling of antibodies involves the same principles and procedures which apply to proteins in general, and the reader is referred to Chapter 5 for a detailed discussion.

4.6.1 Radioiodination of Antibodies

Antibodies may be radioiodinated to high specific activity with ^{125}I by the chloramine-T method (Section 5.3.1). Incorporation of one iodine per IgG molecule corresponds to a specific activity of approximately $12 \mu\text{Ci}/\mu\text{g}$. Experience with affinity-purified polyclonal antibodies from goat, sheep or rabbit indicates that it is realistic to expect at least 20–40% of TCA-precipitable counts to bind to antigen. Presumably, the remaining molecules are damaged by the iodination procedure.

Mouse antibodies have a reputation for being easily damaged by radioiodination. However, a detailed study of the distribution of murine Ia antigens was carried out using mouse alloantibodies labelled with ^{125}I by the lactoperoxidase technique (Goding *et al.*, 1975). Tsu and Herzenberg (1980) were able to radiolabel mouse anti-allotype antibodies using the chloramine-T method. In this case, their combining sites were protected from damage by performing the iodination while the antibody was bound to antigen.

Ballou *et al.* (1979) used the "Iodogen" method (Section 5.3.5) to radiolabel anti-tumour antibodies. There are numerous other reports of the successful use of radioiodinated monoclonal antibodies. However, it would appear that many unpublished failures have also occurred, and that loss of antigen-binding after iodination is a relatively common event (see Nussenzweig *et al.*, 1982).

If a particular monoclonal antibody is damaged by radioiodination using the chloramine-T procedure, a trial of other procedures (Iodogen, lactoperoxidase, or Iodobeads) is worthwhile. All the above methods label tyrosine residues, and failure to retain activity might indicate the presence of tyrosine in the antigen-binding site. The Bolton–Hunter reagent (Section 5.3.4) labels lysine residues, and may be coupled under extremely mild conditions. In some cases, however, even the Bolton–Hunter reagent may cause damage (Nussenzweig *et al.*, 1982). If radioiodination cannot be carried out successfully using any of these methods, one might try a different antibody, a different isotope, or use of ^{125}I-labelled anti-immunoglobulin or staphylococcal protein A (Section 3.10.3). Finally, one might consider conjugation of the antibody with biotin, and use of ^{125}I-labelled avidin as a sandwich reagent (Section 7.3).

4.6.2 Extrinsic Labelling of Antibodies with Tritium and ^{35}S

Although antibodies may be radiolabelled to the highest specific activity with iodine, there are a number of situations where tritium labelling may be useful. The very low energy of tritium ($E_{max} = 18$ keV) allows very precise localization of grains in autoradiographic experiments (see Cuello *et al.*, 1980).

Recently, Tack *et al.* (1980) have shown that antibodies and other proteins may be tritiated to very high specific activities by reductive methylation. The specific activities obtained approached those routinely achieved by radioiodination. The method was applied by Wilder *et al.* (1979) to antibodies and staphylococcal protein A, and was the only successful method of extrinsically labelling the monoclonal anti-dendritic cell antibody of Nussenzweig *et al.* (1982). Practical details are given in Section 5.4.

An alternative procedure involves the use of N-succinimidyl[2,3-^{3}H] propionate (Table 5.1). The compound is available from Amersham at a specific activity of 30–60 Ci/mmol, or about 1–3% of that of the ^{125}I-labelled analogue. It may be useful in situations where the low energy of tritium is an advantage, and where low specific activity is accceptable. A related ^{35}S-labelled compound is also available from Amersham at a specific activity of ~ 1000 Ci/mmol. The compound is known as ^{35}SLR (t-Butoxycarbonyl-L-[^{35}S]methionine-N-hydroxysuccinimide ester). Its catalogue number is SJ.440. Conditions for labelling are exactly as for the Bolton–Hunter reagent (Section 5.3.4).

4.6.3 Biosynthetic Labelling of Monoclonal Antibodies

The biosynthetic incorporation of radiolabelled amino acids into monoclonal antibodies is easily performed. The principles are discussed in detail in Section 5.5.2. If the highest possible specific activity is desired, the use of ^{35}S-methionine (~ 1000 Ci/mmol) or ^{3}H-lysine, arginine, leucine or phenyl-alanine (20–200 Ci/mmol) are recommended (see Galfrè and Milstein, 1981).

It should be noted that ^{35}S-methionine is supplied in aqueous solution containing 0.1% (1.2×10^{-2} M) mercaptoethanol. Myeloma and hybridoma cells are very sensitive to mercaptoethanol, and cannot withstand concentrations of more than $\sim 5 \times 10^{-5}$ M. If higher concentrations of isotope are needed, the methionine must be lyophilized immediately prior to use to remove the mercaptoethanol. Similar considerations apply to amino acids supplied in solutions containing ethanol (see Section 5.5.2).

Typically, 10^{7} hybridoma cells are labelled for 2–5 h in 1–2 ml medium containing 50 μCi isotope per ml. At the end of the labelling period, cells are removed by centrifugation. It is advisable to add a small amount of non-radioactive amino acid at the end of the labelling period. Immunoglobulin will be by far the major labelled protein in the supernatant (Ledbetter *et al.*, 1979), which may often be used without further purification. Specific activi-ties of up to 1000 Ci/mmol may be achieved by biosynthetic incorporation (Cuello *et al.*, 1980).

4.7 Conditions for Stability and Storage of Monoclonal Antibodies

As mentioned repeatedly throughout this book, individual monoclonal anti-bodies may have highly individual characteristics. It is thus to be expected that they may differ greatly in their susceptibility to damage by environment-al factors, and it is impossible to formulate conditions, under which every clonal product would be unconditionally stable. However, adherence to a few simple principles will minimize the chances of damage. If attention is paid to the avoidance of denaturation and proteolysis, the long-term storage of monoclonal antibodies presents few problems.

4.7.1 Denaturation of Antibodies

Denaturation of protein (Kauzman, 1959) is a relative term. It may range from a slight conformational change to a drastic loss of solubility and massive irreversible aggregation. An appreciation of the forces which govern protein folding (Anfinsen, 1973) has led to the understanding that even fully

Table 4.3 Storage of monoclonal antibodies

Form of antibody	Recommended storage[a]
Serum or Ascites	Freeze at $-20°C$, or preferably at $-70°C$, in small aliquots. Long-term storage of serum at 4°C may usually be achieved by addition of an equal volume of saturated ammonium sulphate. Ascites may contain protease activity, and should be frozen.
Culture Supernatant	Storage at 4°C as a sterile solution containing 10 mM sodium azide or 0.005% merthiolate is usually safe, providing infection does not occur. Alternatively, freeze in aliquots, preferably at $-70°C$.
Purified IgG and IgM	Neutral pH; salt concentration 100–200 mM; protein concentration 1–10 mg/ml. Storage at 4°C with 10 mM sodium azide or 0.005% merthiolate is usually safe over long periods, but occasionally proteolytic breakdown occurs. Storage at $-20°C$ in PBS in 50% glycerol is usually safe over long periods (50% glycerol does not freeze at $-20°C$). Alternatively, may be stored frozen at $-70°C$. IgM is particularly susceptible to denaturation by freeze–thaw cycles.
Antibodies conjugated with biotin, fluorochromes, enzymes etc.	Very prone to aggregation by freezing. Store at 4°C as for IgG and IgM. Alternatively, store in 50% glycerol at $-20°C$.

[a]Frozen samples should be stored in multiple small aliquots, and the number of freeze–thaw cycles kept to a minimum. Some domestic freezers have automatic defrost cycles, and some are barely capable of freezing reliably. Repeated freeze–thaw cycles are a potent cause of denaturation.

denatured proteins may sometimes be renatured with full restoration of biological activity. Providing that the disulphide bonds are allowed to re-form correctly, totally denatured ribonuclease may be restored to full enzymic activity (Anfinsen, 1973). These principles have been applied successfully to many other enzymes (Hager and Burgess, 1980).

Recovery of antigen-binding activity by renaturation of extensively denatured antibody in the absence of antigen (Haber, 1964; Whitney and Tanford, 1965) was classical proof that their primary structure was sufficient to specify their final tertiary structure and biological activity. The ability of antibody molecules to recover from extensive denaturation by urea, guanidine and extremes of pH (see also Chapter 6) emphasizes the strong thermodynamic preference for folding into a particular conformation. Polyclonal antisera generally require quite harsh conditions (6–8 M urea, 5–6 M guanidine-HCl, pH < 3 or > 10) before the antigen–antibody bond is disrupted. Once physiological conditions are restored, antibody activity usually returns. However, it remains to be seen how often these generalization will apply to monoclonal antibodies. It may be expected that some clonal products will be irreversibly denatured by such conditions. The subject of the reversibility of the antigen–antibody bond will be discussed in more detail in Chapter 6.

Antibodies may be denatured by other physical processes. Excessive heat should be avoided. Most antibodies will survive heating at 56°C for 30 min but some will not. Denaturation of antibodies by heat is likely to be irreversible. Similarly, frothing of protein solutions is a potent cause of irreversible denaturation. In the case of ovalbumin, denaturation by heat or frothing results in fried eggs and meringues respectively (Cobb, 1974).

Freeze–thaw cycles are also potentially damaging, particularly to IgM and murine IgG3. Some IgG antibodies will survive multiple freeze–thaw cycles, while others will become irreversibly aggregated. Most monoclonal antibodies will survive one or two freeze–thaw cycles, but occasional ones may lose activity. The number of freeze–thaw cycles should be limited by freezing in multiple small aliquots.

4.7.2 Degradation of Antibodies by Proteases

Providing that they are not exposed to proteases, purified monoclonal antibodies may be stored at 4°C for years without significant loss of activity. Proteolysis upon storage may arise from proteases in the antibody source, or perhaps more commonly from microbial contamination. Solutions may be protected from microbial growth by preservatives such as sodium azide (10 mM) or merthiolate (0.005%), although occasional organisms are resistant to these agents. Sterilization by membrane filtration is safer, but more inconvenient.

Although serum contains a number of proteases, they are mostly present in an inactive form (Travis and Salvesen, 1983). Serum contains a number of protease inhibitors, such as α_2-macroglobulin and α_1-antitrypsin. Whole serum may usually be stored for a few weeks at $4°C$ with preservatives. Ascites is more prone to proteolytic breakdown than serum. Bruck *et al.* (1982) have described a simple procedure for obtaining protease-free IgG from ascitic fluid.

In some respects, the requirements for minimization of proteolytic activity (freezing) and minimization of denaturation (not freezing) are contradictory. Proteolytic degradation may be eliminated by lyophilization (freeze-drying), but it would appear that many monoclonal antibodies are irreversibly denatured by the process. Recommended storage conditions for monoclonal antibodies are given in Table 4.3.

References

Anfinsen, C. B. (1973). Principles that govern the folding of protein chains. *Science* **181**, 223–230.

Ballou, B., Levine, G., Hakala, T. R. and Solter, D. (1979). Tumor location detected with radioactively labeled monoclonal antibody and external scintigraphy. *Science* **206**, 844–847.

Böttcher, I., Hämmerling, G. and Kapp, J-F. (1978). Continuous production of monoclonal mouse IgE antibodies with known allergenic specificity by a hybrid cell line. *Nature* **275**, 761–762.

Bourgois, A., Abney, E. and Parkhouse, R. M. E. (1977). Mouse immunoglobulin receptors on lymphocytes: identification of IgM and IgD molecules by tryptic cleavage and a postulated role for cell surface IgD. *Eur. J. Immunol.* **7**, 210–213.

Bruck, C., Portetelle, D., Glineur, C. and Bollen, A. (1982). One-step purification of mouse monoclonal antibodies from ascitic fluid by DEAE Affi-gel blue chromatography. *J. Immunol. Methods* **53**, 313–319.

Cobb, V. (1974). "Science Experiments You Can Eat." Penguin Books, Middlesex, England.

Cuello, A. C., Milstein, C. and Priestly, J. V. (1980). Use of monoclonal antibodies in immunocytochemistry with special references to the central nervous system. *Brain Res. Bull.* **5**, 575–587.

Der Balian, G. P., Slack, J., Clevinger, B. L., Bazin, H. and Davie, J. M. (1980). Subclass restriction of murine antibodies. III. Antigens that stimulate IgG3 in mice stimulate IgG2c in rats. *J. exp. Med.* **152**, 209–218.

Dissanayake, S. and Hay, F. C. (1975). Pepsin digestion of mouse IgG immunoglobulins: subfragments of the Fc region. *Immunochemistry* **12**, 373–378.

Eshhar, Z., Ofarim, M. and Waks, T. (1980). Generation of hybridomas secreting murine reaginic antibodies of anti-DNP specificity. *J. Immunol.* **124**, 775–780.

Ey, P. L., Prowse, S. J. and Jenkin, C. R. (1978). Isolation of pure IgG1, IgG2a and IgG2b immunoglobulins from mouse serum using protein A-Sepharose. *Immunochemistry* **15**, 429–436.

Fischer, K. (1969). "An Introduction to Gel Chromatography." North-Holland, Amsterdam.

Galfrè, G. and Milstein, C. (1981). Preparation of monoclonal antibodies: strategies and procedures. *Meth. Enzymol.* **73**, 3–46.

Garvey, J. S., Cremer, N. E. and Sussdorf, D. H. (1977). "Methods in Immunology", 3rd ed. W. A. Benjamin, Reading, Mass.

Goding, J. W. (1976). Conjugation of antibodies with fluorochromes: modifications to the standard methods. *J. immunol. Methods* **13**, 215–226.

Goding, J. W. (1978). Use of Staphylococcol protein A as an immunological reagent. *J. immunol. Methods* **20**, 241–253.

Goding, J. W. (1980). Structural studies of murine lymphocyte surface IgD. *J. Immunol.* **124**, 2082–2088.

Goding, J. W., Nossal, G. J. V., Shreffler, D. C. and Marchalonis, J. J. (1975). Ia antigens on murine lymphoid cells: distribution, surface movement and partial characterization. *J. Immunogenet.* **2**, 9–25.

Grey, H. M., Sher, A. and Shalitin, N. (1970). The subunit structure of mouse IgA. *J. Immunol.* **105**, 75–84.

Haber, E. (1964). Recovery of antigen specificity after denaturation and complete reduction of disulphides in a papain fragment of antibody. *Proc. natn. Acad. Sci. U.S.A.* **52**, 1099–1106.

Hager, D. A. and Burgess, R. R. (1980). Elution of proteins from sodium dodecyl sulfate-polyacrylamide gels, removed of sodium dodecyl sulfate, and renaturation of enzymatic activity: results with sigma subunit of *Escherichia coli* RNA polymerase, wheat germ DNA topoisomerase, and other enzymes. *Anal. Biochem.* **109**, 76–86.

Herrmann, S. H. and Mescher, M. F. (1979). Purification of the H-2K^k molecule of the murine major histocompatibility complex. *J. biol. Chem.* **254**, 8713–8716.

Jehanli, A. and Hough, D. (1981). A rapid procedure for the isolation of human IgM myeloma proteins. *J. immunol. Methods* **44**, 199–204.

Kauzmann, W. (1959). Some factors in the interpretation of protein denaturation. *Adv. Protein Chem.* **14**, 1–63.

Kehry, M. R., Fuhrman, J. S., Schilling, J. W., Rogers, J., Sibley, C. H. and Hood, L. E. (1982). Complete amino acid sequence of a mouse μ chain: homology among heavy chain constant region domains. *Biochemistry* **21**, 5415–5424.

Komisar, J. L., Fuhrman, J. A. and Cebra, J. J. (1982). IgA-producing hybridomas are readily derived from gut-associated lymphoid tissue. *J. Immunol.* **128**, 2376–2378.

Kunkel, H. G. (1954). Zone electrophoresis. *Meth. biochem. Analysis* **1**, 141–170.

Lamoyi, E. and Nisonoff, A. (1983). Preparation of F(ab′)$_2$ fragments from mouse IgG of various subclasses. *J. immunol. Methods* **56**, 235–243.

Langone, J. J. (1982). Protein A of *Staphylococcus aureus* and related immunoglobulin receptors produced by streptococci and pneumococci. *Adv. Immunol.* **32**, 157–252.

Ledbetter, J. A. and Herzenberg, L. A. (1979). Xenogeneic monoclonal antibodies to mouse lymphoid differentiation antigens. *Immunol. Rev.* **47**, 63–90.

Ledbetter, J. A., Goding, J. W., Tsu, T. T. and Herzenberg, L. A. (1979). A new mouse lymphoid alloantigen (Lgp 100) recognized by a monoclonal rat antibody. *Immunogenetics* **8**, 347–360.

Liu, F-T., Bohn, J. W., Ferry, E. L., Yamamoto, H., Molinaro, C. A., Sherman, L. A., Klinman, N. R. and Katz, D. H. (1980). Monoclonal dinitrophenyl-specific IgE antibody: preparation, isolation and characterization. *J. Immunol.* **124**, 2728–2737.

Lowry, O. H., Rosenbrough, N. J., Farr, A. L. and Randall, R. J. (1951). Protein measurement with the Folin phenol reagent. *J. biol. Chem.* **193**, 265–275.

Matthew, W. D. and Reichardt, L. F. (1982). Development and application of an efficient procedure for converting mouse IgM into small, active fragments. *J. immunol. Methods* **50**, 239–253.

Monthony, J. F., Wallace, E. G. and Allen, D. M. (1978). A non-barbital buffer for immunoelectrophoresis and zone electrophoresis in agarose gels. *Clin. Chem.* **24**, 1825–1827.

Nisonoff, A., Hopper, J. E. and Spring, S. B. (1975). "The Antibody Molecule." Academic Press, New York, San Francisco and London.

Nussenzweig, M. C., Steinman, R. M., Witmer, M. D. and Gutchinov, B. (1982). A monoclonal antibody specific for mouse dendritic cells. *Proc. natn. Acad. Sci. U.S.A.* **79**, 161–165.

Oi, V. T. and Herzenberg, L. A. (1979). Localization of murine Ig-1b and Ig-1a (IgG2a) allotypic determinants detected with monoclonal antibodies. *Molec. Immunol.* **16**, 1005–1017.

Parham, P. (1983). On the fragmentation of monoclonal IgG1, IgG2a and IgG2b from BALB/c mice. *J. Immunol.* **131**, 2895–2902.

Perez-Montfort, R. and Metzger, H. (1982). Proteolysis of soluble IgE-receptor complexes: localization of sites on IgE which interact with the Fc receptor. *Molec. Immunol.* **19**, 1113–1125.

Peterson, E. A. (1970). "Cellulosic Ion Exchangers." North-Holland, Amsterdam.

Radola, B. (1973). Isoelectric focusing in layers of granulated gels. I. Thin-layer isoelectric focusing of proteins. *Biochem. biophys. Acta.* **295**, 412–428.

Rousseaux, J., Biserte, G. and Bazin, H. (1980). The differential enzyme sensitivity of rat immunoglobulin G subclasses to papain and pepsin. *Molec. Immunol.* **17**, 469–482.

Rousseaux, J., Picque, M. T., Bazin, H. and Biserte, G. (1981). Rat IgG subclasses: differences in affinity to protein A-Sepharose. *Molec. Immunol.* **18**, 639–645.

Rousseaux, J., Rousseaux-Prévost, R. and Bazin, H. (1983). Optimal conditions for the preparation of Fab and F(ab')₂ fragments from monoclonal IgG of different rat IgG subclasses. *J. immunol. Methods* **64**, 141–146.

Scopes, R. K. (1982). "Protein Purification." Springer-Verlag, New York, Heidelberg and Berlin.

Secher, D. S., Milstein, C. and Adetugbo, K. (1977). Somatic mutants and antibody diversity. *Immunol. Rev.* **36**, 51–72.

Seppälä, I., Sarvas, H., Péterfy, F., and Mäkelä, O. (1981). The four sub-classes of IgG can be isolated from mouse serum by using protein A-Sepharose. *Scand. J. Immunol.* **14**, 335–342.

Shimizu, A., Watanabe, S., Yamamura, Y. and Putnam, F. W. (1974). Tryptic digestion of immunoglobulin M in urea: conformational lability of the middle part of the molecule. *Immunochemistry* **11**, 719–727.

Stanworth, D. R. and Turner, M. W. (1978). Immunochemical analysis. *In* "Handbook of Experimental Immunology" (D. M. Weir, ed), p. 6.25. Blackwell, Oxford.

Surolia, A., Pain, D. and Khan, M. I. (1982). Protein A: Nature's universal anti-antibody. *Trends biochem. Sci.* **7**, 74–76.

Svasti, J. and Milstein, C. (1972). The disulphide bridges of a mouse immunoglobulin G1 protein. *Biochem. J.* **126**, 837–850.

Tack, B. F., Dean, J., Eilat, D., Lorenz, P. E. and Schechter, A. N. (1980). Tritium labeling of proteins to high specific radioactivity by reductive methylation. *J. biol. Chem.* **255**, 8842–8847.

Tomasi, T. B. and Grey, H. M. (1972). Structure and function of immunoglobulin A. *Prog. Allergy* **16**, 81–213.

Travis, J. and Salvesen, G. S. (1983). Human plasma proteinase inhibitors. *Ann. Rev. Biochem.* **52**, 655–709.

Tsu, T. T. and Herzenberg, L. A. (1980). Solid-phase radioimmunoassays. *In* "Selected Methods in Cellular Immunology" (B. B. Mishell and S. M. Shiigi, eds), pp. 373–397. Freeman, San Francisco.

Watanabe, M., Ishii, T. and Nariuchi, H. (1981). Fractionation of IgG1, IgG2a, IgG2b and IgG3 immunoglobulins from mouse serum by protein A-Sepharose column chromatography. *Japan. J. exp. Med.* **51**, 65–70.

Weiss, J. B. (1976). Preparative block electrophoresis. *In* "Chromatographic and Electrophoretic Techniques", (I. Smith, ed), Vol. 2, pp. 367–377. Heinemann, London.

Whitney, P. L. and Tanford, C. (1965). Recovery of specific activity after complete unfolding and reduction of an antibody fragment. *Proc. natn. Acad. Sci. U.S.A.* **53**, 524–532.

Wilder, R. L., Yuen, C. C., Subbarao, B., Woods, V. L., Alexander, C. B. and Mage, R. G. (1979). Tritium (^{3}H) radiolabeling of protein A and antibody to high specific activity: application to cell surface antigen radioimmunoassays. *J. immunol. Methods* **28**, 255–266.

5   Analysis of Antigens Recognized by Monoclonal Antibodies

Monoclonal antibodies are by far the most highly selective yet versatile of all biochemical isolation tools. Their usefulness in the identification and isolation of particular molecules contained in extremely complex mixtures is unsurpassed. Antibodies can provided the information that a particular structure is present, localize it with extreme accuracy, and allow it to be isolated on an analytical or preparative scale. Subsequent analysis of the structure of the antigen may be made by standard biochemical techniques.

This chapter will discuss the use of monoclonal antibodies in the isolation and structural analysis of antigens. The major emphasis will be on proteins, but carbohydrate antigens will be mentioned briefly.

5.1 Determination of the Biochemical Nature of the Antigen

In general, the naturally occurring antigens are proteins or carbohydrates. Carbohydrates may be present as part of more complex structures such as glycoproteins or glycolipids. Lipids lacking carbohydrate are seldom recognized by antibodies, because they tend to form micelles and membranes, and thus remove themselves from the aqueous environment.

The preliminary steps to determine whether an antigen is a protein or carbohydrate may involve a number of simple tests. Protein antigens are likely to be sensitive to proteases such as pronase or trypsin, destroyed by heating to 100°C, and to survive treatment with periodate. The converse is true for carbohydrate antigens (Layton, 1980; Shapiro and Erickson, 1981). None of these tests is absolutely diagnostic. For example, some proteins are extremely resistant to proteolysis (Handman et al., 1981) or heat (Gullick et al., 1981). Certain amino acids, notably tyrosine and tryptophan, may be destroyed by periodate (Geoghegan et al., 1980). Methionine is also susceptible to oxidation by periodate (Yamasaki et al., 1982). A particular monoclonal antibody may recognize a glycoprotein via either the protein moiety or the carbohydrate prosthetic group. The conformation of a glycoprotein may be influenced by modification or absence of its carbohydrate (Sharon and Lis, 1982). In spite of all these caveats, the overall pattern of the effects of treatment of the antigen with heat, proteases and periodate will often give a hint of the nature of the antigen.

5.1.1 Glycolipid and Other Carbohydrate Antigens

The glycolipids of cell membranes (Hakomori, 1981) are highly immunogenic. When mice are immunized with whole cells from rats or humans, antibodies against glycolipids are commonly produced (Hakomori and Kannagi, 1983; Stern et al., 1978; Young and Hakomori, 1981). While the distribution of individual glycolipid antigens is often confined to certain cell types (Hakomori, 1981; Feizi, 1981; Hakomori, 1984), it is usually difficult to make any biological sense out of their distribution (see Section 5.2).

In many cases, carbohydrate antigens have a highly repetitive polymeric structure, with large numbers of identical antigenic determinants. In these cases, the strength of the "signal" obtained by binding of monoclonal antibodies may be much greater than in cases in which there is only a single determinant per molecule. The multivalent structure of the antigen may also allow the formation of very strong precipitin lines in Ouchterlony analysis (see Section 4.1).

In addition to generating extremely strong signals, the polymeric nature of many carbohydrate antigens facilitates their detection by allowing "two site" immunoradiometric assays (IRMA). In these assays, the antigen is immobilized by a non-radioactive monoclonal antibody attached to a solid surface such as nitrocellulose, and is then detected by ^{125}I-labelled (or enzyme labelled) monoclonal antibody. In other words, the antigen is the "meat in the sandwich" between two monoclonal antibodies. The assay may be used with the two antibodies having the same or different specificity; the only requirement is that both antibodies must be able to bind simultaneously to the same molecule. "Two site" assays of this type allow antigens to be detected and quantitated in very complex mixtures without any need for purification.

The power of such an approach is exemplified by the analysis of the glycoconjugate of Leishmania, a protozoan parasite that grows in macro-

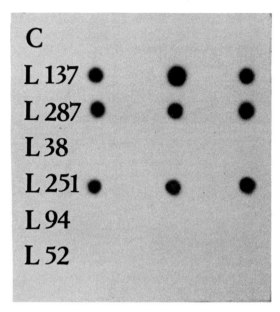

Fig. 5.1 Detection of antigen by a two-site "dot-blot" immunoradiometric assay (IRMA). Nitrocellulose was coated with a monoclonal antibody that recognizes a polymeric carbohydrate antigen of Leishmania. *After saturation of any remaining nonspecific binding sites with 5% nonfat powdered milk in PBS ("BLOTTO", see Index), the antigen-containing mixture (2 μl) was dotted onto the damp membrane. (The membrane must not be allowed to dry until the assay is completed.) Unbound antigen was washed off with BLOTTO, and the bound antigen detected by adding ^{125}I-monoclonal antibody (3×10^5 cpm/ml in BLOTTO). After further washing in BLOTTO, the membrane was autoradiographed at $-70°C$ using an intensifying screen. Typical incubation times are 15–30 min and typical exposure times are 1–4 h. From* Handman *et al. (1984).*

phages. The glycoconjugate is the receptor via which the parasite attaches to and penetrates the macrophage (Handman and Goding, 1985). Detection of the glycoconjugate by conventional biosynthetic labelling with tritiated sugars requires many days of autoradiographic exposure, but a simple nitrocellulose "dot blot" assay based on binding of ^{125}I-labelled monoclonal antibodies allows detection in a few hours (Handman *et al.*, 1984; Handman and Jarvis, 1985; Fig. 5.1).

If it is desired to select for hybridoma clones secreting monoclonal antibodies against glycolipid antigens, the assay of Smolarsky (1980) may be useful. The analysis of the structure of complex carbohydrates and glycolipids is a highly specialized subject, and will not be dealt with in this book. For further information, the reader should consult the reviews of Sharon (1975), Sharon and Lis (1982), Hakomori (1981), Feizi (1981), and Hakomori and Kannagi (1983). Assays for glycolipids are also discussed in Section 3.10.4.

5.2 Cellular Distribution of Antigens Detected by Monoclonal Antibodies

It is not necessary to know the structure of the antigen to exploit the usefulness of monoclonal antibodies. One may use monoclonal antibodies as a probe for identification and classification of cells or other structures on a purely empirical basis. This sort of approach is not without its hazards, however. In several cases, the initial impression that an antigen detected by a particular monoclonal antibody is confined to a functional lineage of cells may be disproven by a more extensive tissue survey.

For example, the monoclonal antibody OKT-9 was originally thought to be specific for a subpopulation of immature human thymocytes (Reinherz *et al.*, 1980). Subsequently, the antigen detected by OKT-9 was found to be present on all cells undergoing proliferation, and was shown to be the receptor for the iron transport protein transferrin (Trowbridge and Omary, 1981; Goding and Burns, 1981; Goding and Harris, 1981; Sutherland *et al.*, 1981).

In some cases, the cellular distribution of a particular antigen can be seen to make biological sense. The association of the OKT-9 antigen with cellular proliferation is easily understood when it is known that it is critically involved in the uptake of iron. Similarly, the restriction of the plasma cell antigen PC-1 to the terminal differentiation phase of B lymphocytes into antibody-secreting cells (Goding and Shen, 1982) would be easily understandable if the PC-1 protein were functionally involved in the process of secretion.

In other instances, the distribution of cellular antigens may be harder to understand. A particular antigen may be found in a wide variety of cell types with no obvious relationship in differentiation lineage or function. Milstein and Lennox (1980) have named these molecules "jumping" differentiation antigens. Springer (1980) has noted that jumping antigens are usually glyco-lipids or glycoproteins with a high carbohydrate content, and that their distribution often changes when a cell moves to a different tissue. Jumping antigens were postulated to be involved in cell migration.

5.3 Radioiodination of Soluble Protein Antigens

The extreme sensitivity of radioisotopic procedures is often essential for the detection of the minute quantities of antigens present in complex biological mixtures. Radiolabelling also allows the addition of extraneous non-radioactive proteins (e.g. antibodies) without their detection in the final readout.

Radioiodination with ^{125}I ($t_{1/2} = 60$ days) is by far the commonest method of labelling soluble proteins (Bolton, 1977). It is inexpensive and simple to

Table 5.1 Procedures for radioiodination of soluble proteins

Method	Exposure to oxidizing agents	Specific activity obtainable	Efficiency	Alteration of native charge	Convenience
Chloramine-T	Yes	High	High	No	+++
Lactoperoxidase	Yes	Moderate	Moderate	No	++
Iodogen	Yes (solid state)	High	High	No	+++
Bolton–Hunter	No	Moderate	Low–moderate[a]	Yes[b]	±[c,d]
Iodobeads	Yes (solid state)	High	Moderate–high	No	+++

[a]Efficiency depends on protein concentration. Typical figures are 5% for 0.1 mg/ml, 10–20% at 1.0 mg/ml, and 50–90% at 10 mg/ml. [b]Loss of one positive charge for each substitution. [c]Reagent is extremely susceptible to hydrolysis, and it is advisable to use one whole vial at a time. [d]A reagent similar to the Bolton–Hunter reagent is N-succinimidyl[2,3-^{3}H]propionate which is available at 30–60 Ci/mmol from Amersham. The specific acitivity of labelled proteins would be much less than the corresponding iodinated proteins.

perform, and results in proteins of high specific activity. The main disadvantage of radioiodination is that it may occasionally damage the protein, resulting in loss of antigenic determinants or other biological activity.

Many of the methods for protein iodination involve oxidizing agents, such as chloramine-T or hydrogen peroxide. These may cause oxidation of methionine to methionine sulphoxide, and tryptophan to oxindole (Salacinski *et al.*, 1981). Other methods, notably the Iodogen method and Bolton–Hunter reagent, avoid these problems, but may introduce problems of their own. The relative merits of the various iodination procedures are listed in Table 5.1.

The susceptibility of individual proteins and antigenic determinants to damage by radioiodination is unpredictable, but may be minimized by attention to detail. Sometimes one method of iodination will damage a protein while another will not. In other cases, all methods of radioiodination may damage the protein (e.g. Nussenzweig *et al.*, 1982), and alternative approaches such a tritium labelling by reductive methylation (Section 5.4) may be needed.

When pure proteins are to be radioiodinated, it is customary to aim for an average substitution of approximately one iodine atom per molecule of protein. If carrier-free ^{125}I is used, the substitution of a single ^{125}I atom results in a specific activity of $\sim 18 \, \mu Ci/\mu g$ for a protein of molecular weight 100 000, or $180 \, \mu Ci/\mu g$ for a protein of molecular weight 10 000.

[One microcurie is equal to 2.2×10^6 disintegrations per minute. The recommended unit is now the Becquerel, which is one disintegration per second. So far, most workers have preferred to use the older unit.]

Substitution of proteins with an average of less than one iodine per molecule will result in a proportion of unlabelled molecules, which merely degrade the sensitivity by competing with labelled molecules. Higher average substitution may result in increased sensitivity at the cost of increased radiation damage. The decay event may damage the antigen. The substitution of one iodine per molecule ensures that once decay has occurred, that molecule will no longer be detected.

If the antigen to be studied is contained within a complex mixture of proteins, it is impossible to predict its specific activity, because the iodination efficiency of each protein will be different. In many practical situations, even the total protein concentration will be unknown.

5.3.1 The Chloramine-T Method

The chloramine-T method (Greenwood *et al.*, 1963) is the most widely used method of protein iodination. The main amino acid to be labelled is tyrosine, although histidine may be iodinated if the pH is greater than 8.0–8.5. The method has the advantages of simplicity and efficiency, and in most cases the degree of damage to the antigen is minimal.

Chloramine-T is an oxidizing agent, and high concentrations may result in damage of the antigen. As a general rule, only 1–10 µg chloramine-T per reaction are necessary, rather than the 100 µg originally used. It is customary to terminate the iodination by addition of the reducing agent sodium meta-bisulphite, but this step may do more harm than good. Termination by addition of tyrosine (final concentration 1 mM) is equally effective, and has no potential for damage to protein.

To prevent exposure to volatile iodine or aerosols, iodinations should always be performed in a fume hood. It is good practice to add a small amount of cold $Na^{127}I$ (final concentration 1 mM) at the end of all iodinations to help terminate the reaction and to minimize adsorption of radioiodide to the glassware.

A number of substances are capable of inhibiting the chloramine-T iodination of proteins. These include reducing agents and thiocyanate ions (George and Schenck, 1983). It is rare to find a protein which will not iodinate. (One such example appears to be ovalbumin.) If difficulty is experienced, it is recommended that the protein be dialysed for 1–2 days against phosphate-buffered saline to remove inhibitors.

The procedure works best if protein concentration is fairly high (> 1.0 mg/ml). The protein may be in Tris-HCl or phosphate buffer, pH 7–8.

Practical procedure

(1) Weigh out chloramine-T powder just before use, and make up to 1.0 mg/ml in distilled water.
(2) Pipette 10 µg protein into a small tube on ice.
(3) Add 10 µl 0.1 M sodium phosphate, pH 7.5, to buffer the NaOH which is always present in the radioactive iodide to prevent oxidation to iodine.
(4) Add desired volume of ^{125}I.
(5) Add 1–10 µl chloramine-T. Mix. (Reaction occurs virtually instantaneously.)
(6) Add 10 µl of a saturated solution of tyrosine in water, to terminate reaction.
(7) Add 2.5 ml phosphate-buffered saline containing 0.1% bovine serum albumin and 10 mM NaN_3; transfer to a disposable PD-10 Sephadex column (Pharmacia) equilibrated with the same buffer. Allow the sample run in; discard effluent. Add 3.5 ml of the same buffer; collect effluent, which contains the iodinated protein, free of unreacted iodide.

Aliquots (typically $1.0 \mu l$) should be removed for direct counting or (preferably) counting after TCA precipitation. Typically, 50–90% of input counts should be incorporated into protein. If the protein concentration is very low (less than $50 \mu g/ml$), the incorporation may be much lower, but in some experiments this may not greatly matter.

5.3.2 TCA Precipitation

After any radiolabelling procedure, it is advisable to measure incorporation by TCA precipitation. If the percentage of total counts in protein is high, liquid-phase precipitation is adequate. However, if the fraction of total counts in protein is low (for example, after cell surface iodination or biosynthetic labelling), more accurate results will be obtained by collection and washing of the precipitate on a filter.

Liquid-phase procedure

(1) Take 1 μl aliquots of labelled protein (triplicate), pipette into an Eppendorf centrifuge tube containing carrier solution ($500 \mu l$ phosphate-buffered saline plus 0.5% fetal calf serum or 0.25 mg/ml bovine serum albumin, and 1 mM KI or 1 mM of the appropriate amino acid if radioactive amino acids are present).
(2) Add $500 \mu l$ 10% TCA. Mix.
(3) Let stand for 30 min at room temperature, or overnight at 4°C. The solution will go very slightly cloudy.
(4) Spin in Eppendorf centrifuge for 5 min ($\sim 10\,000\,\mathbf{g}$).
(5) Remove and save $500 \mu l$ supernatant.
(6) Count the $500 \mu l$ of removed supernatant (S) and the remaining volume (R).
(7) Calculate as follows:

$$\% \text{ TCA precipitable counts} = \frac{R - S}{R + S} \times 100$$

Filter procedure

The procedure requires a side-arm flask connected to a vacuum (water pump) and a filtration apparatus for TCA precipitation (ICN Chemical and Radioisotope Division, 2727 Campus Drive, Irvine, California; Model E8B; cat. no. 803012, 15/16 inch diameter). Also required are Millipore type HA 0.45 μm filters (25 mm diameter; cat. no. HAWP 2500).

(1) Perform steps 1–3 of liquid-phase procedure.
(2) Assemble filtration apparatus with filter in place. Wet filter with carrier solution; apply vacuum.
(3) Add sample to filter.
(4) Wash through with 10 ml 5% TCA.
(5) For ^{125}I, place into tube for counting.
(6) For ^{35}S, ^{14}C or ^{3}H, dry filter under a heat lamp; and place into Triton-based scintillation fluid for counting.

5.3.3 Lactoperoxidase Method

In some cases, the chloramine-T method may result in damage to the antigen due to oxidation. The lactoperoxidase method (Marchalonis, 1969) may prove more gentle. The iodination is almost exclusively confined to tyrosine.
(1) Pipette 10 μl of protein (1.0 mg/ml) into a tube. Add 10 μl 0.1 M Tris-HCl, pH 8, to provide additional buffering.
(2) Add 5 μl lactoperoxidase (0.25 mg/ml).
(3) Add desired volume of ^{125}I. Mix.
(4) Add 10 μl H_2O_2 (diluted 1:30 000 in PBS from 30% stock).
(5) Incubate at room temperature for 10 min.
(6) Terminate reaction, and separate free iodide from protein as for the chloramine-T method.

Uptake of 30–70% of input counts is typical. The most critical parameter is the concentration of H_2O_2. Too little provides insufficient substrate; too much poisons the enzyme. If difficulties are experienced, try varying the concentration of H_2O_2. A 1:1000 dilution of 30% H_2O_2 in phosphate-buffered saline should have an optical density of ~ 0.7 at 230 nm (Phillips and Morrison, 1970).

Some proteins may be damaged by the H_2O_2. The peroxide concentration may be minimized by the use of glucose oxidase to generate continuously micromolar amounts of H_2O_2 in a coupled system (Hubbard and Cohn, 1975). Beads coated with a mixture of glucose oxidase and lactoperoxidase are available commercially ("Enzymobeads"; Bio-Rad, cat. no. 170–6003).

5.3.4 Bolton–Hunter Method

A third method of radioiodination involves the use of N-succinimidyl 3-(4-hydroxy,-5-[^{125}I]iodophenyl) propionate, which reacts with the ε-amino group of lysine (Bolton and Hunter, 1973; Bolton, 1977). The reaction is extremely gentle, as no oxidizing agents are used. The main disadvantages are that the reagent is more expensive than sodium iodide, and it is not practicable to dispense multiple aliquots from a vial of Bolton–Hunter reagent on different days.

The net charge of the protein is decreased by one unit for each modified lysine. The introduction of artefactual charge heterogeneity may be of little importance in many situations, but it should be borne in mind if analysis by two-dimensional gels is contemplated.

The Bolton–Hunter reagent is available commercially at 2000 Ci/mmol or 4000 Ci/mmol (i.e. close to the theoretical maximum specific activities for mono- and di-substituted tyrosine). As is the case for all succinimide esters (see Chapter 7), the Bolton–Hunter reagent is extremely susceptible to hydrolysis (half-life of the order of minutes in alkaline aqueous solution). Iodination of the protein and hydrolysis of the Bolton–Hunter reagent are therefore simultaneous competing reactions. The competition may be biased in favour of protein iodination by a high protein concentration. A concentration of > 1.0 mg/ml is advisable, and 10 mg/ml is preferable (Table 5.1). Extraneous nucleophiles such as free amines (e.g. Tris) or azide ions will inhibit the reaction.

Practical procedure

The Bolton–Hunter reagent is supplied by New England Nuclear in 1.0 mCi units, in 100 μl dry benzene. It should be stored refrigerated, not frozen. Aliquoting is not recommended, because even traces of water result in hydrolysis.

(1) Evaporate the benzene by inserting a needle as an intake for a gentle stream of dry nitrogen or dry air, through the septum of the combi-v-vial just above the surface of the benzene. A charcoal trap is supplied to contain any radioiodine released. Evaporation must be gentle, to concentrate the ester in the apex of the "v" container.

(2) Add the protein in as small a volume and as concentrated form as possible (typically 10 μl of 10 mg/ml). Suitable buffers include borate or phosphate, pH 7.4–8.5. The efficiency is higher at the alkaline end.

(3) Incubate for 1 h at room temperature (New England Nuclear recommends 4°C for up to 18 h for maximal uptake).

(4) Add 10 μl 10 mM ethanolamine, Tris-HCl, glycine or sodium azide to terminate reaction.

(5) Pass over a PD-10 Sephadex column (Section 5.3.1) equilibrated with phosphate-buffered saline plus 0.1% gelatin. (The Bolton–Hunter reagent binds to albumin via hydrophobic interactions.)

Typical uptake of ^{125}I is 5–30% (Table 5.1).

5.3.5 The "Iodogen" Method

Fraker and Speck (1978) have described a novel method of protein iodination which uses the water-insoluble compound 1,3,4,6-tetrachloro-3α,6α-diphenyl glycoluril (Iodogen®, available from Pierce Chemicals). The method has achieved considerable acceptance (Markwell and Fox, 1978; Salacinski *et al.*, 1982). Damage to proteins should be minimal, because they are not exposed to soluble oxidizing agents. The main amino acid to be iodinated is tyrosine.

Iodogen is dissolved in chloroform or dichloromethane and pipetted into borosilicate glass tubes or iodination vials (Walter Starstedt, No. 690 test tubes), and the solvent gently blown off with a stream of dry nitrogen. Iodogen forms a thin coating on the surface of the tube. Removal of the solvent by simple evaporation results in flaking of the coating (Markwell and Fox, 1978). Coated tubes may be stored for at least 6 months at room temperature, protected from light in a dessicator.

The tube should be rinsed with buffer just prior to use, to remove any loose flakes. Iodination of proteins is performed by simply adding the protein to the tube, followed by the desired volume of ^{125}I. Reaction time is typically 5–10 min at room temperature. It is recommended that tubes be coated with not more than $10\,\mu g$ Iodogen per $100\,\mu g$ of protein.

It is often stated that the reaction is terminated by simply removing the contents of the tube. However, it is probably advisable to add an excess (1 mM) of tyrosine, because the active iodous (I^+) ion may persist for a few minutes. In addition, small amounts of Iodogen may become detached from the glass. Unreacted iodide should be removed by gel filtration (Section 5.3.1.).

5.3.6 The "Iodo-beads" Method

Chloramine-T, covalently attached to polystyrene beads, has recently been shown to be an efficient and gentle reagent for protein iodination (Markwell, 1982). The beads are available from Pierce Chemicals under the name "Iodo-beads". The reaction is simple and efficient.

On the day of use, Iodo-beads are washed twice in phosphate-buffered saline, and blotted dry on filter paper. Then, $100\,\mu g$ protein in $500\,\mu l$ phosphate-buffered saline is added, followed by 1 mCi of $Na^{125}I$. The iodination reaction is initiated by addition of one or more Iodo-beads, and allowed to proceed for 15 min at room temperature. The reaction is terminated by removal of the liquid, addition of non-radioactive NaI or tyrosine (1 mM), and gel filtration to remove unreacted iodide.

The reaction volume is not critical, and shaking is evidently not necessary. The reaction is not inhibited by azide, sodium dodecyl sulphate, 8 M urea, or 2% Nonidet P-40, although it is abolished by reducing agents such as mercaptoethanol. The efficiency of incorporation was 35% with one bead, and virtually 100% with five beads.

5.4 Radiolabelling of Soluble Proteins with Tritium by Reductive Methylation

Occasionally, the protein of interest may be inactivated by all of the above methods of radioiodination (e.g. Nussenzweig *et al.*, 1982). The successful alternative procedure involved labelling with tritium by reductive methylation (Tack *et al.*, 1980).

The respective disintegration rates for ^{125}I, ^{3}H and ^{14}C at 100% isotopic abundance are 1.7×10^{4}, 9.8×10^{3} and $4.6 \, Ci/g$. Until recently, radiolabelling with ^{125}I was the only method capable of achieving the high specific activities needed for highly sensitive radioimmunoassay or receptor studies. Tack *et al.* (1980) have now shown that it is feasible to label haemoglobin, complement and immunoglobulins to very high specific activities by reductive methylation.

Advantages of reductive methylation include minimal disruption to the conformation of the protein, preservation of native charge, and long half-life (12 years). Disadvantages include the need to handle extremely large amounts of a chemically unstable radioactive compound, and the additional work involved in use of scintillation methods of detection of tritium.

Practical procedure (after Tack et al., *1980)*

$NaB^{3}H_{4}$ of specific activity 40–60 Ci/mmol was obtained from New England Nuclear upon special request. A quantity corresponding to 500 mCi was weighed out, dissolved in anhydrous methylamine and dispensed in 100 mCi aliquots in dry glass vials. The solvent was removed under vacuum, and nitrogen gas introduced.

[Since the first edition of this book was written, tritiated borohydride has become routinely available from New England Nuclear in a much more convenient form. It is supplied at a specific activity of 70 Ci/mmol, in 25 mCi batches frozen in 1 ml 10 mM NaOH, and may be stored for several months at − 70°C. It should not be frozen and thawed repeatedly, but rather should be stored in small aliquots.]

The protein (5–10 mg/ml) was dialysed against 0.2 M borate, pH 8.9, and 200 µl transfered to 1.0 ml "Reacti-vials" (Kontes Glass, or Pierce). The vials were placed on ice for 1 h, and all subsequent operations were carried out in a well-ventilated fume hood.

The crystalline $NaB^{3}H_{4}$ was dissolved in 0.01 M NaOH to a final concentration of 1.0 Ci/ml just prior to use, and a stock solution of 12.4 M formaldehyde diluted with water to 0.1–0.2 M. The formaldehyde (10–20 µl) and $NaB^{3}H_{4}$ (30–50 µl) were added sequentially to each vial, which was then sealed with a rubber septum and held on ice for 10 min. Protein solutions were removed by needle aspiration through the septum and desalted by gel filtration on disposable Sephadex G-25 columns. (In view of the extremely large quantities of low molecular weight isotope present, it is questionable whether this procedure would be adequate to remove all the unreacted borohydride.)

5.5 Radiolabelling of Cellular Proteins

5.5.1 Cell Surface Radioiodination

By far the easiest way to obtain radiolabelled membrane proteins of high specific activity is via cell surface radioiodination of intact, living cells. The two procedures which are most commonly used are lactoperoxidase-catalysed iodination (Marchalonis *et al.*, 1971) and an adaptation of the Iodogen method (Markwell and Fox, 1978). The efficiency of the two procedures is not greatly different. A typical experiment might start with 10^7 cells and $500\,\mu\text{Ci}$ ^{125}I (i.e. $\sim 10^9$ cpm). About 1% of the counts will be incorporated into protein, and a somewhat larger percentage into lipid.

The mere presence of ^{125}I-labelled material in such experiments does not prove, in itself, that such material was synthesized by the cell. This seemingly obvious point has led many people astray, and the common association of serum albumin has probably been confused with immunoglobulin heavy chains on more than one occasion (Sidman, 1981).

In the same vein, the presence of ^{125}I-labelled protein does not prove that the protein was present on the cell surface. If the recommended conditions for iodination are changed appreciably (e.g. by increasing the iodide concentration), cytoplasmic labelling may occur. Similarly, if there are any dead cells in the population to be labelled, extensive cytoplasmic labelling is unavoidable.

Proof that the label is confined to the cell surface may be obtained in several ways. If the labelled protein can be removed from intact cells by protease treatment, this constitutes good evidence for a surface location (Felsted and Gupta, 1982). Electron microscope autoradiography of labelled cells (Marchalonis *et al.*, 1971; Tartakoff and Vassalli, 1979) is another approach, but the method is cumbersome and technically demanding. A third way of assessing the degree of cytoplasmic labelling is to analyse the whole lysate by two-dimensional (charge-size) polyacrylamide gel electrophoresis. The autoradiograph should be laid over the dried, stained gel, and the spots on the film compared with the stained spots. Only cytoplasmic proteins are sufficiently abundant to be seen by staining. It therefore follows that there should be no correspondence between stained spots and spots on the film. The most prominent stained protein will probably be actin, which is an acidic protein of M_r 43 000. Presence of ^{125}I in actin should be taken as evidence of cytoplasmic labelling.

Assessment of cell viability

If it is crucial that the labelling be confined to the cell surface, the cell population should have very few dead cells ($< 3\%$). Viability may be assessed by the acridine orange/ethidium bromide method (Lee *et al.*, 1975), which is much more accurate and unambiguous than eosin or trypan blue exclusion. Both dyes are potentially carcinogenic, and should be handled with care to avoid ingestion or skin contact.

One drop of cells in phosphate-buffered saline (PBS) is placed on a glass slide, and one drop of PBS containing 1 part per million acridine orange and 1 part per million ethidium bromide is added, followed by a cover slip. Cells are examined by fluorescence microscopy, using filters for fluorescein (Chapter 7). Living cells stain bright green, while dead cells stain bright orange.

Lactoperoxidase-catalysed cell surface iodination

(1) Wash cells three times in **PBS** to remove serum and loosely adsorbed protein. *After washing, transfer cells to a fresh tube to prevent iodination of protein adsorbed to the sides of the tube.*
(2) Resuspend cells ($1–5 \times 10^7$) in $200\,\mu l$ **PBS** (do not alter volume). All steps may be at room temperature, unless otherwise directed.
(3) Just before iodination, dilute $10\,\mu l$ of 30% H_2O_2 in $10\,ml$ PBS (i.e. 1:1000). The optical density of the 1:1000 stock should be about 0.7 at $230\,nm$ (Phillips and Morrison, 1970). Then prepare serial three-fold dilutions in PBS, giving final dilutions of 1:3000; 1:9000 and 1:27000.
(4) Add $50\,\mu l$ of $0.2\,mg/ml$ lactoperoxidase to the cells, then $500\,\mu Ci$ ^{125}I.
(5) At one minute intervals, add successively $10\,\mu l$ of 1:27000; 1:9000; 1:3000 H_2O_2.
(6) One minute after the last addition, wash the cells twice in $10\,ml$ PBS containing $1\,mM$ KI or $1\,mM$ tyrosine to terminate the reaction. (The KI should be freshly prepared to avoid oxidation to I_2, which would kill the cells.)
(7) Solubilize the cells in $300\,\mu l–3.0\,ml$ PBS containing 0.5% Triton X-100 or Nonidet P-40, at $4°C$ for $30–60\,min$ (see Section 5.6). If desired, the solubilization buffer may contain the protease inhibitors EDTA, N-ethyl maleimide and phenylmethyl sulphonyl fluoride ($1\,mM$ of each). The latter two must be made up freshly.

All subsequent steps should be at $4°C$.

(8) Remove nuclei and insoluble debris by centrifugation at $2000–10000\,g$ for $5–10\,min$.

A good iodination should result in 10–40% of the input counts remaining with the cells after washing. Of these, only 1–10% will be TCA-precipitable, indicating incorporation into protein. The remainder will be in free iodide or lipid. TCA precipitations must be performed on membrane filters (Section 5.3.2).

The level of incorporation of ^{125}I into protein (1–3% of input counts) is low, but this is the best that can be achieved. The concentration of enzyme is not very critical. The most important parameter is the concentration of peroxide; too low a concentration results in poor efficiency, while too high a concentration poisons the enzyme and may damage the cells. The increasing pulses of H_2O_2 guarantee that the optimal concentration will be reached, yet the total concentration is not excessive.

If the concentrations of H_2O_2 employed causes problems, continuous micromolar amounts of H_2O_2 may be generated by glucose and glucose oxidase (Hubbard and Cohn, 1975). If cells containing significant amounts of peroxidase are to be labelled, the lactoperoxidase method may result in cytoplasmic labelling. In these cases, the Iodogen method (see below) may be preferred.

Use of "Iodogen" to label cell surface membrane proteins

Markwell and Fox (1978) have shown that the Iodogen method for iodination of soluble proteins (Section 5.3.5) may be adapted to the specific labelling of the externally disposed proteins of cell membranes. The pattern of labelling of proteins is virtually identical to that obtained using the lactoperoxidase technique (Felsted and Gupta, 1982). Advantages of the Iodogen method include the absence of any extraneous added protein or H_2O_2. Tubes may be coated with Iodogen as described in Section 5.3.5. Alternatively, if adherent cells such as fibroblasts are to be labelled, Iodogen may be coated onto a glass cover slip, which is gently floated above the cell monolayer (Markwell and Fox, 1978).

Cells should be washed three times in phosphate-buffered saline to remove extraneous protein. As for the lactoperoxidase method, cell viability must be very high. The Iodogen-coated iodination vial should be rinsed with PBS just prior to use, to remove any loosely attached material. Cells (typically 10^7) are added in 1.0 ml PBS, followed by 500 μCi ^{125}I, and the reaction allowed to proceed for 10 min at room temperature, with occasional agitation.

The cells are then harvested by centrifugation in PBS containing 1 mM sodium iodide, and washed once in the same buffer. Conditions for solubilization are identical to those for the lactoperoxidase technique (see also Section 5.6).

Typical amounts of Iodogen per vial are 5–10 μg. Higher amounts are likely to kill the cells and result in cytoplasmic labelling.

5.5.2 Biosynthetic Incorporation of Radioactive Amino Acids

The choice of amino acid and isotope warrants careful consideration. The aim will usually be to incorporate the greatest number of counts at the least expense. Useful information about the choice of amino acids has been published by Vitetta et al. (1976) and Coligan et al. (1983).

In many cases, ^{35}S-methionine will be the amino acid of choice ($E_{max} = 167 \, KeV$; $t_{1/2} = 87$ days). Its extremely high specific activity (often > 1000 Ci/mmol) and good uptake by cells more than compensates for its relative rarity in proteins. The next highest specific activity amino acids are those labelled with tritium. The maximum specific activities currently available range from 20–200 Ci/mmol. Tritiated amino acids have a radioactive half-life of 12 years, although they usually deteriorate at 1–3% per month. The relatively low energy of tritium ($E_{max} = 18 \, KeV$) was once a serious problem, but the advent of simple fluorographic techniques (Bonner and Laskey, 1974; Chamberlain, 1979; Laskey, 1980, 1984) have made auto-radiography with tritium a trivial matter. Tritium is detected by soaking the gel in a solution containing a scintillant. The scintillant is then precipitated in the gel (by a change of solvent or by drying). The low energy β-emission of tritium is converted into photons with high efficiency, and the film is thus exposed by light rather than direct ionizing radiation. Experimental details and recommendations are given in Section 5.8.3.

Labelling with ^{14}C-amino acids ($t_{1/2} = 5760$ years; $E_{max} = 155 \, KeV$) is seldom justified. Their specific activity (typically 300 mCi/mmol) is much lower than the tritiated amino acids, and they are much more expensive. The gamma-emitting analogue of methionine, ^{75}Se-methionine, has some advantages over ^{35}S-methionine (Gutman et al., 1978), but has not yet seen widespread use. The sensitivity of detection of ^{75}Se is greatly increased by use of intensifying screens (Section 5.8.2), but its extremely high energy makes storage and shielding very problematical.

The uptake and incorporation of amino acids does not exactly parallel their relative abundance in cellular proteins. Good results are obtained with methionine, arginine, leucine, lysine and tyrosine. Even though cysteine can be obtained at as high specific activity as methionine and is usually more abundant, it generally gives poorer labelling. Cysteine receives its sulphur from methionine, and if ^{35}S-cysteine is used, it is a good idea to use ^{35}S-methionine as well.

In some circumstances, use of cysteine and methionine may result in non-biosynthetic incorporation into protein (Gutman et al., 1978; Suissa, 1981). The problem seems to be an unidentified contaminant in the isotope preparations, and is not seen when the proteins are reduced.

Storage and handling of radioactive amino acids

Methionine and cysteine are supplied in aqueous solution containing 0.1% (1.2×10^{-2} M) mercaptoethanol. The maximum concentration of mercapto-ethanol that most cells can tolerate is around 5×10^{-5} M (this corresponds to 50 μCi/ml). Tritiated or ^{14}C-amino acids are usually supplied in water plus 2% ethanol to scavenge free radicals (Evans, 1976). A concentration of 0.2–0.3% ethanol should not be exceeded. If higher concentrations of isotope are required, the ethanol or mercaptoethanol may be removed by lyophiliza-tion. Since these reagents are added to stabilize the amino acid, lyophilization should be performed just prior to labelling, and only in the quantity needed.

^{35}S-methionine and cysteine may be stored at $-70°$C or in liquid nitrogen. When a vial is first opened, the isotope should be aliquoted into small tubes (0.5 mCi/tube). Do not repeatedly freeze and thaw. Tritiated and ^{14}C-amino acids and sugars should be stored at 4°C, protected from light. In general, aqueous solutions of ^{3}H compounds should not be frozen, because molecular clustering by freezing accelerates self radiolysis (Evans, 1976). While the beta-emission of ^{35}S and ^{14}C will not penetrate a thin layer of plastic or glass, the resulting interaction may generate penetrating Brehmsstrahlung radia-tion and cause fogging of adjacent films unless lead shielding is used.

Practical procedure

(1) Prepare medium lacking appropriate amino acid. (Gibco "Selectamine" kit is ideal.)
(2) Add 10% fetal calf serum (preferably dialysed against PBS to remove any free amino acids).
(3) Set up cultures containing 10^6–10^7 cells in 1–2 ml medium containing desired amount of radioactive amino acid (typically 50–100 μCi/ml).
(4) Culture at 37°C for desired period (generally 1–4 h). If the culture is for less than about 4 h, the cells need not be sterile, although gross bacterial contamination must be avoided.
(5) Add non-radioactive amino acid to ~ 1 mM.
(6) Harvest cells by centrifugation. If desired, save supernatant.
(7) Wash cells twice in medium lacking isotope but containing non-radioactive amino acid.
(8) Solubilize cells as for surface iodination.
(9) Check incorporation of isotope by TCA precipitation using a mem-brane (Section 5.3.2).

It is advisable to check that the kinetics of uptake of radioactivity are linear. Non-linear kinetics indicate that something is changing during the culture period (e.g. the cells are dying). Linear kinetics are absolutely essen-tial for "pulse-chase" experiments. The achievement of sufficient incorporation of isotope during pulse-chase exeepriments may require depletion of non-radioactive cellular amino acid pools by pre-incubation for 1–2 h at 37°C in medium lacking the relevant amino acid. The chase may be carried out by addition of the non-radioactive amino acid to a final concentration of ~ 1 mM, which is a vast excess over that of the radioactive species. In the case of long incubations of rapidly metabolising cells, it may be necessary to add small (micromolar) amounts of non-radioactive species, to prevent amino acid starvation.

5.5.3 Biosynthetic Labelling with ^{32}P

Cells should be cultured for 2–4 h in phosphate-free culture medium containing 5% fetal calf serum and 0.5–5.0 mCi carrier-free [^{32}P]-orthophosphate (Radke and Martin, 1979; Radke *et al.*, 1980; Cooper and Hunter, 1981). Labelling is terminated by washing in phosphate-buffered saline. Radioactive phosphate will be incorporated into phosphoproteins, phospholipids, DNA and RNA. The presence of labelled DNA and RNA may cause severe "background" problems in electrophoretic analyses of proteins, and many authors treat the cell lysates with nucleases (e.g. Radke and Martin, 1979; Radke *et al.*, 1980). Cells may receive substantial amounts of irradiation during labelling.

5.5.4 Biosynthetic Labelling of the Carbohydrate Moieties of Glycoproteins and Glycolipids

Biosynthetic labelling of carbohydrate may be accomplished using ^{3}H-mannose, fucose, galactose or glucosamine (Tartakoff and Vassali, 1979; Vasilov and Pleogh, 1982; Melchers,1973). Extensive metabolic conversion to other amino acids is not a severe problem, except in the case of ^{3}H-glucosamine, which may be converted to sialic acid (Sharon and Lis, 1982). Glycoproteins cannot be labelled by addition of ^{3}H-sialic acid to the cultures, because it is not taken up by cells.

The practical details of biosynthetic labelling with radioactive sugars are little different to those for amino acids, except that glucose must be omitted from the medium during labelling. The specific activities that can be achieved are generally very low.

5.5.5 Radioactive Labelling of Carbohydrate by Oxidation Followed by Reduction with Tritiated Borohydride

The externally disposed sugars of glycoproteins and glycolipids of cells may be labelled by oxidation with galactose oxidase (Gahmberg and Hakomori, 1973; Steck and Dawson, 1974; Gahmberg *et al.*, 1976) or periodate (Gahmberg and Andersson, 1977). The specific activities obtainable are fairly low, and certain glycoproteins and glycolipids may be labelled much more strongly than others.

Tritiated borohydride is now available from New England Nuclear in a convenient form. It is supplied at a specific activity of 70 Ci/mmol in 25 mCi vials, frozen in 1 ml 10 mM NaOH, and may be stored for several months at − 70°C. It should not be frozen and thawed repeatedly, but rather should be stored in small aliquots.

Galactose oxidase procedure

The procedure is from Gahmberg *et al.* (1976). Twenty million cells in 1.0 ml Dulbecco's PBS are treated with 5U galactose oxidase (with or without 12.5U neuraminidase) for 1 h at 37°C. They are then washed three times in PBS, and resuspended in 0.5 ml PBS. Tritiated borohydride (0.5 mCi) is then added, and the cells left at room temperature for 30 min. Finally, the cells are washed several times.

Periodate procedure

As an alternative to the use of enzymes, the cell surface carbohydrate may be oxidized with sodium periodate. Providing that the periodate concentration is low, the incubation times are kept short, and the cells kept cold, labelling may be restricted to the cell surface (Gahmberg and Andersson, 1977).

Approximately 3×10^7 mouse lymphocytes are treated with 1 mM sodium periodate in 1.0 ml PBS in the dark on ice for 5 min. Glycerol (200 μl of a 0.1 M solution) is then added to quench the reaction, and the cells are washed three times. They are then treated with tritiated borohydride (0.5 mCi in 0.5 ml PBS) for 30 min at room temperature, and finally washed three times in PBS.

Typical incorporation was $2–4 \times 10^3$ cpm per 10^6 cells (Gahmberg and Andersson, 1977). By comparison, the labelling of a similar number of cells with 0.5 mCi ^{125}I by the lactoperoxidase technique results in typical incorporations of $\sim 10^6$ cpm per 10^6 cells (Section 5.5.1).

5.6 Solubilization of Membrane Proteins

Before the classical techniques of biochemical purification and analysis can be applied to membrane proteins, they must be converted into a water-soluble form. In a few limited and special cases, solubilization of membrane proteins may be achieved by detachment from the membrane using proteolytic cleavage, or relatively minor changes in ionic conditions. In almost all other cases, however, the solubilization of membrane proteins in intact and native form can only be achieved by the use of detergents. Successful isolation of membrane antigens requires an understanding of the forces which hold membranes together, and of the mechanism of action of detergents.

5.6.1. Basic Principles

The cell membrane consists of an essentially fluid bilayer of lipids, arranged with their hydrophobic portions facing inwards and their polar head-groups interacting with the aqueous environment (Singer and Nicolson, 1972). In discussions of membranes, the lumen of intracellular organelles such as the endoplasmic reticulum and Golgi apparatus is considered to be topographically extracellular. Membrane lipids exhibit varying degrees of asymmetry in their disposition; all the carbohydrate of glycolipids and glycoproteins lies on the extracellular face, while phosphatidyl ethanolamine lies mainly on the cytoplasmic face (Rothman and Lenard, 1977). Lateral diffusion of lipids is rapid, but "flip-flop" movement across the membrane is rare.

In marked contrast to lipids, the asymmetrical disposition of membrane proteins is absolute. This asymmetry is a consequence of the fact that most membrane proteins are inserted into the membrane during their synthesis, and once inserted, the energy required to move a polar region of protein across a non-polar lipid bilayer is so great that the process never occurs. Membrane proteins are held in or on the membrane by two distinct mechanisms. Some are attached by electrostatic or other noncovalent interactions, and may be released by relatively small changes in pH or ionic strength. This class is known as "peripheral membrane proteins" (Singer and Nicolson, 1972). Once released, peripheral membrane proteins are usually soluble in water in the absence of detergents. Most, but not all, peripheral membrane proteins lie on the cytoplasmic surface. Peripheral membrane proteins do not span or penetrate the lipid bilayer. A well-known example of a peripheral membrane protein is β_2-microglobulin, which is a subunit of the major histocompatibility antigens, and is noncovalently attached to an extracellular portion of their heavy chains. Isolated β_2-microglobulin is freely soluble in water in the absence of detergents.

The other major class of membrane proteins has been termed "integral", because their removal and solubilization requires disruption of the membrane with detergents. Integral membrane proteins generally possess at least one uninterrupted stretch of ~ 25 hydrophobic amino acids. This region spans or penetrates the lipid bilayer, and its extreme hydrophobicity ensures that the protein remains firmly embedded in the membrane.

Integral membrane proteins may be further subdivided. Class I integral membrane proteins possess a single hydrophobic sequence, which is usually situated close to the C-terminus. They only penetrate the membrane once, and usually (but not always) have their N-terminus outside the cell and the C-terminus inside. Examples include the histocompatibility antigens, glycophorin and membrane immunoglobulin. Class II integral membrane proteins span the membrane more than once, and often many times. Either terminus may be inside or outside the cell. This class of protein includes many pumps and channels, such as the anion channel protein (band 3) of human erythrocytes (Sabban *et al.*, 1981) and bacteriorhodopsin, a light-activated proton pump (Engelman and Zaccai, 1980).

In addition, a minority of integral membrane proteins possess covalently attached fatty acid (Schlesinger, 1981). The role of the fatty acid is not clear, but it would appear to be embedded in the lipid bilayer. In the case of the Thy-1 antigen, which lacks a hydrophobic amino acid sequence, covalent lipid is responsible for membrane attachment (Tse *et al.*, 1985).

5.6.2 Solubilization of Membrane Proteins by Detergents

Membrane solubilization by detergents has been reviewed in detail (Helenius and Simons, 1975; Helenius *et al.*, 1979). The essential points are as follows. Detergents are amphiphilic molecules which exist in aqueous solution as monomers and micelles. The micelles consist of aggregates of 2–100 monomers, with their hydrophobic portions buried in the centre and their hydrophilic portions at the surface. At low detergent concentrations, most detergent molecules exist as monomers. With increasing detergent concentration, the concentration of monomers rises until at a poorly defined concentration called the *critical micelle concentration*, the monomer concentration ceases to rise, and further increase in detergent concentration results from an increase in micelle concentration. The micelle size is largely independent of detergent concentration, but is influenced to a variable extent by the type of detergent, and salt concentration and the pH.

Solubilization of integral membrane proteins occurs by replacement of the planar lipid bilayer with a micelle of detergent (Helenius and Simons, 1975). The detergent micelle binds to the hydrophobic transmembrane sequence, with the hydrophilic part of the detergent facing outwards. Non-ionic and weakly ionic detergents do not interact to any significant extent with the hydrophilic cytoplasmic or extracellular portions of membrane proteins, nor with the majority of water-soluble proteins.

It is the monomer concentration which determines the solubilizing power. Thus, the concentration of detergent should always exceed the critical micelle concentration, so that the monomer concentration is as high as possible (Helenius *et al.*, 1979). The use of lower concentrations is fraught with the risk of incomplete solubilization and a wide variety of resultant artefacts. Concentrations much higher than 10–20 times the critical micelle concentration are best avoided, because there is no increase in solubilizing power, and the effects of impurities in the detergent (Ashani and Catravas, 1980) may become significant. [More highly purified grades of Triton X-100 suitable for membrane research have recently become available from Calbiochem and Boehringer.]

The other major requirement for solubilization concerns the total mass of detergent. Membrane lipid and detergent may be regarded as competing with each other for the hydrophobic regions of membrane proteins, so the total mass of detergent should be at least ten times the total mass of cell lipid. This requirement is easily satisfied in most analytical experiments, in which the mass of membrane lipid may be considered negligible. However, the total mass of detergent should be carefully considered when large-scale purifications are planned.

Removal of detergent from membrane proteins usually results in uncontrolled aggregation and precipitation. It is therefore essential that buffers should contain an adequate concentration of detergent at all stages during their isolation and handling.

5.6.3 Choice of Detergent

The detergents that have been found useful for membrane solubilization may be divided into three broad groups — non-ionic, weakly ionic and strongly ionic. As a general rule, the order given correlates with increasing solubilizing power, but also with increasing disruption of protein–protein interactions and denaturation.

A great deal of knowledge concerning use of detergents has been obtained empirically, and there is a need for individualization of choice of detergent for solubilization of a particular membrane protein. Although hundreds of different detergents might be considered, the majority of membrane proteins are adequately solubilized by Triton X-100 or the closely related Nonidet P-40. In some cases, other detergents will need to be tried. The newer detergents, such as the zwitterionic sulphobetaines (Gonenne and Ernst, 1978) and CHAPS (Hjelmeland, 1980) have been claimed to be especially effective, although the question of whether increased solubilization power can be achieved without a concomitant increase in denaturing ability has not yet been resolved.

Non-ionic detergents

By far the most widely used detergent in membrane solubilization is Triton X-100. Nonident P-40 is virtually identical in structure. Triton X-100 has a very low critical micelle concentration ($\sim 3 \times 10^{-4}$ M or 0.02%). It is a very effective membrane solubilizer, but has minimal effect on protein–protein interactions and leaves the nucleus intact. Antigen–antibody interactions are unaffected.

A typical protocol for solubilization is as follows. To $1-5 \times 10^7$ cells, add 0.5–2.0 ml 0.5% Triton X-100 in PBS, and mix gently. Leave on ice for 15–60 min, then remove nuclei and debris by centrifugation. For many applications, a low-speed spin (say 3000 g for 10 min) is sufficient. For rigorous demonstration that solubilization has been achieved, it is necessary to spin at 100 000 g for 30–60 min.

Removal of Triton X-100 by dialysis is extremely slow, due to its low critical micelle concentration, and alternative detergent removal methods using hydrophobic beads (Holloway, 1973) may result in drastic loss of membrane protein. A newer non-ionic detergent, octyl glucoside (Baron and Thompson, 1975) may be substituted for Triton X-100. It has a very high critical micelle concentration (~ 25 mM) and is easily removed by dialysis (Helenius *et al.*, 1979).

Bile salts

A second class of detergents in common use are the bile salts. The most widely used is sodium deoxycholate, which is more effective than Triton X-100 in solubilizing certain proteins, such as the Thy-1 antigen (Barclay *et al.*, 1975).

Deoxycholate has a greater ability to disrupt protein–protein interactions, and may sometimes denature proteins. It will lyse the nucleus, causing release of DNA. The pKa of deoxycholate is 6.2, and it forms an insoluble gel at a pH of 7.2 or lower. Deoxycholate is also precipitated by divalent cations. Unlike Triton X-100, deoxycholate does not absorb light appreciably at 280 nm.

Antigen–antibody interactions are usually, but not always preserved. Herrman and Mescher (1979) found that the monoclonal anti-H-2K antibody 11-4.1 failed to bind antigen in the presence of deoxycholate. It appears that deoxycholate causes a significant conformational change in the antigen (Herrman *et al.*, 1982).

Sodium dodecyl sulphate

Sodium dodecyl sulphate is an example of a "strong" ionic detergent. It is highly denaturing, and very effective at disrupting protein–protein interactions. It is a very rare protein which cannot be solubilized in sodium dodecyl sulphate. Removal of sodium dodecyl sulphate from proteins is difficult, but can be achieved by precipitating the protein in 90% acetone or methanol at $-20°C$ (see Section 8.1.4). The SDS will remain in solution. The protein may sometimes be renatured by transfer into 6 M guanidine-HCl containing 1 mM dithiothreitol, followed by dilution into physiological buffer (Hager and Burgess, 1980).

Most antigen–antibody bonds are disrupted by sodium dodecyl sulphate, although occasionally it is possible to carry out immunoprecipitation procedures if a large excess of Triton X-100 is included. Presumably, the sodium dodecyl sulphate is incorporated into Triton X-100 micelles, lowering its effective concentration. Antigens denatured by sodium dodecyl sulphate are capable of eliciting surprisingly strong antibody responses when injected into animals (Stumph *et al.*, 1974; Tjian *et al.*, 1975; Lane and Robbins, 1978; Carroll *et al.*, 1978; Granger and Lazarides, 1979). (See Section 8.1.4).

5.7 Isolation of Radiolabelled Antigens by Immunoprecipitation

In addition to providing an exquisitely sensitive basis for its detection, radiolabelling of the antigen has the major attraction that non-radioactive proteins such as antibodies may be added without detection in the final readout (scintillation counting or autoradiography). In other words, radioactive antigen may be specifically precipitated by non-radioactive antibody. The antigen–antibody precipitates may be collected by centrifugation, washed free of material which is not bound to antibody, and the antigen recovered and analysed (Fig. 5.2). This approach, which was pioneered by Schwartz and Nathenson (1971), has been widely adopted to isolate hundreds of different antigens.

The attractions of immunoprecipitation include simplicity, flexibility and extreme sensitivity. It is feasible to isolate and analyse 10–30 different antigens in one experiment. The minimum quantity of antigen detectable depends mainly on the specific activity of the radiolabelled antigen. If ^{125}I-labelled antigen is used, detection in the picogram–nanogram range may be achieved without difficulty.

The main disadvantage of immunoprecipitation is that it may occasionally create ambiguity. If a particular molecular entity is precipitated by a monoclonal antibody, the possibility may exist that the antigenic detereminant recognized is not on that molecule, but rather on another molecule that is

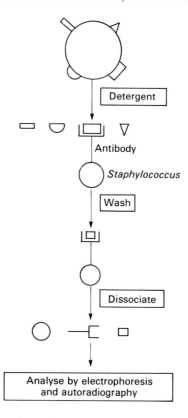

Fig. 5.2 *Isolation of antigens by immunoprecipitation.*

physically attached. The second molecule could escape detection by being non-radioactive, running off the end of a polyacrylamide gel, or being of a class of molecule that escaped detection in the analytical system used. For example, if one used an anti-β_2-microglobulin antibody to isolate HLA antigens, and analysed the proteins on a 7.5% acrylamide gel, a single band of molecular weight 45 000 would be seen. The "real" antigen would have escaped detection by running off the end of the gel. Provided that one is aware of the problem and approaches immunoprecipitation intelligently, the method will be found to be very useful. The problem of identification of the polypeptide which actually contains the relevant antigenic determinant may sometimes be solved by "Western" blots (Section 5.8.4).

The use of biosynthetic labelling rather than surface iodination of cells places much greater demands on the specificity of the immunoprecipitation system, because the proportion of TCA-precipitable counts incorporated into any one protein will be a much smaller fraction of the total counts. If the protein of interest is known to be glycosylated (as are the majority of membrane and secretory proteins), preliminary fractionation on lectin columns may provide cleaner results. Lentil lectin (Hayman and Crumpton, 1972) is popular because its specificity for mannose allows most (but not all) glycoproteins to bind, and its affinity is low enough to allow efficient elution by competing sugars. The volume of the matrix need only be 50–500 μl per 10^7–10^8 cells. It is important to appreciate that any one lectin will not bind all the various modified forms of carbohydrates of glycoproteins, and the recovery is generally low.

It is important to appreciate that antibodies are not the only proteins in serum that can bind to other proteins. In particular, the iron transport protein transferrin binds to cell surface receptors. The possibility of artefacts due to transferrin has been suggested (Goding and Burns, 1981), and a case has been documented (Harford, 1984). There are many other examples of serum proteins that bind to cells.

In summary, success in immunoprecipitation depends very largely on having strong, specific antisera or monoclonal antibodies, together with highly radioactive and soluble antigens. If these requirements are met, it is unlikely that the remaining steps will present difficulties.

Immunoprecipitation analysis of membrane proteins may be considered as occurring in four distinct phases: binding of the antibody; precipitation; washing and elution.

5.7.1 Binding of Antibody

For most practical purposes, antibodies bind almost equally well at 37°, room temperature and 4°C. It is advisable to perform all steps at 4°C, however, to minimize the chance of proteolytic degradation. For the same reason, work should be performed as rapidly as possible.

It is preferable to perform the precipitation step on the same day as the labelling step, because freezing and thawing of the antigen-containing mixture may cause protein denaturation and aggregation, or disruption of protein–protein interactions (Moosic et al., 1980). If it is impossible to avoid freezing, the antigen should be snap-frozen in a dry ice–ethanol bath and stored at − 70°C. The extract should always be centrifuged after thawing to remove any insoluble denatured proteins.

The amount of antiserum required will depend on a number of factors. If the antibody is added in large excess, incubation times may be kept short (30–60 min) and precipitation will often be quantitative. However, it is often not clear how much antibody constitutes an excess, especially in early stages of experimentation. As a rough guide, typical amounts of strong polyclonal antisera for quantitative precipiation of individual membrane antigens from 10^7 cells range from 5–50 μl. Corresponding figures for monoclonal antibodies are in the range 0.1–1.0 μl ascites fluid or serum, and 20–200 μl culture supernatant.

The length of time of incubation at 4°C with the antiserum is not very critical. For strong polyclonal antisera used in excess, 30–60 min is usually adequate. Occasionally, weak or low-affinity antisera may require longer to reach equilibrium. Some authors recommend overnight incubations. There is little evidence that this is necessary if the antibody is in large excess.

Usually, the incubation will be carried out at physiological salt concentration and pH (150 mM salt, pH 7.2–7.4). Occasionally, individual monoclonal antibodies may precipitate spontaneously in the cold (cryoglobulins) or at low ionic strength (euglobulins). Some monoclonal antibodies may fail to bind when seemingly minor changes in pH or salt are made (Herrman and Mescher, 1979).

5.7.2 Precipitation

The extremely small mass of antigen is usually insufficient to allow a precipitate to form. Even if the mass of antigen were sufficient, monoclonal antibodies may not always allow the formation of the three-dimensional lattice which is necessary for precipitation (Chapter 2). It is therefore virtually universal practice to increase the mass of the precipitate by addition of anti-immunoglobulin "second" antibody or protein A-containing staphylococci (Kessler, 1981; Fig. 5.2).

If the first step is mouse antibody, the second step might be goat or rabbit anti-mouse immunoglobulin. If the first antibody is a conventional polyclonal antiserum, it will usually be necessary to add 5–15 μl of second antibody for each microlitre of first antibody. A somewhat higher ratio of second: first antibody may be needed if the first antibody is serum or ascites from hybridoma-bearing mice. If the first antibody is hybridoma supernatant, one might need roughly 20 μl second antibody per millilitre culture fluid. These figures should be regarded as guidelines only, and will vary depending on immunoglobulin concentrations in the first antibody, and the antibody concentration in the second antiserum. Incubation with the second antibody should proceed for at least 1–2 h, and preferably overnight, to allow a large lattice to form.

More recently, it has become common practice to use a solid-phase second step, such as heat-killed and fixed staphylococci (Kessler, 1975, 1976, 1981) or protein A-Sepharose (Pharmacia). The use of solid-phase precipitation has many advantages. The total amount of IgG in the final pellet is much less, resulting in less overloading of polyacrylamide gels and less nonspecific precipitation. Much shorter incubation times are possible, as the binding of immune complexes to staphylococci or protein A-Sepharose is virtually instantaneous. After adding the staphylococci or beads and mixing for a few seconds, washing may be commenced.

The quantity of solid-phase adsorbent required may be calculated from the following information. Typical IgG-binding capacity of staphylococci is 1.0 mg per 100 μl packed bacteria (Johnsson and Kronvall, 1974). The same volume of protein A-Sepharose (Pharmacia) will bind 2 mg IgG. The IgG concentration in immune serum or serum from hybridoma-bearing mice is ∼ 10 mg/ml. Antibody levels in culture fluid are typically 10–100 μg/ml. It is convenient to use a slight excess of bacteria so that one may be sure that all the IgG in solution will bind. The use of an excess of bacteria also avoids the need for individualizing the conditions for each new antibody. Typically, one might use 1.0 μl hybridoma serum followed by 50 μl of a 10% suspension of staphylococci or 25 μl of a 10% suspension of protein A-Sepharose.

It is often necessary to "preclear" the cell lysate by adding staphylococci or protein A-Sepharose, and then removing them prior to adding antibodies, to deplete the antigen-containing solution of molecules which bind non-specifically to the matrix.

Not all forms of IgG bind to protein A (Chapter 4). Even in situations where the major IgG subclass does not bind, surprisingly good recoveries of immune complexes may be found (Kessler, 1975). Alternatively, a "second antibody" which binds protein A may be added, followed by staphylococci. Since the development of a large three-dimensional lattice is not required, an incubation of 1 h at 4°C is adequate for the second antibody.

There are a number of other forms of beads which might be considered for use as solid phase adsorbents for antigen or immune complexes. These include Affigel 10 and Immunobeads (Bio-Rad),Covaspheres (Covalent Technology Corp., 3941 Research Park Drive, Ann Arbor, Michigan) and numerous others. However, these beads have not been widely used for immunoprecipitation, and may exhibit varying degrees of nonspecific binding. As a general rule, beads with significant numbers of charged groups or hydrophobic "spacer arms" are likely to have high levels of nonspecific binding.

5.7.3 Washing

After immune complexes have been bound to the solid phase, unbound material must be washed away. The two main points that require consideration are the amount of washing and the composition of the wash buffer.

Washing is accomplished by addition of a convenient volume of buffer (see below), followed by centrifugation. Staphylococci require centrifugation at 3000–5000 g for 10 min to be pelleted, although lower forces and shorter times may be satisfactory if the bacteria are highly aggregated. Protein A-Sepharose requires less than 400 g for 2–3 min.

Each wash should dilute the soluble phase by a factor of approximately 100-fold. The degree of purification of the desired antigen should be approximately equal to the dilution factor, assuming no loss of antigen or nonspecific binding of contaminants to the solid phase. After two to three washes, the main limiting factor is likely to be nonspecific binding of contaminants, and little is gained by further washing.

It is important to realize that many monoclonal antibodies are of low affinity, and in some cases excessive washing may result in severe loss of antigen. If no antigen is precipitated, the number of washes should be decreased, and the washes should be carried out as rapidly as possible.

Composition of the wash buffer

The earliest studies used isotonic buffers at neutral pH, containing 0.5% Triton X-100 to maintain solubility of membrane proteins. In recent years, it has become apparent that modified wash buffers may lower the nonspecific binding to staphylococci.

Nonspecific binding of staphylococci is highly dependent on pH and salt concentration, suggesting a predominantly electrostatic mechanism. The background is worst at acidic pH and low salt, suggesting that the bacteria act as a cation exchanger. This would be consistent with loss of positive charges during formaldehyde fixation.

Fortunately, alkaline pH tends to stabilize the binding of immunoglobulins to protein A (Ey *et al.*, 1978), and the strength of interaction seems to be independent of salt concentration over a wide range. Good results have been found using a wash buffer consisting of 50 mM Tris-HCl, pH 8.3, with 0.6 M NaCl and 0.5% Triton X-100 (Goding and Herzenberg, 1980). Addition of bovine serum albumin or ovalbumin to the wash buffer may also lower the background by saturating nonspecific protein adsorption sites, but care should be taken to choose materials without protease contamination. Other variations of the wash buffer have been listed by Kessler (1981). It must be emphasized, however, that certain monoclonal antibodies may fail to bind after apparently minor changes (Herrman and Mescher, 1979).

5.7.4 Elution of Antigen from Immune Complexes

Elution of antigen from antibody will generally require denaturing conditions. Many different agents are suitable (MacSween and Eastwood, 1981). The major constraint will usually be the subsequent analytical step.

If analysis is to consist of SDS-polyacrylamide gel electrophoresis, the dry pellet should be resuspended in 30–150 μl SDS sample buffer, placed in a boiling water bath for 1–5 min, and the staphylococci removed by centrifugation. It is usual to load 30–50 μl per gel. The remainder may be kept frozen for subsequent analysis.

If the next step is isoelectric focusing or non-equilibrium pH gradient electrophoresis (NEPHGE), elution is performed by the addition of 200 μl of a buffer containing 9.5 M urea, 2% pH 3–10 Ampholines, 0.5% Triton X-100 and 50 mM dithiothreitol. Heating is both unnecessary and undesirable, as it will result in carbamylation of proteins and artefactual charge heterogeneity (Anderson and Hickman, 1979). The bacteria are removed by centrifugation as previously.

In some cases, it may be desired to maintain as much of the native state of the antigen as possible. If the antigen has a single proteolytic cleavage site, it is sometimes possible to liberate a fragment by gentle proteolysis of the precipitate (Goding, 1980). When different monoclonal antibodies of the same antigen are used, this method may allow the release of individual portions of the antigen and allow topographical mapping (Section 5.9).

5.8 Electrophoretic Methods for Analysis of Protein Antigens

5.8.1 SDS-polyacrylamide Gel Electrophoresis

Polyacrylamide gel electrophoresis in the presence of sodium dodecyl sulphate (SDS-PAGE) is perhaps the most widely used single method of protein analysis. It was introduced by Shapiro *et al.* in 1967. When proteins are heated to 100°C for 2–5 min in the presence of SDS and reducing agents, they unfold and bind $\sim$ 1.4 grams SDS per gram of protein. This corresponds to approximately one SDS molecule for each two amino acids, although the exact mechanism of binding is still poorly understood. There is probably still a considerable degree of secondary structure, and models in which the SDS–protein complexes are shown as elongated rods with negative charges buffered along them are over-simplified. SDS binding imparts a very strong negative charge to the protein, dominating its native charge. Thus, the charge:mass ratio becomes constant for virtually all proteins. Under these conditions, the electrophoretic mobility in acrylamide is inversely proportional to the logarithm of the molecular weight (Weber and Osborne, 1969).

In 1970, Laemmli combined SDS-polyacrylamide gel electrophoresis with the discontinuous ("disc") buffer system of Ornstein (1964) and Davis (1964). The Ornstein–Davis system exploits the differing mobilities of chloride and glycine ions at pH 6.8 to generate a moving boundary that gathers the sample into an extremely narrow band in a short upper "stacking" gel with negligible sieving, prior to separation or "unstacking" of the proteins in the lower resolving gel. The width of the sample entering the resolving gel is thus virtually independent of the initial sample volume. The Laemmli system is

Table 5.2 Solutions for SDS-polyacrylamide gel electrophoresis

Solution	Composition	Recipe
Sample buffer	62 mM Tris-HCl, pH 6.8 0.2% SDS, 50 mM dithiothreitol, 10% glycerol	To 400 ml distilled water, add 3.8 g Trizma base, 50 ml glycerol and 11.5 g SDS. Titrate carefully to pH 6.8. Add 3.9 g dithiothreitol, and make to 500 ml. Store at 4°C.
Lower gel buffer	1.5 M Tris-HCl, pH 8.8, 0.4% SDS	To 900 ml deionised distilled water, add 182 g Trizma base and 4.0 g SDS. Titrate to pH 8.8 with conc. HCl. then make up 1 l. Store at 4°C.
Upper gel buffer	0.5 M Tris-HCl, pH 6.8, 0.4% SDS	To 400 ml deionized distilled water, add 30 g Trizma base and 2.0 g SDS. Titrate to pH 6.8 with conc. HCl, then make up to 500 ml. Store at 4°C.
Running buffer (10X stock)	25 mM Tris, 190 mM glycine pH 8.3, 0.1% SDS when diluted 1:10	To 10 l distilled water, add 303 g Trizma base, 1440 g glycine and 100 g SDS. Do not titrate. Store at room temperature.

30% Acrylamide stock	bis:acrylamide = 1:36	Weigh out 300 g acrylamide, 8.2 g N,N'-methylene-bis-acrylamide. Add deionized distilled water to 1027 ml. Filter through Whatman No. 1 paper, store at 4°C, protected from light. Acrylamide is a neurotoxin; do not breathe dust or allow to touch skin. Do not mouth pipette.
10% Ammonium persulphate		To 5 ml deionized distilled water, add 0.5 g ammonium persulphate. Store at 4°C, and make fresh solution weekly. Store ammonium persulphate crystals in dessicator. Ammonium persulphate concentration is important, and compound is unstable.
N,N,N',N'-tetramethylethylenediamine (TEMED)		Store at 4°C.

thus capable of extremely high resolution. In view of its importance, some of its features will now be described in more detail.

Theory of the discontinuous buffer system

The Ornstein–Davis buffer system works as follows. The sample buffer is Tris-HCl pH 6.8, and is followed by Tris-glycine pH 8.3 in the running buffer. When the current is applied, the negatively charged glycinate ions start to move into the Tris-HCl sample buffer. At pH 6.8, however, glycinate ions have virtually no net charge, because their amino and carboxyl groups are both fully ionized. Glycinate ions therefore trail behind the fully ionized chloride ions, but their tendency to fall behind is counteracted by the fact that this would generate a zone of higher resistance, causing a greater field strength and their consequent acceleration. The result is that a sharp moving boundary is formed, with chloride ions at its leading edge and glycinate at its trailing edge.

Now, the large protein–SDS complexes (and the marker dye bromphenol blue) have a mobility less than that of the small fully ionized chloride ions, but greater than that of the virtually uncharged glycinate ions. Thus, as the moving boundary passes through the sample, proteins and bromphenol blue are gathered into the extremely narrow gap between the chloride and glycinate ions, and enter the resolving gel as a very narrow band, regardless of the initial sample volume. Once the boundary enters the resolving gel, the pH rises to 8.8. The glycinate ions become negatively charged again, and overtake the protein. The proteins then migrate according to their size.

Effect of reduction

If proteins are heated in SDS *without* reducing agents, they usually bind less than 1.4 g SDS per gram of protein (Pitt-Rivers and Impiombato, 1968). This might be expected to cause the proteins to move more slowly than when reduced, due to decreased charge. In practice, unreduced polypeptides that contain intra-chain disulphide bonds generally migrate somewhat more *rapidly* when unreduced (Peterson *et al.*, 1972; Kaufman and Strominger, 1982; Allore and Barker, 1984). This result may be due to a more extended shape when the protein is allowed to unfold after reduction, and to the fact that the mass of the detergent itself causes significant sieving effects (Kubo *et al.*, 1979). Molecular weight estimates of unreduced proteins are therefore generally less reliable than those of reduced proteins. The bands are also often more diffuse in unreduced gels.

Effect of glycosylation

The presence of carbohydrate on glycoproteins causes them to migrate more slowly than the corresponding non-glycosylated protein. If the amount of carbohydrate is small (less than 5% of the protein molecular weight), the mobility of the glycoprotein corresponds approximately to its total molecular weight (protein plus carbohydrate). However, the retardation due to carbohydrate is disproportionately great for low percentage gels, and the molecular weight estimation of glycoproteins on SDS gels is not very accurate.

Effect of modifications of the charge of the protein on mobility in SDS-polyacrylamide gel electrophoresis

To a first approximation, the binding of SDS completely dominates the charge of proteins, and also causes extensive unfolding. However, it is apparent that when the same protein is compared before and after modifications that affect charge but have little or no effect on size, there is often a detectable change in mobility in SDS gels.

For example, when proteins are reduced and then S-carboxymethylated with iodoacetic acid, they acquire one additional negatively charged carboxyl group for each cysteine residue. Bovine serum albumin (M_r 68 000) has 17 cysteine residues (Brown, 1975). When reduced, it runs at 68 000, but after reduction and S-carboxymethylation, it runs at $\sim 80 000$.

Similarly, mouse β_2-microglobulin has two allelic forms (Michaelson *et al.*, 1980; Goding and Walker, 1980). The *a* allele has aspartic acid at position 85, while the *b* allele has alanine. The *a* allele moves a little more slowly on SDS gels. Extensively carbamylated proteins also move more slowly (Anderson and Hickman, 1979), as do phosphorylated proteins (Wegener and Jones, 1984).

Thus the general trend is that, other things being equal, acquisition of increased negative charge causes proteins to migrate a little more slowly in SDS-polyacrylamide gel electrophoresis.

Practical procedure

(1) Assemble apparatus. Add $100 \mu l$ 0.1% bromphenol blue to upper tank.
(2) Select desired acrylamide concentration; prepare gel mixtures according to Table 5.3. Mix well; add ammonium persulphate and TEMED just before pouring.
(3) Pour lower gel; overlay by spraying with a fine mist of 0.1% SDS in

Table 5.3 Recipes for SDS-polyacrylamide gel electrophoresis (1 gel = 16 ml)

M_r range	% acrylamide	Deionized distilled water (ml)	Lower gel buffer (ml)	30% acrylamide (ml)	10% ammonium persulphate[a] (μl)	TEMED (μl)
70 000–200 000	5	9.3	4.0	2.7	40	20
40 000–150 000	7.5	8.0	4.0	4.0	30	15
20 000–100 000	10	6.7	4.0	5.3	25	12.5
10 000–70 000	12.5	5.3	4.0	6.7	20	10
8 000–50 000	15	4.0	4.0	8.0	15	10

[a]Adjust volume to allow polymerization in 30–45 min at room temperature.

water; allow to polymerize (should take 45 min). Leave for a further hour or (preferably) overnight.

(4) Remove liquid by suction.

(5) Pour stacking gel just before use (Table 5.4).

(6) Insert comb; wait for polymerization (20–30 mins).

(7) Remove comb; suck out excess liquid.

(8) Heat sample (in sample buffer) in boiling water bath for 2–5 mins.

(9) Load sample. (Length of sample must be less than length of stacking gel, as measured from bottom of well to main gel.)

(10) Overlay sample with running buffer.

(11) Run at 20 mA, constant current (for 0.8 mm thick gels), with anode (positive) at bottom, until bromophenol blue line reaches bottom (3–4 h).

(12) Turn off current; remove gel.

(13) The procedure for subsequent handling at the gel will depend on whether it is desired to stain for total protein, to process for autoradiography when radioactivity is present, or possibly both. The type of treatment will also depend on the nature of the isotope present (see below).

Staining for total protein

Place the gel into stain (0.1% Coomassie blue in 40% methanol, 10% acetic acid) for at least 1 h. Destain in 12% ethanol, 7% acetic acid.

Sensitivity of total protein staining may be increased approximately 100-fold by silver staining. I recommend the procedure of Morrisey (1981).

Use of intensifying screens for ^{125} and ^{32}P

The use of intensifying screens greatly increases the sensitivity of detection of ^{125}I and ^{32}P (Laskey, 1980, 1984). If the correct combination of film and screen is used, a protein containing 1000 counts/min will give a dark band with overnight exposure. High-energy beta or gamma radiation from the gel passes through the X-ray film and strikes the intensifying screen, causing the release of photons which expose the film. Each disintegration causes the release of multiple photons, resulting in an improvement of sensitivity of 10–30 fold, but the increase is only obtained at − 70°C because of the instability of activated silver halide crystals at higher temperatures (Laskey 1980, 1984). The screens are only effective for ^{32}P, ^{75}Se and ^{125}I, because their disintegration energy is sufficient to penetrate the film and the protective coating of the screen (Fig. 5.3).

It is important to appreciate that the maximum sensitivity is only achieved

Table 5.4 Recipes for stacking gels (1 gel = 5.0 ml)

	Distilled water (ml)	Upper gel buffer (ml)	30% acrylamide (ml)	urea (g)	10% ammonium persulphate (μl)	TEMED (μl)
Without urea	2.95	1.25	0.8	–	15	5
With urea (~ 4 M)	2.3	1.25	0.8	1.35	10	5

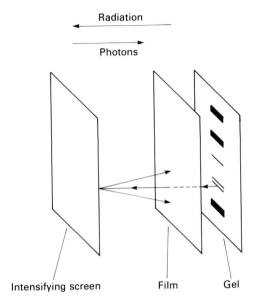

Fig. 5.3 Use of intensifying screens for autoradiography. High-energy beta or gamma radiation from the gel pass through the X-ray film and strike the intensifying screen, causing the release of multiple photons which expose the film. The gel is usually dried before autoradiography. Drying the gel gives a permanent record for long-term storage, and also gives a sharper image.

with certain types of screens and films (Laskey, 1980, 1984). Recommended screens are Dupont Cronex "Lightning Plus" (calcium tungstate), which emit blue light. It is therefore essential to use a blue-sensitive film, such as Agfa Curix RP-2 or Fuji RX. The highest sensitivity is obtained with Kodak X-Omat AR (XAR) film, but this film is considerably more expensive.

If strict linear quantitation is needed, the films should be "pre-flashed" with a brief pulse of light from a domestic photoflash and appropriate filters (Laskey, 1980). Pre-flashing increases the sensitivity of detection of the very weakest signals, but has no effect on stronger signals. If strict linear quantitation is not needed (as is often the case), pre-flashing can be omitted.

Intensifying screens are compatible with Coomassie blue stained gels. Note that screens are completely ineffective for ^{35}S, ^{14}C and ^{3}H, because the energy of these isotopes is too low to penetrate the film and the protective coating of the screen.

Detection of ^{3}H, ^{14}C and ^{35}S by impregnation of the gel with organic scintillants

^{35}S and ^{14}C may be detected by direct autoradiography at room temperature. There is no increase in sensitivity for direct autoradiography at $-70°$C. The gels may be stained with Coomassie blue. *Direct autoradiography cannot be used for ^3H*, because its energy is too low to emerge from the gel or penetrate the gelatin coating of the X-ray film.

The efficiency of detection of weak beta emitters such as ^3H, ^{14}C and ^{35}S is increased by impregnating the gel with organic scintillants which capture the radiation with high efficiency and convert it into photons, which are capable of leaving the gel (Laskey, 1980, 1984). The increase in sensitivity of detection of ^3H is increased enormously. (As mentioned above, direct auto-radiography is useless for ^3H). The increase in sensitivity for ^{14}C and ^{35}S depends on the thickness of the gel. For 0.8 mm gels, the improvement ~ 3 fold, while for thicker gels it is considerably greater.

Several different scintillants are available. In my opinion, the most satis-factory is "Amplify" (Amersham). The gel is simply soaked in "Amplify" for 30 min, placed on Whatman 3 MM paper and immediately dried on a gel drier (80°C). An alternative product is "Enhance" (New England Nuclear), which is used in a similar way, but the fluor must be precipitated in the gel by soaking in water for 30–60 min prior to drying. The fluor used in "Enhance" is rather volatile, and gels must be dried at 60°C rather than the 80°C of most gel driers, to prevent loss by sublimation. In addition, patchy loss or inactivation of the fluor of "Enhance" often causes "graininess" of the image. In my opinion, it is not necessary to fix the proteins in the gel prior to use of either product, providing they are processed as soon as electro-phoresis is finished.

Fluorographic detection of ^3H, ^{35}S and ^{14}C may also be accomplished by impregnating the gel with sodium salicylate (Chamberlain, 1979). The use of salicylate is much more economical than "Amplify" or "Enhance", but the resolution is slightly inferior. The gel is rinsed in distilled water for 10–20 min, then soaked in 1 M sodium salicylate for 30–60 min, and then dried. If the gel has been soaked in a solution containing acid, residual acid may cause partial precipitation of the fluor. If this is encountered, slightly more extensive washing in water prior to salicylate may be needed. The gel may be dried at 80°C.

Regardless of which fluor is used, fluorography is only effective at $-70°C$ or below (Laskey 1980, 1984). As for intensifying screens, linear quantitation requires pre-flashing, although the consequences of not pre-flashing are only apparent for extremely faint bands. Note that the staining of gels with Coomassie blue lowers on the sensitivity when the gels are impregnated with fluor (Higgins and Dahmus, 1982). This is apparently due to quenching of the fluors rather than direct absorption of the blue light, because Coomassie blue does not absorb light significantly at the relevant emission wavelengths of the fluors.

Drying acrylamide gels

To dry the gel, place it on a piece of kitchen plastic ("Glad-Wrap", "Saran-Wrap" or equivalent) smoothed out on bench. Cover with a piece of Whatman 3 MM paper. Trim edges with scissors. Dry on a gel dryer (Bio-Rad model 224 or equivalent) attached to a good water pump or an oil vacuum pump. If the latter is used, a cold trap using dry-ice and ethanol is essential to prevent water from entering the pump and destroying it. Note that once drying has started, if the vacuum is lost, even momentarily, the gel will shatter into hundreds of pieces. Drying takes 30–60 min, depending on the vacuum and gel thickness.

Alternatively, the gel may be dried with virtually no equipment at all, using the following procedure. Take two sheets of cellophane (or Bio-Rad dialysis membranes, cat. no. 165-0922, which are much more expensive), and wet them in water. Lay one sheet onto a glass plate, and lay the gel on top of it, and smooth out any bubbles. Then, lay the second sheet over the gel. Make a "frame" around the edge using thin strips of plastic or wood, held in place with fold-back paper clips (Fig. 5.4). This frame prevents the cellophane from moving as it dries. Leave to dry at room temperature for 24–48 h. Remove clips and strips, and trim cellophane from edges. This procedure is suitable for all forms of fluorography, or for photography. The gels should be stored in a book to prevent curling.

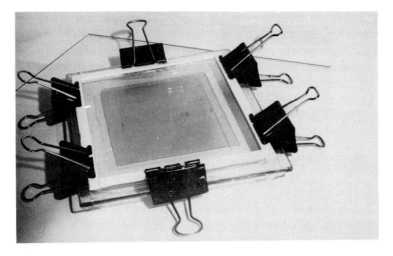

Fig. 5.4 Method of drying acrylamide gels between cellophane sheets. The resulting dried gel is ideal for photography of Coomassie blue or silver-stained proteins, or can be autoradiographed. A similar method has been described by Juang et al. (1984).

Setting up for autoradiography

Identification of the gel and alignment of the autoradiograph with stained bands is facilitated by marking the gel with adhesive labels and writing on them with radioactive ink. Use an ordinary fountain pen (cartridge pens are ideal), and add a few microcuries of any non-volatile ^{14}C or ^{35}S-containing compound to the ink. (Try $1.0\,\mu Ci/ml$).

The "cassettes" used in clinical practice are convenient but very expensive. Equally satisfactory results are obtained by using light-proof plastic bags (or discarded light-proof envelopes of films). Plastic bags may be made by folding and taping black plastic sheeting. It is important that the film be in intimate contact with the gel, or else the image will be blurred. Fold over the top of the envelope, and clamp between two boards with paper clips. The use of steel sheets (1 mm thick) will shield the radiation of ^{125}I.

Acrylamide poisoning

Acrylamide is a neutrotoxin (Kuperman, 1958). It must never be pipetted by mouth, or allowed to contact the skin. Always wear a mask and gloves when weighing the powder.

Use gloves when handling the poured gels. While it is true that the *polymerized* gel is harmless, it is not widely appreciated that "polymerized" gels virtually always contain some unreacted monomer. The gels should therefore be handled with care.

Symptoms of acrylamide poisoning include those of peripheral neuropathy, and in severe cases, brain damage. Symptoms include numbness and weakness in hands, feet, arms or legs, tingling sensation in arms or legs, increased sweating and peeling of skin of hands. In more severe cases, there may be clumsiness, unsteadiness on the feet and difficulties with micturition. Recovery generally occurs after cessation of exposure, but may be very slow (months to years) and may never be complete (McCollister *et al.*, 1964; Garland and Patterson, 1967; Kesson *et al.*, 1977).

5.8.2 Two-dimensional (Charge, Size) Electrophoresis

The combination of isoelectric focusing (IEF) and SDS-PAGE results in an extremely high resolution system which is capable of separating almost all cellular proteins from each other (O'Farrell, 1975). As originally described, the method was only suitable for acidic proteins, but these comprise the great majority of cellular proteins.

A later modification of the technique which allows analysis of basic

Table 5.5 Recipes for isoelectric focusing (IEF) and non-equilibrium pH gradient electrophoresis

Solution	Composition	Recipe
IEF lysis buffer	9.5 M urea, 2% Triton X-100, 2% Ampholines, 50 mM dithiothreitol	28.5 g urea, 1.0 ml Triton X-100, 2.0 ml pH 5–7 Ampholines, 0.5 ml pH 3.5–10 Ampholines, 390 mg dithiothreitol, deionised distilled water to 50 ml. Store in 200 μl aliquots at $-70°C$.
NEPHGE gels (10)	—	2.75 g urea, 0.67 ml 30% acrylamide stock 1.0 ml 10% Triton X-100, 1.0 ml deionized distilled water, 250 μl pH 3.5–10 Ampholines. Mix until *all* urea is dissolved (do not heat). Add 7.0 μl 10% ammonium persulphate and 4.5 μl TEMED. Mix. Pour gels. Overlayer with water until polymerized, then remove water and overlayer with IEF lysis buffer followed by water.
IEF gels (10)	—	Same as NEPHGE gels, except use 200 μl pH 5–7 Ampholines and 50 μl pH 3.5–10 Ampholines.
30% Acrylamide stock	bis:acrylamide = 1:17	28.4 g acrylamide, 1.6 g N,N′-methylene-bis-acrylamide, deionized distilled water to 100 ml. Filter through Whatman No. 1 paper; store at 4°C protected from light.
10% Triton X-100		10 ml Triton X-100 plus 90 ml deionized distilled water. Stir until homogeneous.
Anode solution	10 mM orthophosphoric acid	0.7 ml 85% orthophosphoric acid in 1 l deionized distilled water
Cathode solution	20 mM NaOH	1.6 g NaOH pellets in 2 l deionized distilled water (always make up freshly). (For IEF, boil water for 10 min; add NaOH in 5 ml water, boil again for 5 min. Allow to cool.)

proteins utilizes *non-equilibrium pH gradient electrophoresis* (NEPHGE), in which the separation process is fundamentally very similar to IEF, but the duration is shorter. Acidic proteins become virtually stationary at their isoelectric points. Basic proteins are well resolved from each other, but do not stop moving (O'Farrell *et al.*, 1977). NEPHGE analysis is capable of resolving all but the most acidic and basic cellular proteins. Garrels (1979) has described a number of modifications and refinements to the original system.

Most secretory and externally disposed membrane proteins are glycosylated. When glycoproteins are analysed on two-dimension gels, they do not run as discrete spots, but as fuzz smears or "families" of spots of similar M_r but differing in unitary steps of charge (e.g. Ledbetter *et al.*, 1979; Fig. 5.3). This heterogeneity is at least partly a reflection of their variable carbohydrate content (Ledbetter and Herzenberg, 1979).

Isoelectric focusing (IEF)

Gels are run in 150 mm long, 2 mm inside diameter tubes. The tubes must be soaked in chromic acid, washed, soaked in KOH-saturated ethanol, and rinsed thoroughly in distilled water prior to use.

(1) Cap bottom of tubes with Parafilm. Place on corrugated cardboard around a bottle; hold in place with a rubber band.

(2) Make up gel mixture (Table 5.5), and pour gels, leaving space for sample (20–200 µl) at top. Overlayer with distilled water. After polymerization ($\sim$ 45 min), leave for a further 45 min, then flick out water and overlayer gel with IEF lysis buffer (20 µl) followed by distilled water. Gels may be run immediately, or left for 24 h.

(3) When ready to start, remove overlayer by flicking, and load gels into standard tube gel apparatus, with phosphoric acid in bottom tank (anode).

(4) Overlayer with 20 µl IEF lysis buffer, followed by NaOH cathode solution. Pre-run for 15 min at 200V, 30 min at 300V, and 30 min at 400V (anode at bottom).

(5) Turn off current, remove cathode buffer and overlayer, and apply samples in IEF lysis buffer. Overlayer with a small volume of IEF lysis buffer slightly diluted with water, followed by NaOH cathode solution.

(6) Run at 300–400V (constant voltage) for a total of 4800 volt-hours, then increase voltage to 800V for 1 h.

(7) Turn off power; remove gels from tubes with 1.0 ml tuberculin syringe with plastic tubing attached. Apply presure to bottom of gels; if gels are hard to extrude, try using SDS sample buffer instead of air in syringe.

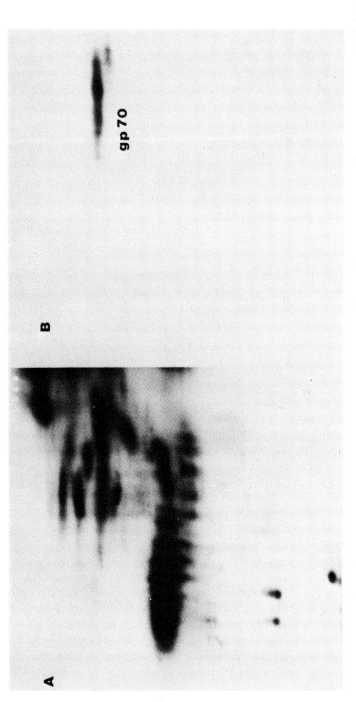

Fig. 5.5 Two-dimensional polyacrylamide gel electrophoresis of membrane proteins of the T-cell lymphoma EL-4. Membrane proteins were radiolabelled with ^{125}I by the lactoperoxidase technique, solubilized in Triton X-100, and analysed by non-equilibrium pH gradient electrophoresis (right to left) followed by SDS-polyacrylamide gel electrophoresis (top to bottom). Acidic proteins lie to the right. A: Whole extract. B: Murine leukaemia virus envelope protein gp 70, isolated from EL-4 cells by immunoprecipitation. Note that gp 70 is visible in the whole extract.

(8) Equilibrate each gel with 5 ml SDS sample buffer (Table 5.2) for 1–2 h, with gentle rocking at room temperature.

(9) Gels may be snap-frozen in SDS sample buffer using a dry ice–ethanol bath any time after 30 min, and equilibration finished just prior to running second dimension.

(10) Pour second dimension SDS gel, preferably on the day prior to use.

(11) Pour stacking gel for second dimension, 30 min before equilibration is due to finish. Use a straight Teflon sheet instead of a comb, or use combs upside-down. While gel is polymerizing, set up a boiling water bath, and tanks for second dimension. Place 0.2 g agarose (Seakem HGT(P)) in 10 ml SDS sample buffer, heat until dissolved.

(12) When stacking gel is polymerized, suck out excess liquid. Insert a small piece of Teflon between the plates at one end, to provide a well for molecular weight standards.

(13) Add 1–2 ml hot agarose, and quickly lie first dimension gel onto stacking gel. Leave agarose to set for 5 min. Remove Teflon piece; load molecular weight standards.

(14) Fill reservoirs with SDS running buffer (Table 5.2). Remove bubbles from under plate. Add 100 μl 0.1% bromphenol blue to upper reservoir.

(15) Run at 20 mA per gel, with anode at bottom, exactly as for one-dimensional gels.

Non-equilibrium pH gradient electrophoresis (NEPHGE)

The gels are set up exactly as for IEF, except that all Ampholines are pH 3.5–10 (Table 5.5), the pre-run is omitted, and the cathode (NaOH) is at the bottom. Gels are run at 500V (constant voltage) for 5 h, and extruded by applying pressure to the lower end. It is not necessary to boil the cathode buffer.

Calibration and alignment of two-dimensional gels

Molecular weight standards for SDS gels are available commercially as kits of purified proteins. Suitable proteins include myosin (200 000); β-galactosidase (116 000), phosphorylase (95 000), bovine serum albumin (68 000), ovalbumin (43 000), beef heart lactate dehydrogenase (30 000), soybean trypsin inhibitor (20 000) and cytochrome C (13 000). Inconsistencies of ~ 10% in molecular weight estimations between laboratories are very common, especially for glycoproteins.

The measurement of isoelectric points is complicated by the fact that pH measurements in the presence of high concentrations of urea may have large errors (O'Farrell, 1975). The published values for isoelectric points of proteins are often in poor agreement. Two published values for the isoelectric point of the human receptor for transferrin differ by almost one pH unit (Bleil and Bretscher, 1982; Felsted and Gupta, 1982).

In many respects, a more useful way to compare results between individual gels is to incorporate well-characterized non-radioactive proteins into the sample as internal standards. Suitable standards include ovalbumin (M_r 43,000; pI = 4.6) and bovine serum albumin (M_r 68 000; pI = 4.9). Commercial isoelectric point standard kits have proven disappointing. The use of carbamylated protein standards (Anderson and Hickman, 1979) holds some promise, and would be especially useful in conjunction with proteins of well-characterized isolectric points. Such kits are now available from Pharmacia ("Carbamylyte" Kits).

Alignment of the autoradiograph with the gel is facilitated by marking the gel with a fountain pen containing ink to which a few microcuries of any non-volatile ^{14}C compound has been added. This also allows identification of each film with the gel and experiment number.

5.8.3 Trouble-shooting Acryalamide Gels

The complexity of acrylamide gel electrophoresis is not very great, but there are a number of things that can go wrong. The following is a list of common problems, and suggestions for their remedy.

Poor polymerization

Polymerization is very temperature-sensitive, and is much slower on cold days. In the winter, the gels may fail to polymerize if the laboratory is not adequately heated. Polymerization is also inhibited by heavy metal ions, especially copper, other impurities in the water or reagents, and contaminants from the glass, combs, spacers and tubing. New combs, spacers and tubing may need "conditioning" by several "dummy" uses until they are ready. Try to avoid contact of acrylamide and buffers with the inserts in the tops of bottles. Gel tubes must be rinsed *very* throroughly after ethanol–KOH or chromic acid cleaning.

Ammonium persulphate is unstable; it is hygroscopic and breaks down in aqueous solution. Store the crystals in a dessicator at room temperature. They should be free-running and dry. I find that a 10% stock solution of ammonium persulphate is sufficiently stable at 4°C for at least 1 week, but many authors make it up fresh each time, or store the solution frozen in small aliquots.

High background on autoradiographs

Include an excess of non-radioactive iodine or amino acid after labelling, to dilute out its specific activity and "compete out" any tendency to stick nonspecifically. If labelling proteins with ^{32}P, there may be background due to DNA or RNA. This may be eliminated by use of appropriate nucleases.

If the whole cell extract or the whole of an *in vitro* translation mix is loaded onto a gel, there will be a large amount of unincorporated isotope. This may diffuse out into the stain, destain or fluor solution, and can then diffuse back into the gel, causing the whole of the outline of the gel to be black. The solution is simple. Wash the gel thoroughly with several changes of destain or water prior to adding the fluor solution or drying.

Diffuse uneven background is often due to stray radiation. Check freezer or lab for radiation. Use 1 mm steel sheets outside gels to shield them during autoradiography.

Coomassie blue staining faint

The dye solution may be used repeatedly, but eventually becomes less effective. This is probably due to contamination with SDS from gels rather than the dye being "used up". The SDS probably competes with the dye for the protein. The solution is to make up fresh dye. To prevent contamination of the dye with SDS, and to achieve more reproducible staining, it may be a good idea to rinse the gel for 10–30 min in destain prior to staining.

Dye precipitates on surface of gel

Filter dye solution through filter paper before use. Dye may precipitate if alcohol or acetic acid is lost by evaporation. Keep gel fully immersed at all times; drying causes precipitation. Precipitates can be removed by gentle wiping with paper tissues; the gel is strengthened and tearing prevented by soaking it in 100% methanol for a few minutes prior to wiping. It is then transferred back into destain.

Poor autoradiographs

There *must* be intimate contact between gel and film. Are the recommendations concerning film, screens and fluors being followed exactly?

Replace developer monthly. The correct safelight for Kodak X-omat AR film is Kodak 6B (cat. no. 1521541). Check for light leaks. Remember that fluorography and intensifying screens only work at $-70°C$.

Sometimes, a coarse granular image occurs when "Enhance" is used. The cause appears to be excessive heating and patchy loss of fluor. This problem is not seen with "Amplify". Gels treated with "Enhance" must be dried at 60°C. Gels treated with "Amplify" can be dried at 80°C.

Wavy bands

Excessive heating is the most likely culprit. Use lower current. Remember that heating is proportional to the *square* of the current or voltage. Other causes include uneven polymerization, which may be caused by inadequate mixing, air bubbles, chemical contaminants, movement or vibration during polymerization, or uneven room heating. Do not use too much agarose to hold first dimension gel in place (no more than 2 ml).

Gels brittle, milky or soft

Inadequate polymerization or incorrect concentration of acrylamide or bis. Milky gels arise from too much bis; soft gels from not enough. Make up new ammonium persulphate.

Double or broad bands in SDS gels; failure of stacking

The length of the sample must be less than the distance between the bottom of the sample well and the top of the resolving gel. Pour a longer stacking gel. Note that the dye marker is always fuzzy in gels with more than 11–12% acrylamide.

If the sharp blue dye marker line does not form, it probably means that one of the buffers is incorrectly made up. Check all buffers, by substitution with new ones if necessary. A conductivity meter is a great help in locating incorrectly made buffers. The pH of the buffers must be correct. Many pH electrodes give large errors with Tris. Is your electrode suitable for Tris? Is the pH meter working properly? Remember that Tris has a large temperature coefficient.

The ionic composition and pH of the sample should be close to that of sample buffer.

Gels run too fast or too slow

Wrong composition or pH of buffer, or (less likely) faulty current or voltage measurement. Check pH of lower gel buffer.

Cracking of gel during drying

Providing the vacuum is not interrupted during drying, 0.8 mm thick gels should not present any difficulties. Thicker gels may crack more easily. The problem may be eased somewhat by soaking the gel in 55% methanol, 2% glycerol overnight after destaining. The gel will shrink considerably, but is then more resistant to cracking. Other possible causes include excessive heat, poor quality acrylamide and loss of vacuum.

Incomplete reduction

Dithiothreitol (DTT) is a better reducing agent than mercaptoethanol, and less susceptible to oxidation by air. Nonetheless, DTT can deteriorate over a period of time, and would probably be best stored in a concentrated solution in aliquots at $-70°C$. Addition of the charged reducing agent sodium thioglycollate (1 mM) to the upper tank buffer of SDS gels provides a reducing environment within the gel during electrophoresis.

Poor isoelectric focusing or NEPHGE

Excessive salt in sample. Acrylic acid contamination in acrylamide (deionize with mixed bed resin such as Bio-Rad AG501-x8). Urea concentration too low. Gel tubes not adequately rinsed before use.

Crumbling of basic end of NEPHGE gels

A common problem. The collapse seems to be due to the combination of high electric field strength (due to depletion of ampholytes) and high pH. See Tanaka (1981) and Tanaka *et al.* (1982) for an interesting discussion. Try deionizing the acrylamide. Wait 5–10 min after turning off current before extruding gel. (Broadening of bands will be negligible). Extrude gently.

First dimension gel falls off during run

This is only a problem if it occurs during the first 30 min of electrophoresis. Try a purer grade of agarose. (I use Seakem HGT(P), which is the strongest available). Try a higher percentage agarose.

Artefactual charge heterogeneity in IEF and
NEPHGE

Heating proteins in urea will result in artefactual charge heterogeneity, due to carbamylation of lysines (Anderson and Hickman, 1979). The urea should be good quality (preferably "ultra-pure"). Urea solutions should be made up freshly or stored at $-70°C$. They must not be heated.

Protein overload

Will result in distorted bands, smearing due to incomplete solubility, and may result in physical weakening of the first dimension gel of two-dimensional systems.

Current rises during IEF or NEPHGE; no focusing

Electrodes are reversed! The anode (positive) must be at the acidic end.

5.8.4 Peptide Mapping by Limited Proteolysis

Proteins often consist of a series of compact and protease-resistant "domains" joined by short amino acid sequences which are more susceptible to proteolysis. Partial proteolytic cleavage of native proteins may therefore yield large fragments which can provide useful information about the structure of the intact molecule.

Frequently, high-resolution electrophoretic analysis of antigens immunoprecipitated by monoclonal antibodies reveals multiple spots. Peptide mapping may help decide whether they represent different modified forms of the same basic sequence (glycosylated, phosphorylated or degraded by protease), or distinct sequences of a multi-subunit structure.

Peptide mapping is often useful in conjunction with monoclonal antibodies, as a way of testing relatedness between two similar proteins. For example, a protein consisting of two apparently identical disulphide-bonded M_r 95 000 polypeptides is precipitated from proliferating human cells by the monoclonal antibody OKT-9. The receptor for transferrin has a similar structure. Peptide maps of the protein bound by OKT-9 were identical to maps of a transferrin-binding protein of the same molecular weight and subunit structure, proving that OKT-9 recognizes the transferrin receptor (Goding and Burns, 1981).

Many proteases are active in the presence of SDS and reducing agents, and even when nonspecific proteases are used to digest partially denatured substrates, the resulting breakdown pattern is highly reproducible and characteristic of each individual protein (Cleveland *et al.*, 1977). SDS-polyacrylamide gel electrophoresis of the proteolytic fragments can therefore be used as a simple and powerful way of assessing relatedness of proteins. Analysis of fragments is usually carried out on one-dimensional gels, although two-dimensional analysis has also been used (Hoh *et al.*, 1979; Whalen *et al.*, 1979).

The enzymes most commonly used include staphylococcal V8 protease (which cleaves at glutamic and aspartic acid), and the more nonspecific proteases papain, chymotrypsin, pronase, subtilisin and thermolysin. Trypsin has been used only rarely, and at very high concentrations, presumably due to inactivation by SDS and reducing agents. In a few cases, even SDS-treated proteins are highly resistant to proteolysis. In these cases, digestion in 4M urea will usually result in adequate cleavage (Handman *et al.*, 1981).

Gullick *et al.* (1981) used monoclonal antibodies to immunoprecipitate proteolytic fragments of the acetylcholine receptor. Interestingly, many fragments were still recognizable by monoclonal antibodies after heating to 100°C in 2% SDS followed by dilution into 0.1% SDS and 0.5% Triton X-100.

Practical procedure

If the polypeptide is available in solution, digestion may be carried out in the liquid phase. If it has been isolated by immunoprecipitation, it may be solublized by heating in SDS sample buffer at 100°C for 2–5 min. The solid phase should be removed by centrifugation, and the solution allowed to cool prior to adding the protease.

Typical conditions are 0.1–50 μg/ml protease at 20°C for 30–90 min, but should be adjusted to give a good range of breakdown products. Digestion may be terminated by heating to 100°C, but this is not essential, as the sample may be loaded immediately onto the analytical gel. If two-dimensional gels are used, it is probably wise to remove the SDS by acetone precipitation (Hager and Burgess, 1980), prior to resuspension in IEF lysis buffer. NEPHGE and IEF gels will tolerate small amounts of SDS, especially if a large excess of Triton X-100 is present.

A very useful variant involves cutting out protein bands from polyacrylamide gels and eluting the protein electrophoretically, together with added protease, into the stacking gel of a 15% SDS gel (Handman *et al.*, 1981; Goding and Burns, 1981; Wiegers and Dernick, 1981; Goding, 1982). The stacking process allows the protease and its substrate to be brought together. The proteins may be stained or radioactive, and the gel spot may be wet (in which case it should be equilibrated with SDS sample buffer) or dried. The presence of "Enhance" scintillant does not seem to influence digestion. If the spot is from a dried gel, it should be placed directly into the sample well of a 15% Laemmli gel and rehydrated for 1 h with sample buffer containing protease (1–50 $\mu g/ml$), then overlaid with running buffer in the usual way. As the bromphenol blue dye approaches the main gel, the current is turned off for 30–90 min, to allow digestion to take place in the stacking gel. Protease-resistant polypeptides may be digested more readily if 4M urea is incorporated into the stacking gel (Handman *et al.*, 1981; Table 5.4).

5.8.5 Peptide Mapping by Chemical Cleavage

In the last few years, the Cleveland peptide mapping system has been adapted to use chemical cleavage rather than proteases. The advantages of chemical cleavage include less need to individualize conditions for each protein, and a wider choice of points of cutting. Perhaps the most useful of these procedures involves N-chlorosuccinimide, which cuts mainly at tryptophan (Lischwe and Ochs, 1982). Tryptophan is uncommon, so fragments are large. In addition, it is one of the most highly conserved amino acids, so the fragmentation tends to emphasize similarities rather than differences.

Other chemical cleavage methods include hydroxylamine, which cuts at asparagine–glycine bonds (Saris *et al.*, 1983); dilute acid, which cuts at aspartyl–proline bonds (Rittenhouse and Marcus, 1984), and cyanogen bromide, which cuts at methionine (Nikodem and Fresco, 1979; Lam and Kasper, 1980; Lonsdale-Eccles *et al.*, 1981).

In the next few sections, I will describe adaptations of these methods that have been derived in my laboratory. The method involving N-chlorosuccinimide is preferred because it gives excellent results virtually every time, and the reagent is inexpensive and of low toxicity. The acid cleavage method generates a very small number of large fragments (sometimes none), and is also extremely simple The cyanogen bromide method involves the use of a very toxic cleavage reagent, and should only be used when all other methods fail.

Peptide mapping with N-chlorosuccinimide (NCS)

(1) On the day of the experiment, make up a solution of acetic acid/urea/water (AUW) by taking 10 ml glacial acetic acid, 10 g urea and 10 ml H_2O.

(2) Identify and cut out desired spot from gel (keep spot as small as possible, preferably less than 2 mm in width).

(3) Rehydrate spot in 3 ml AUW for 10 min at room temperature, with occasional agitation.

(4) Suck out liquid, and remove paper backing.

(5) Transfer slice to fresh 3 ml AUW.

(6) Rotate on vertical wheel 20 min.

(7) Prepare 10 ml AUW containing 15 N-Chlorosuccinimide (20 mg NCS per 10 ml).

(8) Transfer gel slice to 3 ml NCS solution.

(9) Rotate on wheel 20 min at room temperature.

(10) Suck out liquid.

(11) Add 10 ml 1.0 M Tris-HCl, pH 8.0 to neutralize acid.

(12) Rotate on wheel for 10–20 min.

(13) Suck out liquid. Replace with 10 ml reducing SDS sample buffer.

(14) Pour stacking gel onto a 15% SDS gel, with teeth of comb upwards to generate a flat surface. (Better results are obtained with gradient gels, such as 10–15% acrylamide).

(15) Suck out liquid from gel slice. Load slice onto stacking gel, taking care to avoid bubbles under it.

(16) Overlay with sample buffer, then running buffer.

(17) Run the gel in the usual way (no interruption of current).

Peptide mapping by cleavage of aspartyl–proline bonds in dilute acid

The method is based on that of Rittenhouse and Marcus (1984) with slight modifications. These authors used imidazole buffers in the stacking gel and sample buffer, but in my hands Tris-HCl is satisfactory providing the width of the gel slice is kept small.

(1) Cut out slice from dried gel. Rehydrate in 1.5 ml 15 mM HCl in water.

(2) Remove paper backing.

(3) Place sample in a boiling water bath for 10–20 min.

(4) Suck out acid. Replace with 1 ml SDS sample buffer. Change the sample buffer 2–3 times over 30 mins until pH rises to ~ 6.8 (pH paper). (It may be possible to simplify this step).

(5) Go to step 13 of previous procedure.

[It is also possible to cleave polypeptides in wet gels after Coomassie blue staining. Simply add 1 ml destain, place in a boiling water bath for 10–20 mins, then go to step 11 of the previous procedures.]

Peptide mapping by CNBr cleavage

(1) Rehydrate dried gel slice in 70% formic acid (FA) for 1–5 min.

(2) Remove paper (discard).

(3) Equilibrate gel slice in 5 ml FA 20 min on wheel at room temperature (RT).
(4) Make up CNBr in DMF in a screw-cap *glass* vial. (DMF dissolves plastic). (Weigh vial, then add estimated 500 mg CNBr, then tightly cap tube, then weigh again. Then add same number of μl DMF as mg CNBr. This will make a solution of $\sim$ 588 mg/ml).
(5) Take 340 μl CNBr, add to 5 ml FA, containing gel slice. (Final conc. 40 mg/ml).
(6) Rotate on wheel 1.5h at RT.
(7) Remove liquid (*see below for disposal of CNBr waste*).
(8) Wash $\times$ 2 (20 min/wash) in 10 ml 10% acetic acid (or D.W.).
(9) Go to step 11 of the N-chlorosuccinimide procedure.

[CNBr is *extremely toxic*, and must be handled with great care. It should only be handled in a fume hood, and should be stored in a tightly capped bottle within a second bottle, at 4°C or below. Waste containing CNBr should be placed into a large excess of sodium hypochlorite solution for 24 h, prior to disposal.]

5.8.6. "Western" Blots

Immunoprecipitation analysis as described in earlier portions of this chapter has some fundamental limitations. It is seldom possible to know with certainty whether a radioactive band on a gel represents the polypeptide recognised by the antibody, or whether it is precipitated because it is physically attached to another (possibly non-radioactive) molecule which bears the antigenic determinant. A second problem with immunoprecipitation is that it may be difficult to radiolabel the antigen to sufficiently high specific activity.

These problems can sometimes be overcome by probing the proteins with antibodies *after* electrophoretic separation (Burnette, 1981). The procedure is often known as "Western" blotting (reviewed by Gershoni and Palade, 1983). The heterogeneous mixture of non-radioactive proteins is separated by electrophoresis in a polyacrylamide gel, and the proteins eluted electrophoretically by a transverse electric field onto a membrane which binds protein tightly. (Nitrocellulose is now the most popular membrane.) The membrane is then probed with a radioactive antibody, washed and autoradiographed.

Practical procedure

After electrophoresis, the gel is removed from the apparatus and placed in a dish containing 20% methanol in 20 mM Tris base, 150 mM glycine, pH $\sim$ 8. The methanol prevents the gel from shrinking or expanding. A sandwich is then built up, consisting of a perforated Plexiglass support, a porous poly-ethylene sheet (Bel-Art) or Scotch-Brite scouring pads, three sheets of heavy filter paper (Whatman 3MM), the gel, the membrane, more filter paper, a porous pad and a second perforated support sheet (Fig. 5.6). All components should be wetted in buffer, and special care must be taken to avoid trapping air bubbles between the gel and the nitrocellulose membrane. The membrane must not be touched with the fingers at any stage.

The whole assembly is held together with rubber bands, and placed in a tank containing buffer and platinum electrodes. Suitable tanks are available commercially, but they are very expensive. A simple plastic box or bucket would be perfectly adequate and much cheaper.

The current must be applied with the nitrocellulose membrane on the anode side of the gel. The field strength may be determined empirically, but typical values are 0.6–0.8 V/mm for 16–24 h (Burnette, 1981). Excessive current may result in overheating and distorted bands. If possible, transfer should take place in a cold room.

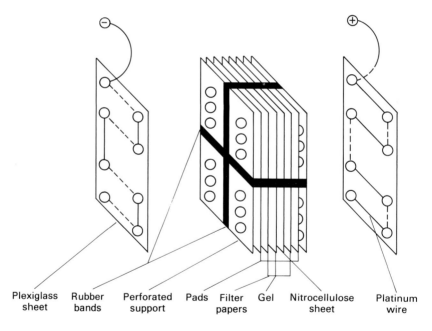

| Plexiglass sheet | Rubber bands | Perforated support | Pads | Filter papers | Gel | Nitrocellulose sheet | Platinum wire |

Fig. 5.6 "Western" blotting. The polyacrylamide gel containing the sample is overlaid with a sheet of nitrocellulose, and sandwiched between filter papers, kitchen scouring pads and perforated Perspex (Plexiglass) supports. The whole sandwich is held together by rubber bands, and submerged in a buffer consisting of 20 mM Tris base, 150 mM glycine and 20% methanol in water. The methanol prevents the gel from shrinking or expanding. An electric field is applied such that the nitrocellulose is on the anode side of the gel. Proteins in the gel are electrophoretically transferred to the nitrocellulose, to which they bind.

Some variability in the efficiency of transfer has been noted. In general, large proteins ($M_r > 100\,000$) may require higher field strengths and longer transfer times. Erickson *et al.* (1982) have shown that the addition of 0.1% SDS to the transfer buffer improves the transfer of high molecular weight proteins. An additional source of variability is the brand and batch of the nitrocellulose. Some brands have been treated with a non-ionic detergent, which inhibits protein binding. Washing the membrane in distilled water or transfer buffer prior to use often improves the transfer.

Following transfer, the membrane is removed from the gel, washed in 150 mM NaCl, 10 mM Tris-HCl, pH 8.0, containing 5% bovine serum albumin (wash buffer), to saturate remaining protein-binding sites. The amounts of bovine serum albumin needed to saturate the membrane are surprisingly large, but attempts to use less seem to result in higher "background". Batteiger *et al.* (1982) have shown that the detergent Tween 20 is equally effective. It is then placed in a dish containing the antibodies (typical concentration 1–50 μg/ml). After 30–60 min, the membrane is removed, washed in buffer, and placed in the same buffer containing 10^5 cpm/ml of ^{125}I-labelled staphylococcal protein A or affinity-purified anti-immunoglobulin. After a further 30–60 min, the membrane is removed, washed extensively, and processed for autoradiography using intensifying screens (Fig. 5.3). If peroxidase-labelled antibody is used, the readout may be made by ELISA (see Gershoni and Palade, 1983).

The potential sensitivity of Western blotting is extremely high. Burnette (1981) has shown that is is easily capable of detecting murine leukemia virus proteins from as few as 1000 cells.

Use of nonfat powdered milk ("BLOTTO") to block nitrocellulose in Western blots

The problem of blocking "nonspecific" binding of proteins to nitrocellulose has already been mentioned. Recently, it has been shown that nonfat powdered milk (Bovine Lacto Transfer Technique Optimizer or "BLOTTO") is a very effective substitute for bovine serum albumin (Johnson *et al.*, 1984). "BLOTTO" consists of 5% (w/v) nonfat powdered milk in PBS plus 0.01% Antifoam A (Sigma) and 0.001% merthiolate as preservative. If the BLOTTO is used on the day that it is made, the merthiolate is unnecessary. The Antifoam is also optional.

Results using "BLOTTO" are generally much better than those using other blockers, and the cost is much less than BSA. It seems likely that this method will become very widely used. BLOTTO may also substitute for BSA in other immunological procedures such as radioimmunoassays.

*Western blots with nonspecific polyclonal
antisera*

If the relevant antigen is available in pure form, or if it has detectable enzymic activity, it is possible to adapt the Western blot so that the antigen may be identified even when the antiserum contains numerous irrelevant antibodies (Muilerman *et al.*, 1982; van der Meer *et al.*, 1983). The gel is run and blotted as usual, and probed with the nonspecific antiserum. Then, instead of anti-immunoglobulin or staphylococcal protein A, it is probed with ^{125}I-labelled pure antigen or the enzyme-containing mixture. After washing, the antigen is detected by autoradiography or by enzyme assay. The fact that antibodies are symmetrical (with two identical binding sites) means that any antibodies that have only one site bound to the nitrocellulose have one "free" site which allows the labelled antigen or enzyme to bind. Only the subpopulation of "specific" antibodies are thus detected.

*Use of Western blots with monoclonal
antibodies*

It is usually considered that proteins which have been heated to 100°C in SDS plus reducing agents are totally denatured. This view may not be strictly correct. It was found that immunoglobulin γ-chains isolated from SDS gels and subjected to limited proteolysis in SDS-containing buffers were cleaved almost exclusively at regions between domains (Goding, 1982). The existence of many additional potential cleavage sites was revealed by the substantially larger number of breakdown products when digestion was performed in 4 M urea.

The conformation of the protein after it has been transferred to nitro-cellulose is not known, nor is the precise mechanism of binding to the membrane. It would seem likely that the protein would be electrophoretically "stripped" of bound SDS, which would continue to the anode. The protein might thus regain more of its native configuration.

It has been known for many years that the reactivity of immune serum made against native proteins is usually much weaker when tested on denatured proteins (Arnon, 1973). However, antisera against the native protein will almost always contain at least some clonal products which recognize the denatured protein, and vice versa. It is this fact that allows the Western technique to function.

In marked contrast to polyclonal antibodies, monoclonal antibodies against the native protein may or may not recognize the denatured product, in an all-or-none fashion. It may be expected that many clones (perhaps the majority) will fail to recognize the denatured antigen. Published information on this point is somewhat sparse, but it would be expected that the Western technique would work much more reliably with polyclonal antibodies.

Goldstein *et al.* (1982) produced a monoclonal antibody against cyto-megalovirus, which detected an M_r 80 000 protein in Western blots. Interest-ingly, the antibody did not precipitate any protein in standard immuno-precipitation system. Whether this failure was due to sensitivity of the imm-une complex to the high salt concentration and reducing agent present in the wash buffer, a lack of methionine residues in the antigen, or other reasons, was not ascertained (see Herrman and Mescher, 1979). It seems unlikely that the antigen was unduly sensitive to denaturation, because the antibodies were capable of binding to antigens that had been fixed in methanol (Goldstein *et al.*, 1982). Barbour *et al.* (1982) were able to use the Western technique with a considerable proportion of monoclonal antibodies against variable proteins of *Borrelia hermsii*. Parham *et al.* (1982) found three out of fifteen mono-clonal anti-HLA antibodies worked O'Connor and Ashman (1982) found four out of five monoclonal anti-*Salmonella* antibodies detected protein in Western blots.

*Recovery of antibody, antigen and re-use of
Western blots*

Antibody may be eluted off the nitrocellulose-immobilized protein by treat-ment with pH 2.2–2.5 glycine-HCl, preferably in the presence of 0.1–1.0% BSA (Erickson *et al.*, 1982; Legocki and Verma, 1981). The nitrocellulose-immobilized protein remains firmly attached to the nitrocellulose. Indeed, it cannot be removed by SDS or deoxycholate, although it is efficiently eluted by Triton X-100, Nonidet P-40 or octyl glycoside (see Lin and Kasamatsu, 1983). The general rule seems to be that non-ionic detergents are good blockers and eluters, while anionic detergents neither block nor elute, perhaps because of repulsion from the negatively charged paper. The bound protein can also sometimes be recovered by dissolving the nitrocellulose in dimethyl sulphoxide, and may be used as antigen for immunization (Knudsen, 1985).

5.9 Topographical Analysis of Proteins by Monoclonal Antibodies

Monoclonal antibodies usually recognize single discrete sites on the surface of protein antigens. They may therefore be used as very precise probes for the topography of proteins.

Some of the principles involved are illustrated by studies on lymphocyte membrane IgD. Murine IgD exhibits genetic polymorphism, first detected by the presence of anti-IgD antibodies in antisera made in C57B1/6 mice against CBA lymphocytes (Goding *et al.*, 1976). Subsequently, monoclonal antibodies were produced against IgD allotypic determinants (Pearson *et al.*, 1977; Oi *et al.*, 1978).

Treatment of intact cells with trypsin abolished the binding of monoclonal antibody 11–6.3, but did not affect the binding of antibody 10–4.22 (Kessler *et al.*, 1979). Antibody 11–6.3 was found to bind to the Fab portion of IgD (Kessler *et al.*, 1979) while antibody 10–4.22 bound to the Fc portion (Goding, 1980). These results proved that IgD was attached to the membrane via its Fc portion.

When the anti-Fc monoclonal antibody was used to immunoprecipitate IgD from detergent lystates of cells, a Fab′ portion of IgD could be released from the precipitates by gentle proteolysis with staphylococcal V8 protease. The Fab′ fragment consisted of an M_r 40 000 heavy chain fragment (Fd′) disulphide-bonded to an intact light chain. Conversely, when antibodies against the Fab portion of IgD were used for immunoprecipitation, a fragment consisting of two disulphide-bonded M_r 20 000 heavy chain fragments was released from the precipitate by V8 protease. These results proved that the only inter-heavy chain disulphide bonds in IgD must reside in the C-terminal 20 000 dalton portion (Goding, 1980). This result was vindicated by subsequent sequence studies (Tucker *et al.*, 1980; Cheng *et al.*, 1982).

Finally, the use of monoclonal antibodies to isolate well-defined large proteolytic fragments of IgD under mild conditions allowed an analysis of their detergent-binding properties. It was found that the Fc portion of membrane IgD bound large amounts of non-ionic detergent, while the Fab did not (Goding, 1980). This result, which was consistent with anchorage of IgD by its Fc portion, strongly suggested that membrane IgD was an intrinsic membrane protein. Sequence data subsequently revealed the presence of an extremely hydrophobic segment of amino acids close to the C-terminus (Cheng *et al.*, 1982).

This type of approach may be used to build up a topographic picture of protein antigens, providing information about their orientation, attachments, ligand binding sites and carbohydrate-attachment sites. It may be particularly useful for membrane proteins, because they may possess topographical "landmarks" such as carbohydrate (always extracellular), covalent lipid (presumably close to the lipid bilayer), and phosphorylated amino acids (always intracellular) (Omary and Trowbridge, 1980, 1981; Schneider *et al.*, 1982).

5.10 Use of Antibodies in the Production and Identification of Cloned DNA Sequences

5.10.1 General Comments

The "average" protein has a molecular weight of about 50 000, and consists of about 500 amino acids. If these were encoded without interruption, a typical gene would be $500 \times 3 = 1500$ base pairs in length. However, the great majority of genes in higher organisms are much larger, because they are made up of discontinuous segments. These segments are termed *exons* and *introns*. Exons are those sequences that remain in mature messenger RNA (mRNA). Introns, or intervening sequences, are removed during RNA maturation. The result is that typical genes are 3–50 kilobases in length, and occasionally as large as 200 kilobases.

The first decision in any cloning experiment is therefore whether to attempt to clone genomic DNA, or DNA copied from mRNA via reverse transcriptase (cDNA). The factors that influence this decision are beyond the scope of this book (see Maniatis *et al.*, 1982, Glover, 1984, for discussion). In brief, genomic cloning requires vectors capable of accepting large DNA inserts (lambda phage or cosmids). The great complexity of genomic DNA means that genomic cloning usually requires screening of larger numbers of clones than may be the case for cDNA cloning. On the other hand, cDNA cloning requires isolation of mRNA, which demands a certain level of technical competence. The cloning of cDNA also requires a larger number of manipulations. In contrast to genomic cloning, the nucleotide sequence of cDNA clones usually allows unambiguous prediction of the full protein sequence, because the introns have been removed.

The cloning strategy for any individual gene should be individualized to exploit whatever special characteristics are available. In the case of cDNA cloning, these might include regultory properties such as differential mRNA expression in various tissues or cells, or response to stimuli.

Antibodies are now widely used in gene cloning. Some examples of cloning strategies involving antibodies are given in the following sections. It must be emphasized that the examples given are by no means exhaustive, and that the most appropriate strategy for any individual gene is best approached on a case by case basis.

5.10.2 Hybrid Selection, in Vitro Translation and Immunoprecipitation

If single-stranded DNA from a pool of cDNA clones is bound to nitro-cellulose, the presence of clones containing sequences complementary to a desired mRNA can be established by the following procedure. Messenger RNA is incubated with the cDNA-coated nitrocellulose. After washing to remove unbound mRNA, the bound mRNA is eluted and used to direct protein synthesis in a cell-free translation system (e.g. reticulocyte lysate). The identity of any candidate polypeptides is then established by immuno-precipitation and gel electrophoresis (see Section 5.7). When a "positive" pool is found, each member of the pool is tested individually, until the desired clone is isolated. The approach is basically "divide and conquer".

This approach was used by Parnes *et al.* (1981), who isolated 9-10S poly-(A)$^+$ mRNA from mouse liver, and showed that it was enriched for sequences which directed the translation of β_2-microglobulin. The mRNA was then used to direct the synthesis of cDNA, which was cloned into the Pst 1 site of the plasmid pBR322. Approximately 100 pools of 14 cDNA clones were made. DNA from each pool was extracted and bound to nitrocellulose membranes. The immobilized DNA was then used to select mRNA encoding β_2-microglobulin, as detected by *in vitro* translation and immuno-precipitation. Four positive pools were found, and the plasmids from these pools tested individually. Screening required hundreds of *in vitro* trans-lations, but succeeded in isolating three non-sibling clones.

This approach is laborious and technically difficult. The amount of screen-ing required may be significantly reduced if the mRNA is unusually small (as in this case), or unusually large. Sucrose gradient centrifugation of the mRNA may give up to 10-fold enrichment in favourable cases (see also Stearne *et al.*, 1985).

5.10.3 Enrichment of Polysomes with Antibodies

A major step forward in the use of antibody for gene cloning was made by Shapiro and Young (1981). These authors isolated polysomes from trypano-somes, incubated them with antibody to the trypanosome variable surface antigen, and passed the complexes over protein A-Sepharose. The unbound complexes were washed through, and the mRNA encoding the trypanosome variable surface antigen eluted with EDTA, which disrupts the structure of ribosomes. The elution was therefore very gentle, and the eluted RNA was highly enriched.

Korman *et al.* (1982) used this approach to isolate mRNA for HLA-DR antigens using a monoclonal antibody, and constructed a cDNA library from it. They screened with ^{32}P cDNA (enriched, and non-enriched as control) and isolated an HLA-DR clone by differential hybridization.

A similar approach was used by Oren and Levine (1983) to isolate a cDNA clone for the p53 tumour antigen, and by Schneider *et al.* (1983), to isolate a cDNA clone encoding the human transferrin receptor. In the latter case, polyclonal antibodies were used.

The approach of antibody-enrichment of polysomes is technically difficult, because the isolation and affinity purification of polysomes must be done without degradation of the mRNA by ribonucleases. In skilled hands, and with a good deal of luck, it can work very well.

5.10.4 Direct Identification of Proteins Expressed in Bacteria

There are now many examples of successful identification of cloned genes by direct analysis of polypeptides synthesized in bacteria. In the majority of cases, polyclonal antibodies were used, and these would be expected to be more likely to detect denatured, non-glycosylated or fragmented proteins (see Chapter 8).

Both plasmid and phage vectors may be used. The approach is feasible for both genomic DNA and cDNA, although the latter has been more common. The big attraction of antibody screening is simplicity. The disadvantages are uncertain reliability and low efficiency.

The approach may fail because the antibodies do not recognize the protein in the form synthesized in bacteria, or because the desired protein is toxic for *E. coli*, or because foreign proteins are often rapidly degraded in *E. coli*. These variables are almost impossible to predict, and depend both on the gene itself and the properties of the host and vector.

The immunological identification of cloned sequences also depends on the cloned sequence being in the correct reading frame (1 in 3 chance) and the correct orientation (1 in 2 chance). Thus, it is to be expected that only about 1 in 6 clones containing the desired sequence will be detected. The problem is most severe for very rare clones. [It must be pointed out that occasionally one finds correct expression of a polypeptide in spite of its being in the "wrong" reading frame. These instances are probably due to internal initiation of protein synthesis.]

Helfman *et al.* (1983) successfully identified cDNA clones encoding tropomyosin using polyclonal rabbit antibodies. They isolated mRNA from chicken stomachs and gizzards, and cloned cDNA into the plasmid pUC8. Bacterial colonies were lysed by suspending nitrocellulose filters in chloroform vapour, and then placing them in a buffer containing 50 mM Tris-HCl, pH 7.5, 10 mM NaCl, 5 mM $MgCl_2$, 3% bovine serum albumin, 1 μg/ml DNAse and 40 μg/ml lysozyme. Filters were washed in saline, and incubated for 1 h with a 1:40 dilution of rabbit anti-tropomyosin antibody in 3% bovine serum albumin. After extensive washing, they were incubated for 1 h with 5 × 10^6 cpm of ^{125}I-labelled anti-rabbit immunoglobulin in 3% bovine serum albumin, washed again, dried and autoradiographed, using intensifying screens. Control experiments showed that less than 1 ng of antigen could be detected.

The pUC8 library contained 9 000 independent clones. This is a very small number, and would only allow detection of very abundant cDNA species. Nonetheless, two positive colonies were detected. One was verified by showing that it directed the synthesis of an M_r 17 000 protein that reacted specifically with anti-tropomyosin antibody on Western blots. The purified plasmid also selected mRNA that, when translated *in vitro*, gave rise to a protein that co-migrated with tropomyosin on two-dimensional gels.

A similar approach was used by Godson *et al.* (1983), who isolated a *Plasmodium knowlesi* circumsporozoite antigen cDNA clone by screening a pBR322 cDNA library with a monoclonal antibody. The antigen was found to have a remarkable repetitive structure that greatly facilitated its detection. The unusual structure of the antigen may have been crucial in its detection, and it would be unwise to assume that the procedure is generally applicable to more common non-repetitive antigens.

More recently, numerous other plasmid expression vectors have been described. These include the vectors of Rüther and Müller-Hill (1983) which allow cloning in all three reading frames, and have the potential for easy enzymic readout. Those of Stanley and Luzio (1984) have the additional advantage that insolubility of the fusion protein protects it against proteolytic breakdown.

The main disadvantage of plasmid vectors is their low cloning efficiency. If the desired mRNA is of low abundance, it may be difficult or impossible to construct a plasmid library of adequate size to ensure detection of the corresponding cDNA clone. The problem of efficiency is exacerbated by the additional requirement for the correct frame and orientation for antibody recognition.

In order to overcome the limited efficiency of plasmid cloning, lambda phage vectors suitable for cDNA have been developed. The *in vitro* packaging of DNA into phage particles allows much higher transformation efficiency (typically 10^6–10^7 clones per μg cDNA).

At the time of writing, the most popular vector is lambda gt11 (see Young *et al.*, 1985). A detailed account of its use is given by Huynh *et al.* (1985). In some cases, expression of the desired polypeptide has been detected with monoclonal antibodies (e.g. Young *et al.*, 1985; Goridis *et al.*, 1985). However, the majority of successful reports of gene isolation with lambda gt11 have used polyclonal antibodies, and it is to be expected that monoclonal antibodies would work only in a minority of cases (see Chapter 8).

The use of antibodies to detect expression of cloned genes in *E. coli* is thus very attractive. Many genes have been cloned using both polyclonal and monoclonal antibodies. However, there have been many unpublished failures, and it would be wrong to think that the system is general. However, the use of expression vectors is currently undergoing rapid development, and it is likely that there will be continuing improvements.

5.10.5 Transfection of Genes for Cell Surface Antigens into Eucaryotic Cells, and Selection of Transformants by Antibody

When certain cells, such as NIH3T3 fibroblasts, are incubated with high molecular weight genomic DNA, a small proportion take up the DNA and express its genes. A few of these cells will integrate the foreign DNA into their own genome, and continue to express it in a stable long-term fashion. The expression of a particular gene may be detected by antibodies against its product. With repeated cycles of transfection, it is possible to isolate individual genes.

Kavathas and Herzenberg (1983) have shown that monoclonal antibodies may be used in conjunction with the fluorescence-activated cell sorter (Section 7.2) to identify and isolate mouse 3T3 fibroblasts which have been transfected with human DNA, and which express human cell surface antigens. Kühn *et al.* (1984) used this type of approach to isolate genomic clones encoding the human transferrin receptor. Transfection into eucaryotic cells has the major advantage that the expressed proteins may be expected to be virtually identical in conformation to the original protein.

Littman *et al.* (1985) have adapted the selection procedure to eliminate the need for a fluorescence-activated cell sorter. Mutant mouse L cells lacking functional thymidine kinase (tk$^-$) were cotransfected with $20\,\mu$g human genomic DNA and $100\,\mu$g cloned thymidine kinase. Transformants with the tk$^+$ phenotype were selected by growth in HAT medium (Section 2.8.1). The resulting colonies were incubated with monoclonal antibodies to the human lymphocyte surface antigen T8, washed, and then exposed to sheep-erythrocytes coated with anti-mouse immunoglobulin. Colonies expressing the T8 gene formed rosettes that were visible to the naked eye, and could be subcultured.

In general, human genes can be detected in mouse DNA by hybridization with the human–specific *Alu* sequences which lie close to or within most human genes. In this case, however, *Alu* sequences were lacking, and the gene for T8 was isolated by subtractive hybridization.

It would seem that the approach of Littman *et al.* should allow the isolation of virtually any heterologous gene that can be transferred and expressed in mouse L cells. In the case of genes for proteins that are not expressed at the cell surface, detection by antibody would require replicating of colonies, because the immunological detection of cytoplasmic antigens requires lysis of the cell.

5.10.6 Purification of Protein by Affinity Chromatography on Monoclonal Antibody, and Use of Synthetic Oligonucleotides Based on Partial Protein Sequences

Under conditions of high salt concentration and low temperature, stable hybrids can be formed between complementary DNA strands that are as short as 14 bases. In "6xSSC" (i.e. $0.9\,$M NaCl, $90\,$mM citrate, pH 7.0), the minimum melting temperature of short hybrids is given by the formula:

$$t_m = (G + C) \times 4° + (A + T) \times 2°C$$

where $(G + C)$ is the total number of G and C, and $(A + T)$ is the total number of A + T residues.

The greater contribution of G or C residues to the stability of the hybrid is explained by the fact that a G–C pair involves three hydrogen bonds, while an A–T pair involves only two.

To give a concrete example, consider the sequence:

ACGTTAGCGAATGA.

$$T_m = 6 \times 4°C + 8 \times 2°C$$

$$= 40°C$$

If such a sequence were used as a probe for isolating a given gene, it would remain hybridized to the desired clone after washing in 6xSSC, providing the temperature was below about 40°C.

How long should an oligonucleotide probe be? Most successful probes are at least 14 bases in length. At this length, a single mismatch will usually cause complete loss of hybridization, especially if the mismatch is towards the middle. With longer probes ($\geqslant$ 25–35 bases), a greater degree of mismatch may be tolerated. Longer probes also have greater specificity (see below).

Let us now consider the use of such a probe to screen a large cDNA library. How selective will a short oligonucleotide probe be? The probability that an individual probe of length n bases will be exactly complementary to a randomly chosen sequence of the same length is 1 in 4^n. In other words, a particular probe of length 14 bases would be exactly complementary to one clone within a hyptothetical library consisting of $4^{14} = 2.7 \times 10^8$ random clones, each of 14 bases in length.

More realistically, if we wished to screen a library of 10^6 clones of average length 1 000 bases, the library would contain the equivalent of $10^6 \times 10^3 \div 14 = 0.71 \times 10^8$ "random" 14 mer sequences, and few if any "false positives" would be expected. On the other hand, a library of 10^7 clones of average length 10 000 bases would contain the equivalent of $10^7 \times 10^4 \div 14 = 7.1 \times 10^9$ random 14 mer sequences, and we would expect $7.1 \times 10^9 \div 2.7 \times 10^8 = 26$ perfectly matched clones to occur by chance alone.

The hypothetical examples given above assumed that we knew the exact sequence needed for probing the library. Unfortunately, the "real-life" situation is more complicated. The degeneracy of the genetic code means that for most amino acids there will be several possible codons, and although some codons are used more often than others, we cannot predict with certainty which will be used in a particular case.

Table 5.6 shows the genetic code in reverse. It may be seen that only two amino acids(methionine and tryptophan) are encoded by single codons.

Table 5.6 Reverse genetic code

		1	2	3	1	2	3
ALA	A	G	C	X			
ARG	R	C	G	X	A	G	A G
ASN	N	A	A	T C			
ASP	D	G	A	T C			
CYS	C	T	G	T C			
GLN	Q	C	A	A G			
GLU	E	G	A	A G			
GLY	G	G	G	X			
HIS	H	C	A	T C			
ILE	I	A	T	CT A			
LEU	L	C	T	X	T	T	A G
LYS	K	A	A	A G			
MET	M	A	T	G			
PHE	F	T	T	T C			
PRO	P	C	C	X			
SER	S	T	C	X	A	G	T C
THR	T	A	C	X			
TRP	W	T	G	G			
TYR	Y	T	A	T C			
VAL	V	G	T	X			

This table displays the genetic code as a function of individual amino acids. The left-hand columns indicate the standard three-letter and one-letter abbreviations for each amino acid. The columns marked 1, 2 and 3 indicate the first, second and third base positions.

It may be seen that only two amino acids (methionine and tryptophan) are encoded by unique codons. Arginine, leucine and serine each have six possible codons. The remaining amino acids have 2–4 possible codons.

X = any base.

Arginine, leucine and serine are each encoded by six possible codons. The remaining amino acids have 2–4 codons.

If we can determine a short stretch of protein sequence, preferably one in which there are five or more amino acids encoded by four or fewer codons, we can design *mixed oligonucleotide probes* that encompass all the possibilities. Such probes may consist of as many as 256 different sequences. The larger the number of sequences in the mixture, the smaller the fraction of radioactivity in the "correct" sequence. This "dilution" of radioactivity is seldom a problem, as the hybridization signals are usually very strong. A more serious problem is that such highly degenerate probes increase the risk of detecting "false positives". Consider the example given earlier (a library of 10^6 clones of average length 1000 bases), and assume that instead of a single probe sequence, 256 different sequences were present. The chance of a perfect match with a randomly occurring 14 mer is increased 256-fold, to 1 in 10^6. Our library still contains 0.71×10^8 "equivalent 14 mer sequences", and thus we can expect 71 "false positives". The desired clone would be only one of these.

The probability of obtaining the correct clone may be greatly increased if two non-overlapping or only slightly overlapping probes are used (see Stearne *et al.*, 1985, for an example). The chances of obtaining the correct clone are also greatly increased by the use of longer probes. Indeed, recent advances in oligonucleotide chemistry have made the synthesis of 30–40 mers routine. Such long probes are quite tolerant of mismatches, and it is feasible to choose arbitrarily the most commonly used codon for all positions. The "long probe" approach has been very successful, and may soon render short mixed probes obsolete (see Ebina *et al.*, 1985).

Screening libraries with oligonucleotide probes is undoubtedly the most reliable method for gene cloning. If the correct protein has been purified, and if sufficient reliable sequence can be obtained, success in cloning is virtually guaranteed. On the negative side, the procedure is laborious, and requires access to both protein sequencing and oligonucleotide synthesis facilities. However, the bulk of the work in sequencing of protein involves the initial purification, and only limited sequence information is needed. The minimum amount of sequence is 5 contiguous amino acids, each of which is encoded by four or fewer codons.

This sequence can be obtained from any part of the protein. In general, the common options would be the amino terminus or a randomly chosen peptide. This choice may be influenced by at least two factors, Firstly, the amino terminus may be "blocked" to sequencing by acetylation, cyclization or other chemical modification. A second problem exists concerning the use of amino terminal sequences for the design of oligonucleotide probes. This region is encoded by the 5′ end of the mRNA, which is often under-represented in cDNA libraries primed with oligo–dT (van Driel *et al.*, 1985). This "3′ bias" may be severe for large mRNA species, but may be overcome by constructing "randomly primed" cDNA libraries (Ebina *et al.*, 1985; van Driel *et al.*, 1985).

Affinity chromatography using monoclonal antibodies may greatly facilitate the protein purification. The special requirements for protein sequencing are described in Section 6.2.5. If further purification is needed, preparative SDS-polyacrylamide gel electrophoresis provides high resolution and recovery. Details of elution of proteins from preparative SDS gels are given in Section 8.2.

5.10.7 Authentication of Clones

In all cloning experiments, it is essential to verify that the correct clone has been obtained. The verification procedure is necessary to eliminate "false positives" arising as a result of ambiguities in the screening procedure, such as those due to unexpected antibody reactivities or highly degenerate oligonucleotide probes. In order to be certain, authentication should be performed using procedures that are independent of those used to obtain the clones in the first place.

Verification could include checks on the presence of hybridizing mRNA of the appropriate size and abundance in expressing cells, but not in non-expressing cells. It could include hybridization of the cloned gene with an independent oligonucleotide probe (e.g. from a different peptide). Correct prediction of amino acid sequences lying outside the region used for design of the probe, or the ability of the cloned gene to transfer expression (detected by monoclonal antibodies), would constitute strong evidence. Finally, the cloned DNA might be transferred into an expression system (e.g. SV–40 based vectors in monkey COS cells) and tested for the ability to direct the synthesis of a protein with the expected biological properties.

References

Allore, R. J. and Barber, B. H. (1984). A recommendation for visualizing disulfide bonding by one-dimensional sodium dodecyl sulfate-polyacrylamide gel electrophoresis. *Anal. Biochem.* **137**, 523–527.

Anderson, N. L. and Hickman, B. J. (1979). Analytical techniques for cell fractionation. XXIV. Isoelectric point standards for two-dimensional electrophoresis. *Anal. Biochem.* **93**, 312–320.

Arnon, R. (1973) Immunochemistry of enzymes. *In* "The Antigens" (M. Sela, ed) Vol. 1, pp 88–159. Academic Press, New York.

Ashani, Y. and Catravas, G. N. (1980). Highly reactive impurities in Triton X-100 and Brij 35: Partial characterization and removal. *Anal. Biochem.* **109**, 55–62.

Barbour, A. G., Tessier, S. L. and Stoenner, H. G. (1982). Variable major proteins of *Borrelia hermsii*. *J. exp. Med.* **156**, 1312–1324.

Barclay, A. N., Letarte-Muirhead, M. and Williams, A. F. (1975). Purification of the Thy-1 molecule from rat brain. *Biochem. J.* **151**, 699–706.

Baron, C. and Thompson, T. E. (1975). Solubilisation of bacterial membrane proteins using alkyl glycosides and dioctanoyl phosphatidylcholine. *Biochim. biophys. Acta* **382**, 276–285.

Batteiger, B., Newhall, W. J. and Jones, R. B. (1982). The use of Tween 20 as a blocking agent in the immunological detection of proteins transferred to nitrocellulose membranes. *J. immunol. Methods* **55**, 297–307.

Bleil, J. D. and Bretscher, M. S. (1982). Transferrin receptor and its recycling in HeLa cells. *EMBO J.* **1**, 351–355.

Bolton, A. E. (1977). "Radioiodination Techniques," (Review 18). Amersham International Limited, Buckinghamshire, England.

Bolton, A. E. and Hunter, W. M. (1973). The labelling of proteins to high specific activity by conjugation to a ^{125}I-containing acylating agent. *Biochem. J.* **133**, 529–538.

Bonner, W. M. and Laskey, R. A. (1974). A film detection method for tritium-labelled proteins and nucleic acids in acrylamide gels. *Eur. J. Biochem.* **46**, 83–88.

Brown, J. R. (1975). Structural origins of mammalian albumin. *Fed. Proc* **35**, 2141–2144.

Burnette, W. N. (1981). "Western Blotting": Electrophoretic transfer of proteins from sodium dodecyl sulfate-polyacrylamide gels to unmodified nitrocellulose and radiographic detection with antibody and radioiodinated protein A. *Anal. Biochem.* **112**, 195–203.

Carrol, R. B., Goldfine, S. M. and Mehero, J. A. (1978). Antiserum to polyacrylamide gel-purified simian virus 40 T antigen. *Virology* **87**, 194–198.

Chamberlain, J. P. (1979). Fluorographic detection of radioactivity in polyacrylamide gels with the water-soluble fluor, sodium salicylate. *Anal. Biochem.* **98**, 132–135.

Cheng, H.-L., Blattner, F. R., Fitzmaurice, L., Mushinski, J. F. and Tucker, P. W. (1982). Structure of genes for membrane and secreted murine IgD heavy chains. *Nature* **296**, 410–415.

Cleveland, D. W., Fischer, S. G., Kirschner, M. W. and Laemmli, U. K. (1977). Peptide mapping by limited proteolysis in sodium dodecyl sulfate and analysis by gel electrophoresis. *J. biol. Chem.* **252**, 1102–1106.

Coligan, J. E., Gates, F. T., Kimball, E. S. and Maloy, W. L. (1983). Radiochemical sequence analysis of biosynthetically labeled proteins. *Meths. Enzymol.* **91**, 413–434.

Cooper, J. A. and Hunter, T. (1981). Changes in protein phosphorylation in Rous sarcoma virus-transformed chicken embryo cells. *Molec. Cell. Biol.* **1**, 165–178.

Davis, B. J. (1964). Disc electrophoresis. II. Method and application to human serum proteins. *Ann. N.Y. Acad. Sci.* **121**, 404–427.

Ebina, Y., Ellis, L., Jarnagin, K., Edery, M., Graf, L., Clausner, E., Ou, J., Masiarz, F., Kan, Y. W., Goldfine, I. D., Roth, R. A. and Rutter, W. J., 1985. The human insulin receptor cDNA: The structural basis for hormone-activated transmembrane signalling. *Cell* **40**, 747–758.

Engelman, D. M. and Zaccai, G. (1980). Bacteriohodopsin as an inside-out protein. *Proc. natn. Acad. Sci. U.S.A.* **77**, 5894–5898.

Erickson, P. F., Minier, L. N. and Lasher, R. S. (1982). Quantitative electrophoretic transfer of polypeptides from SDS polyacrylamide gels to nitrocellulose sheets: a method for their re-use in immunoautoradiographic detection of antigens. *J. immunol. Methods* **51**, 241–249.

Evans, E. A. (1976). "Self-decomposition of Radiochemicals." (Review 16). Amersham Corporation, Illinois.

Ey, P. L., Prowse, S. J. and Jenkin, C. R. (1978). Isolation of pure IgG1, IgG2a and IgG2b immunoglobulins from mouse serum protein A-Sepharose. *Immunochemistry* **15**, 429–436.

Feizi, T. (1981). Carbohydrate differentiation antigens. *Trends biochem. Sci.* **6**, 333–335.

Felsted, R. L. and Gupta, S. K. (1982). A comparison of K-562 and HL-60 human leukemic cell surface membrane proteins by two-dimensional electrophoresis. *J. biol. Chem.* **257**, 13211–13217.

Fraker, P. J. and Speck, J. C. (1978). Protein and cell membrane iodinations with a sparingly soluble chloroamide, 1,3,4,6-tetrachloro-3α, 6α-diphenylglycoluril. *Biochem. biophys. Res. Commun.* **80**, 849–857.

Gahmberg, C. G. and Hakomori, S. (1973). External labeling of cell surface galactose and galactosamine in glycolipid and glycoprotein of human erythrocytes. *J. biol. Chem.* **248**, 4311–4317.

Gahmberg, C. G. and Andersson, L. C. (1977). Selective radioactive labeling of cell surface sialoglycoproteins by periodate-tritiated borohydride. *J. biol. Chem.* **252**, 5888–5894.

Gahmberg, C. G., Häyry, P. and Andersson L. C. (1976). Characterization of surface glycoproteins of mouse lymphoid cells. *J. Cell. Biol.* **68**, 642–653.

Garland, T. O. and Patterson, M. W. H. (1967). Six cases of acrylamide poisoning. *Brit. Med. J.* **4**, 134–138.

Garrels, J. I. (1979). Two-dimensional gel electrophoresis and computer analysis of proteins synthesized by clonal cell lines. *J. biol. Chem.* **254**, 7961–7977.

Geoghegan, K. F., Dallas, J. L. and Feeney, R. E. (1980). Periodate inactivation of ovotransferrin and human serum transferrin. *J. biol. Chem.* **255**, 11429–11434.

George, S. and Schenck, J. R. (1983). Thiocyanate inhibition of protein iodination by the chloramine-T method and a rapid method for measurement of low levels of thiocyanate. *Anal. Biochem.* **130**, 416–419.

Gershoni, J. M. and Palade G. E. (1983). Protein blotting: principles and applications. *Anal. Biochem.* **131**, 1–15.

Glover, D. M., (1984). "Gene Cloning: The Mechanics of DNA Manipulation." Chapman and Hall, London and New York.

Goding, J. W. (1980). Structure studies of murine lymphocyte surface IgD. *J. Immunol.* **124**, 2082–2088.

Goding, J. W. (1982). Asymmetrical surface IgG on MOPC-21 plasmacytoma cells contains one membrane heavy chain and one secretory heavy chain. *J. Immunol.* **128**, 2416–2421.

Goding, J. W. and Herzenberg, L. A. (1980). Biosynthesis of lymphocyte surface IgD in the mouse. *J. Immunol.* **124**, 2540–2547.

Goding, J. W. and Walker, I. D. (1980). Allelic forms of β_2-microglobulin in the mouse. *Proc. natn. Acad. Sci. U.S.A.* **77**, 7395–7399.

Goding, J. W. and Burns, G. F. (1981). Monoclonal antibody OKT-9 recognizes the receptor for transferrin on human acute lymphocytic leukemia cells. *J. Immunol.* **127**, 1256–1258.

Goding, J. W. and Harris, A. W. (1981). Subunit structure of cell surface proteins: Disulfide bonding in antigen receptors, Ly-2/3 antigens and transferrin receptors of murine T and B lymphocytes. *Proc. natn. Acad. Sci. U.S.A.* **78**, 4530–4534.

Goding, J. W. and Shen, F.-W. (1982). Structure of the murine plasma cell alloantigen PC-1: Comparison with the receptor for transferrin. *J. Immunol.* **129**, 2636–2640.

Goding, J. W., Warr, J. W. and Warner, N. L. (1976). Genetic polymorphism of IgD-like cell surface immunoglobulin in the mouse. *Proc. natn. Acad. Sci. U.S.A.* **73**, 1305–1309.

Godson, G. N., Ellis, J., Svec, P., Schlesinger, D. H. and Nussenzwig, V. (1983). Identification and chemical synthesis of a tandemly repeated immunogenic region of *Plasmodium knowlesi* circumsporozoite protein. *Nature* **305**, 29–33.

Goldstein, L. C., McDougall, J., Hackman, R., Meyers, J. D., Thomas, E. D. and Nowinski, R. C. (1982). Monoclonal antibodies to cytomegalovirus: rapid identification of clinical isolates and preliminary use in diagnosis of cytomegalovirus pneumonia. *Infect. Immun.* **38**, 273–281.

Gonenne, A. and Ernst, R. (1978). Solubilization of membrane proteins by sulfobetaines, novel zwitterionic detergents. *Anal. Biochem.* **87**, 28–38.

Goridis, C., Hirn, M., Santoni, M. J., Gennarini, G., Deagostini-Bazin, H., Jordan, B. R., Kiefer, M. and Steinmetz, M. (1985). Isolation of mouse N-CAM-related cDNA: detection and cloning using monoclonal antibodies. *EMBO. J.* **4**, 631–635.

Granger, B. L. and Lazarides, E. (1979). Desmin and vimentin coexist at the periphery of the myofibril Z disc. *Cell* **18**, 1053–1063.

Greenwood, F. C., Hunter, W. M. and Glover, J. S. (1963). The preparation of ^{131}I-labelled human growth hormone of high specific radioactivity. *Biochem. J.* **89**, 114–123.

Gullick, W. J., Tzartos, S. and Lindstrom, J. (1981). Monoclonal antibodies as probes of acetylcholine receptor structure. I. Peptide mapping. *Biochemistry* **20**, 2173–2180.

Gutman, G. A., Warner, N. L., Harris, A. W. and Bowles, A. (1978). Use of [^{75}Se]selenomethionine in immunoglobulin biosynthetic studies. *J. immunol. Methods* **21**, 101–109.

Hager, D. A. and Burgess, R. R. (1980). Elution of proteins from sodium dodecyl sulfate-polyacrylamide gels, removal of sodium dodecyl sulfate, and renaturation of enzymatic activity: results with sigma subunit of Escherichia coli RNA polymerase, wheat germ topoisomerase and other enzymes. *Anal. Biochem.* **109**, 76–86.

Hakomori, S. I. (1981). Glyhcosphingolipids in cellular interaction, differentiation and oncogenesis. *A. Rev. Biochem.* **50**, 733–764.

Hakomori, S. (1984). Glycosphingolipids as differentiation-dependent, tumor-associated markers and as regulators of cell proliferation. *Trends biochem. Sci.* **9**, 453–458.

Hakomori, S. and Kannagi, R. (1986). Carbohydrate antigens in glycolipids and glycoproteins. *In* "Handbook of Experimental Immunology" (D. M. Weir, L. A. Herzenberg, C. C. Blackwell and L. A. Herzenberg, eds) 4th ed. Blackwell, Edinburgh (**5**, 329–336).

Handman, E. and Goding, J. W. (1985). The *Leishmania* receptor for macrophages is a lipid-containing glycoconjugate. *EMBO J.* (in press).

Handman, E., Mitchell, G. F. and Goding, J. W. (1981). Identification and characterization of protein antigens of Leishmania tropica isolates. *J. Immunol.* **126**, 508–512.

Handman, E., Greenblatt, C. L. and Goding, J. W. (1984). An amphipathic sulphated glycoconjugate of Leishmania: Characterization with monoclonal antibodies. *EMBO J.* **3**, 2301–2306.

Handman, E., and Jarvis, H. M. (1985). Nitrocellulose-based assays for the detection of glycolipids and other antigens: Mechanism of binding to nitrocellulose. *J. immunol. Methods* **83**, 113–123.

Harford, J. (1984). An artefact explains the apparent association of the transferrin receptor with a *ras* gene product. *Nature* **311**, 673–675.

Hayman, M. J. and Crumpton, M. J. (1972). Isolation of glycoproteins from pig lymphocyte plasma membrane using *Lens culinaris* phytohaemagglutinin. *Biochem. biophys. Res. Commun.* **47**, 923–930.

Helenius, A. and Simons, K. (1975). Solubilization of membranes by detergents. *Biochem. biophys. Acta* **415**, 29–79.

Helenius, A., McCaslin, D. R., Fries, E. and Tanford, C. (1979). Properties of detergents. *Meth. Enzymol.* **56**, 734–749.

Helfman, D. M., Feramisco, J. R., Fiddes, J. C., Thomas, G. P. and Hughes, S. H. (1983). Identification of clones that encode chicken tropomyosin by direct immunological screening of a cDNA expression library. *Proc. natn. Acad. Sci. U.S.A.* **80**, 31–35.

Herrmann, S. H. and Mescher, M. F. (1979). Purification of the H-2K^k molecule of the murine major histocompatibility complex. *J. biol. Chem.* **254**, 8713–8716.

Herrmann, S. H., Chow, C. M. and Mescher, M. F. (1982). Proteolytic modifications of the carboxyl-terminal region of H-2K^k. *J. biol. Chem.* **257**, 14181–14186.

Higgins, R. C. and Dahmus, M. E. (1982). Tritium/PPO gel fluorographic efficiency is reduced by Coomassie blue staining. *Electrophoresis* **3**, 214–216.

Hjelmeland, L. M. (1980). A nondenaturing zwitterionic detergent for membrane biochemistry: design and synthesis. *Proc. natn. Acad. Sci. U.S.A.* **77**, 6368–6370.

Hoh, J. F. Y., Yeoh, G. P. S., Thomas, M. A. W. and Higginbotham, L. (1979). Structural differences in the heavy chains of rat ventricular myosin isoenzymes. *FEBS Lett.* **97**, 330–334.

Holloway, P. W. (1973). A simple procedure for removal of Triton X-100 from protein samples. *Anal. Biochem.* **53**, 304–308.

Hubbard, A. L. and Cohn, Z. A. (1975). Externally disposed plasma membrane proteins. I. Enzymatic iodination of mouse L cells. *J. Cell. Biol.* **64**, 438–460.

Huynh, T. V., Young, R. A. and Davis, R. W. (1985). Construction and screening cDNA libraries in λgt10 and λgt11. *In*: "DNA Cloning: A Practical Approach." Vol. 1, pp 49–78. IRL Press, Oxford and Washington, D.C.

Johnson, D. A., Gautsch, J. W., Sportsman, J. R. and Elder, J. H, (1984). Improved technique utilizing nonfat dry milk for analysis of proteins and nucleic acids transferred to nitrocellulose. *Gene Anal. Techniques* **1**, 3–8.

Johnsson, S. and Kronvall, G. (1974). The use of protein A-containing *Staphylococcus aureus* as a solid phase anti-IgG reagent in radioimmunoassays as exemplified in the quantitation of α-fetoprotein in normal human adult serum. *Eur. J. Immunol.* **4**, 29–33.

Juang, R-H., Chang, Y-D., Sung, H-Y. and Su, J-C. (1984). Oven-drying method for polyacrylamide gel slab packed in cellophane sandwich. *Anal. Biochem.* **141**, 348–350.

Kaufman, J. F. and Strominger, J. L. (1982). HLA-DR light chain has a polymorphic N-terminal region and a conserved immunoglobulin-like C-terminal region. *Nature* **297**, 694–697.

Kavathas, P. and Herzenberg, L. A. (1983). Stable transformation of mouse L cells for human membrane T cell differentiation antigens, HLA and β_2-microglobulin: selection by fluorescence-activated cell sorting. *Proc. natn. Acad. Sci. U.S.A.* **80**, 524–528.

Kessler, S. W. (1975). Rapid isolation of antigens from cells with a staphylococcal protein A-antibody adsorbent: Parameters of the interaction of antibody-antigen complexes with protein A. *J. Immunol.* **115**, 1617–1624.

Kessler, S. W. (1976). Cell membrane antigen isolation with the staphylococcal protein A-antibody adsorbent. *J. Immunol.* **117**, 1482–1490.

Kessler, S. W. (1981). Use of protein A-bearing staphylococci for immunoprecipitation and isolation of antigens from cells. *Meth. Enzymol.* **73**, 442–459.

Kessler, S. W., Woods, V. L., Finkelman, F. D. and Scher, I. (1979). Membrane orientation and location of multiple and distinct allotypic determinants of mouse lymphocyte IgD. *J. Immunol.* **123**, 2772–2778.

Kesson, C. M., Baird, A. W. and Lawson, D. H. (1977). Acrylamide poisoning. *Postgrad. Med. J.* **53**, 16–17.

Knudson, K. (1985). Proteins transferred to nitrocellulose for use as immunogens. *Anal. Biochem.* **147**, 285–288.

Korman, A. J., Knudsen, P. J., Kaufman, J. F. and Strominger, J. L. (1982). cDNA clones for the heavy chain of HLA-DR antigens obtained after immunopurification of polysomes by monoclonal antibody. *Proc. natn. Acad. Sci. U.S.A.* **79**, 1844–1848.

Kubo, K., Isemura, T. and Takagi, T. (1979). Electrophoretic behaviour of micellar and monomeric sodium dodecyl sulfate in polyacrylamide gel electrophoresis with reference to those of SDS-protein complexes. *Anal. Biochem.* **92**, 243–247.

Kühn, L. C., McClelland, A. and Ruddle, F. H. (1984). Gene transfer, expression, and molecular cloning of the human transferrin receptor gene. *Cell* **37**, 95–103.

Kuperman, A. S. (1958). Effects of acrylamide on the central nervous system of the cat. *J. Pharmacol. exp. Therap.* **123**, 180–192.

Laemmli, U. K. (1970). Cleavage of structural proteins during the assembly of the head of the bacteriophage T4. *Nature* **227**, 680–685.

Lam, K. S. and Kasper, C. B. (1980). Sequence homology analysis of a heterogeneous protein population by chemical and enzymic digestion using a two-dimensional sodium dodecyl sulfate-polyacrylamide gel system. *Anal. Biochem.* **108**, 220–226.

Lane, D. P. and Robbins, A. K. (1978). An immunochemical investigation of SV40 T antigens. I. Production, properties and specificity of a rabbit antibody to purified simian virus 40 large-T antigen. *Virology* **87**, 182–193.

Laskey, R. A. (1980). The use of intensifying screens or organic scintillators for visualizing radioactive molecules resolved by gel electrophoresis. *Meth. Enzymol.* **65**, 363–371.

Laskey, R. A. (1984). "Radioisotype Detection by Fluorography and Intensifying Screens." (Review 23). Amersham International Ltd. Buckinghamshire, England.

Layton, J. E. (1980). Anti-carbohydrate activity of T cell-reactive chicken anti-mouse immunoglobulin antibodies. *J. Immunol.* **125**, 1993–1997.

Ledbetter, J. A. and Herzenberg, L. A. (1979). Xenogenic monoclonal antibodies to mouse lymphoid differentiation antigens. *Immunol. Rev.* **47**, 63–90.

Ledbetter, J. A., Goding, J. W., Tsu, T. T. and Herzenberg, L. A. (1979). A new mouse lymphoid alloantigen (Lgp100) recognized by a monoclonal rat antibody. *Immunogenetics* **8**, 347–360.

Lee, S.-K., Singh, J. and Taylor, R. B. (1975). Subclasses of T cells with different sensitivities to cytotoxic antibody in the presence of anesthetics. *Eur. J. Immunol.* **5**, 259–262.

Legochi, R. P. and Verma, D. P. S. (1981). Multiple immunoreplica technique: screening for specific proteins with a series of different antibodies using one polyacrylamide gel. *Anal. Biochem.* **111**, 385–392.

Lin, W. and Kasamatsu, H. (1983). On the electrotransfer of polypeptides from gels to nitrocellulose membranes. *Anal. Biochem.* **128**, 302–311.

Lischwe, M. A. and Ochs, D. (1982). A new method for partial peptide mapping using N-chlorosuccinimide/urea and peptide silver staining in sodium dodecyl sulfate-polyacrylamide gels. *Anal. Biochem.* **127**, 453–457.

Littman, D. R., Thomas, Y., Maddon, P. J., Chess, L. and Axel, R., (1985). The isolation and sequence of a gene encoding T8: A molecule defining functional classes of T lymphocytes. *Cell* **40**, 237–246.

Lonsdale-Eccles, J. D., Lyndley, A. M. and Dale, B A. (1981). Cyanogen bromide cleavage of proteins in sodium dodecyl sulphate/polyacrylamide gels. *Biochem. J.* **197**, 591–597.

McCollister, D. D., Oyen, F. and Rowe, V. K. (1964). Toxicology of acrylamide. *Toxicol. Appl. Pharmacol.* **6**, 172–181.

MacSween, J. M. and Eastwood, S. L. (1981). Recovery of antigen from staphylococcal protein A-antibody adsorbents. *Meth. Enzymol.* **73**, 459–471.

Maniatis, T., Fritsch, E. F., and Sambrook, J. (1982). "Molecular Cloning: A Laboratory Manual." Cold Spring Harbour Laboratory, New York.

Marchalonis, J. J. (1969). An enzymic method for the trace iodination of immunoglobulins and other proteins. *Biochem. J.* **113**, 299–305.

Marchalonis, J. J., Cone, R. E. and Santer, V. (1971). Enzymic iodination: A probe for cell surface proteins of normal and neoplastic lymphocytes. *Biochem. J.* **124**, 921–927.

Markwell, M. A. K. (1982). A new solid-state reagent to iodinate proteins. I. Conditions for the efficient labelling of antiserum. *Anal. Biochem.* **125**, 427–432.

Markwell, M. A. K. and Fox, C. F. (1978). Surface-specific iodination of membrane proteins of viruses and eucaryotic cells using 1,3,4,6-tetrachloro-3α,6α-diphenylglycoluril. *Biochemistry* **17**, 4807–4817.

Melchers, F. (1973). Synthesis, surface deposition and secretion of immunoglobulin M in bone marrow-derived lymphocytes before and after mitogenic stimulation. *Transplant. Rev.* **14**, 76–130.

Michaelson, J., Rothenberg, E. and Boyse, E. A. (1980). Genetic polymorphism of murine β_2-microglobulin detected biochemically. *Immunogenetics* **11**, 93–95.

Milstein, C. and Lennox, E. (1980). The use of monoclonal antibody techniques in the study of developing cell surfaces. *Curr. Top. dev. Biol.* **14**, 1–32.

Moosic, J. P., Nilson, A., Hämmerling, G. J. and McKean, D. J. (1980). Biochemical characterization of Ia antigens. I. Characterization of the 31K polypeptide associated with I-A subregion Ia antigens. *J. Immunol.* **125**, 1463–1469.

Morrissey, J. H. (1981). Silver stain for proteins in polyacrylamide gels: A modified procedure with enhanced uniform sensitivity. *Anal. Biochem.* **117**, 307–310.

Muilerman, H. G., ter Hart, H. G. J. and Van Dijk, W. V. (1982). Specific detection of inactive enzyme protein after polyacrylamide gel electrophoresis by a new enzyme-immunoassay method using unspecific antiserum and partially purified active enzyme: application to rat liver phosphodiesterase I. *Anal. Biochem.* **120**, 46–51.

Nikodem, V. and Fresco, J. R. (1979). Protein fingerprinting by SDS-gel electrophoresis after partial fragmentation with CNBr. *Anal. Biochem.* **97**, 382–386.

Nussenzweig, M. C., Steinman, R. M., Witmer, M. D. and Gutchinov, B. (1982). A monoclonal antibody specific for mouse dendritic cells. *Proc. natn. Acad. Sci. U.S.A.* **79**, 161–165.

O'Connor, C. G. and Ashman, L. K. (1982). Application of the nitrocellulose transfer technique and alkaline phosphatase conjugated anti-immunoglobulin for determination of the specificity of monoclonal antibodies to protein mixtures. *J. immunol. Methods* **54**, 267–271.

O'Farrell, P. H. (1975). High resolution two-dimensional electrophoresis of proteins. *J. biol. Chem.* **250**, 4007–4021.

O'Farrell, P. Z., Goodman, H. M. and O'Farrell, P. H. (1977). High resolution two-dimensional electrophoresis of basic as well as acidic proteins. *Cell* **12**, 1133–1142.

Oi, V. T., Jones, P. P., Goding, J. W., Herzenberg, L. A. and Herzenberg, L. A. (1978). Properties of monoclonal antibodies to mouse Ig allotypes, H-2, and Ia antigens. *Curr. Topics Microbiol. Immunol.* **81**, 115–129.

Omary, M. B. and Trowbridge, I. S. (1980). Disposition of T200 glycoprotein in the plasma membrane of a murine lymphoma line. *J. biol. Chem.* **255**, 1662–1669.

Omary, M. B. and Trowbridge, I. S. (1981). Biosynthesis of the human transferrin receptor in cultured cells. *J. biol. Chem.* **256**, 12888–12892.

Oren, M. and Levine, A. J. (1983). Molecular cloning of a cDNA specific for the murine p53 cellular tumor antigen. *Proc. natn. Acad. Sci. U.S.A.* **80**, 56–59.

Ornstein, L. (1964). Disc electrophoresis I. Background and theory. *Ann. N.Y. Acad. Sci.* **121**, 321–349.

Parham, P., Androlewicz, M. J., Brodsky, F. M., Holmes, N. J. and Ways, J. P. (1982). Monoclonal antibodies: purification fragmentation and application to structural and functional studies of class I MHC antigens. *J. immunol. Methods* **53**, 133–173.

Parnes, J. R., Velan, B., Felsenfeld, A., Ramanathan, L., Ferrini, U., Apella, E. and Seidman, J. G. (1981). Mouse β_2-microglobulin cDNA clones: A screening procedure for cDNA clones corresponding to rare mRNAs. *Proc. natn. Acad. Sci. U.S.A.* **78**, 2253–2257.

Pearson, T., Galfrè, G., Ziegler, A. and Milstein, C. (1977). A myeloma hybrid producing antibody specific for an allotypic determinant on "IgD-like" molecules of the mouse. *Eur. J. Immunol.* **7**, 684–690.

Peterson, P. A., Cunningham, B. A., Berggard, I. and Edelman, G. M. (1972). β_2-microglobulin — a free immunoglobulin domain. *Proc. natn. Acad. Sci. U.S.A.* **69**, 1697–1702.

Phillips, D. R. and Morrison, M. (1970). The arrangement of proteins in the human crythrocyte membrane. *Biochem. biophys. Res. Commun.* **40**, 284–289.

Pitt-Rivers, R. and Impiombato, F. S. A. (1968). The binding of sodium dodecyl sulfate to various proteins. *Biochem. J.* **109**, 825–830.

Radke, K. and Martin, G. S. (1979). Transformation by Rous sarcoma virus: effects of src expression on the synthesis and phosphorylation of cellular polypeptides. *Proc. natn. Acad. Sci. U.S.A.* **76**, 5212–5216.

Radke, K., Gilmore, T. and Martin, G. S. (1980). Transformation of Rous sarcoma virus: a cellular substrate for transformation-specific protein phosphorylation contains phosphotyrosine. *Cell* **21**, 821–828.

Reinherz, E. L., Kung, P. C., Goldstein, G., Levey, R. H. and Schlossman, S. F. (1980). Discrete stages of human intrathymic differentiation: analysis of normal thymocytes and leukemic lymphoblasts of T lineage. *Proc. natn. Acad. Sci. U.S.A.* **77**, 1588–1592.

Rittenhouse, J. and Marcus, F. (1984). Peptide mapping in polyacrylamide gel electrophoresis after cleavage at aspartyl-prolyl bonds in sodium dodecyl sulfate-containing buffers. *Anal. Biochem.* **138**, 442–448.

Rothman, J. E. and Lenard, J. (1977). Membrane asymmetry. *Science* **195**, 743–753.

Rüther, U., Müller-Hill, B., (1983). Easy identification of cDNA clones. *EMBO J.* **2**, 1791–1794.

Sabban, E., Marchesi, V., Adesnik, M. and Sabatini, D. D. (1981). Erythrocyte membrane protein band 3: biosynthesis and incorporation into membranes. *J. Cell Biol.* **91**, 637–646.

Salacinski, P. R. P., McLean, C., Sykes, J. E. C., Clement-Jones, V. V. and Lowry, P. J. (1981). Iodination of proteins, glycoproteins, and peptides using a solid-phase oxidizing agent, 1,3,4,6-tetrachloro-3α,6α-diphenyl glycoluril (Iodogen). *Anal. Biochem.* **117**, 136–146.

Saris, C. J. M., van Eeenbergen, J., Jenks, B. G. and Bloemers, H. P. J. (1983). Hydroxylamide cleavage of proteins in polyacrylamide gels. *Anal. Biochem.* **132**, 54–67.

Schlesinger, M. J. (1981). Proteolipids. *A. Rev. Biochem.* **50**, 193–206.

Schneider, C., Sutherland, R., Newman, R. and Greaves, M. (1982). Structural features of the cell surface receptor for transferrin that is recognized by the monoclonal antibody OKT9. *J. biol. Chem.* **257**, 8516–8522.

Schneider, C., Kurkinen, M. and Greaves, M. (1983). Isolation of cDNA clones for the human transferrin receptor. *EMBO J.* **2**, 2259–2263.

Schwartz, B. D. and Nathenson, S. G. (1971). Isolation of H-2 alloantigens solubilized by the detergent NP-40. *J. Immunol.* **107**, 1363–1367.

Shapiro, A. L., Vinuela, E. and Maizel, J. B. (1967). Molecular weight estimation of polypeptide chains by electrophoresis in SDS-polyacrylamide gels. *Biochem. biophys. Res. Commun.* **28**, 815–820.

Shapiro, M. and Erickson, R. P. (1981). Evidence that the serological determinant of H-Y antigen is carbohydrate. *Nature* **290**, 503–505.

Shapiro, S. Z. and Young, J. R. (1981). An immunochemical method for mRNA purification. *J. biol. Chem.* **256**, 1495–1498.

Sharon, N. (1975). "Complex Carbohydrates. Their Chemistry, Biosynthesis, and Functions." Addison-Wesley Publishing Company, Reading, Mass.

Sharon, N. and Lis, H. (1982). Glycoproteins. *In* "The Proteins" (H. Neurath and R. L. Hill, eds), pp. 1–144. Academic Press, New York.

Sidman, C. L. (1981). Lymphocyte surface receptors and albumin. *J. Immunol.* **127**, 1454–1458.

Singer, S. J. and Nicolson, G. L. (1972). The fluid mosaic model of the structure of cell membranes. *Science* **175**, 720–731.

Smolarsky, M. (1980). A simple radioimmunoassay to determine the binding of antibodies to lipid antigens. *J. immunol. Methods* **38**, 85–93.

Springer, T. A. (1980). Cell-surface differentiation in the mouse. Characterization of "jumping" and "lineage" antigens using xenogeneic rat monoclonal antibodies. *In* "Monoclonal Antibodies" (R. H. Kennett, T. J. McKearn and K. B. Bechtol, eds), pp. 185–217. Plenum Press, New York.

Stanley, K. K. and Luzio, J. P. (1984). Construction of a new family of high efficiency bacterial expression vectors: identification of cDNA clones coding for liver proteins. *EMBO J.* **3**, 1429–1434.

Stearne, P. A., Pietersz, G. A. and Goding, J. W. (1985). cDNA cloning of the murine transferrin receptor: Sequence of trans-membrane and adjacent regions. *J. Immunol.* **134**, 3474–3479.

Steck, T. L. and Dawson, G. (1974). Topographical distribution of complex carbohydrates in the erythrocyte membrane. *J. biol. Chem.* **249**, 2135–2142.

Stern, P., Willison, K., Lennox, E., Galfrè, G., Milstein, C., Secher, D., Zeigler, A. and Springer, T. (1978). Monoclonal antibodies as probes for differentiation and tumor associated antigens: A Forssman specificity on teratocarcinoma stem cells. *Cell* **14**, 775–783.

Stumph, W. E., Elgin, S. C. R. and Hood, L. E. (1974). Antibodies to protein dissolved in sodium dodecyl sulfate. *J. Immunol.* **113**, 1752–1756.

Suissa, M. (1981). Nonenzymatic labelling of proteins by preparations of [^{35}S]-methionine. *Anal. Biochem.* **115**, 67–71.

Sutherland, R., Delia, D., Schneider, C., Newman, R., Kemshead, J. and Greaves M. (1981). Ubiquitous cell-surface glycoprotein on tumor cells is proliferation-associated receptor for transferrin. *Proc. natn. Acad. Sci. U.S.A.* **78**, 4515–4519.

Tack, B. F., Dean, J., Eilat, D., Lorenz, P. E. and Schechter, A. (1980). Tritium labelling of proteins to high specific activity by reductive methylation. *J. biol. Chem.* **255**, 8842–8847.

Tanaka, T. (1981). Gels. *Scient. Am.* **244**, 124–133.

Tanaka, T., Nishio, I., Sun, S-T. and Veno-Nishio, S. (1982). Collapse of gels in an electric field. *Science* **218**, 467–469.

Tartakoff, A. and Vassalli, P. (1979). Plasma cell immunoglobulin M molecules. Their biosynthesis, assembly, and intracellular transport. *J. Cell Biol.* **83**, 284–299.

Tjian, R., Stinchcomb, D. and Losick, R. (1975). Antibody directed against bacillus subtilis and σ factor purified by sodium dodecyl sulfate slab gel electrophoresis. *J. biol. Chem.* **250**, 8824–8828.

Trowbridge, I. S. and Omary, M. B. (1981). Human cell surface glycoprotein related to cell proliferation is the receptor for transferrin. *Proc. natn. Acad. Sci. U.S.A.* **78**, 3039–3043.

Tse, A. G. D., Barclay, A. N., Watts, A., and Williams, A. F. (1985). A glycophospholipid tail at the carboxyl terminus of the Thy-1 glycoprotein of neurons and thymocytes. *Science* **230**, 1003–1008.

Tucker, P. W., Liu, C.-P., Mushinski, J. F. and Blattner, F. R. (1980). Mouse immunoglobulin D: Messenger RNA and genomic DNA sequences. *Science* **209**, 1353–1360.

van der Meer, J., Dorssers, L. and Zabel, P. (1983). Antibody-linked polymerase assay on protein blots: a novel method for identifying polymerases following SDS-polyacrylamide gel electrophoresis. *EMBO J.* **2**, 233–237.

van Driel, I. R., Wilks, A. F., Pietersz, G. A. and Goding, J. W. (1985). Murine plasma cell membrane antigen PC-1: Molecular cloning of cDNA and analysis of expression. *Proc. natn. Acad. Sci. U.S.A.* **82**, 8619–8623.

Vasilov, R. G. and Pleogh, H. L. (1982). Biosynthesis of murine IgD: heterogeneity of glycosylation. *Eur. J. Immunol.* **12**, 804–813.

Vitetta, E. S., Capra, J. D., Klapper, D. G., Klein, J. and Uhr, J. W. (1976). The partial amino sequence of an H-2K molecule. *Proc. natn. Acad. Sci. U.S.A.* **73**, 905–909.

Weber, K. and Osborne, M. (1969). The reliability of molecular weight determinations by dodecyl sulfate-polyacrylamide gel electrophoresis. *J. biol. Chem.* **244**, 4406–4412.

Wegener, A. D. and Jones, L. R. (1984). Phosphorylation-induced mobility shift in phospholamban in sodium dodecyl sulfate-acrylamide gels. *J. biol. Chem.* **259**, 1834–1841.

Whalen, R. G., Schwartz, K., Bouveret, P., Sell, S. M. and Gros, F. (1979). Contractile protein isozymes in muscle development: Identification of an embryonic form of myosin heavy chain. *Proc. natn. Acad. Sci. U.S.A.* **76**, 5197–5201.

Wiegers, K. I. and Dernick, R. (1981). Peptide maps of labelled poliovirus proteins after two-dimensional analysis by limited proteolysis in sodium dodecyl sulfate. *Electrophoresis* **2**, 98–104.

Yamasaki, R. B., Osuga, D. T. and Feeney, R. E. (1982). Periodate oxidation of methionine in proteins. *Anal. Biochem.* **126**, 183–189.

Young, R. A., Mehra, V., Sweetser, D., Buchanan, T., Clark-Curtiss, J., Davis, R. W. and Bloom, B. R. (1985). Genes for the major protein antigens of the leprosy parasite *Mycobacterium leprae*. *Nature* **316**, 450–452.

Young, W. W. and Hakomori, S. (1981). Therapy of mouse lymphoma with monoclonal antibodies. *Science* **211**, 487–489.

6 Affinity Chromatography Using Monoclonal Antibodies

Affinity chromatography is a method of fractionation which exploits the biospecific binding of a particular molecule to a second molecule, often termed the "ligand" (reviewed by Cuatrecasas and Anfinsen, 1971; Lowe and Dean, 1974; Parikh and Cuatrecasas, 1975; Ruoslahti, 1976; Lowe, 1979; Chaiken *et al.*, 1983). The technique is extremely powerful. Purification factors of 2000–20 000-fold are often possible, and it is sometimes possible to achieve purification to homogeneity in a single step.

Immobilized antibodies and antigens have been used as affinity reagents for many years (Campbell *et al.*, 1951; Wofsy and Burr, 1969; Ruoslahti, 1976), but the method suffered from problems of low binding capacity, harsh elution conditions, and specificity limited by the quality of the antibodies. As a result, antibody immunoadsorbents did not achieve the widespread usage that might have been expected.

The advent of monoclonal antibodies has revolutionized affinity chromatography. In theory at least, it is now possible to produce affinity columns of any desired specificity, with high capacity and very mild elution conditions (Herrman and Mescher, 1979; Parham, 1979, 1983; Secher and Burke, 1980; Stallcup *et al.*, 1981; Dalchau and Fabre, 1982; Turkewitz *et al.*, 1983; Mescher *et al.*, 1983).

6.1 Preparation of Immobilized Antibodies

6.1.1 Choice of an Affinity Matrix and Coupling Reaction

The ideal affinity matrix would have negligible nonspecific adsorption, lack charged groups, and be capable of binding antibody in a leakproof manner with full preservation of activity. So far, beaded agarose has come closest to meeting this ideal. In practice, the great majority of immunoadsorbents are based on this material.

Many different coupling procedures are available (Table 6.1). By far the most popular is the cyanogen bromide method (Axèn *et al.*, 1967; March *et al.*, 1974). Activation of agarose by cyanogen bromide is simple and inexpensive, but it involves working with a volatile and toxic chemical. It is now possible to obtain pre-activated agarose as a stable lyophilized powder (CNBr-activated Sepharose 4B; Pharmacia). The binding capacity of the reconstituted gel will remain high for a period of months to years, provided that the powder is kept dry. The cost of the commercial product is not excessive when the usual small columns are constructed, but if columns of more than 50 ml are contemplated, activation with CNBr in the laboratory should be considered.

The main disadvantages of CNBr-activated agarose stem from the isourea linkage (Wilchek *et al.*, 1975) between the gel and the amino groups of lysine. This bond introduces an extra charge, causing the gel to act as an ion exchanger at low salt concentrations. In addition, very slow leakage of the protein from the column occurs over a period of months to years (Tesser *et al.*, 1974; Lowe, 1979). Leakage is accelerated by raised temperature and nucleophiles such as primary amines or proteins (Wilchek *et al.*, 1975). Kowal and Parsons (1980) have shown that treatment of the affinity matrix with the protein cross-linker glutaraldehyde ($\sim 0.05\%$) greatly decreases the rate of leakage. It would appear prudent to store the columns at $4°C$, at neutral or slightly acidic pH. There may be theoretical grounds for avoiding the nucleophiles Tris and azide, although many workers have not found them to be a problem. A suitable buffer would be phosphate-buffered saline containing 0.005% merthiolate. In spite of these problems, CNBr-activated agarose remains the most popular affinity matrix.

Proteins may also be coupled to agarose which has been derivatized by spacer arms with N-hydroxysuccinimide ester at their distal ends (Cuatrecasas and Parikh, 1972). Succinimide esters are very susceptible to nucleophilic attack by the ε-amino groups of lysine, resulting in the displacement of N-hydroxysuccinimide and the formation of a stable amide bond between the protein and the spacer arm. A slight practical disadvantage of these gels is that the progress and efficiency of coupling of protein cannot be followed by ultraviolet absorption, because N-hydroxysuccinimide also absorbs strongly. The chemistry of this very useful reaction will be discussed in Chapter 7.

Table 6.1 Properties of coupling methods for affinity chromatography

	CNBr[a]	N-hydroxysuccinimide[b]	Carbonyldiimidazole[c]	Toluene sulphonyl chloride
Ease of preparation of affinity matrix	+	−	+++	+++
Ease of binding of protein	+++	+++	+++	+++
Charge-free linkage[d]	no	yes	yes	no
Stability of linkage[e]	±	+++	+++	+++
Spacer arm[f]	no	yes	no	no

[a]Available commercially as "CNBr-activated Sepharose 4B" (Pharmacia). [b]Available commercially as "Affigel 10" (Bio-Rad) or "Activated CH-Sepharose 4B" (Pharmacia). [c]Available commercially as "Reacti-Gel (6X)" (Pierce). [d]Charged linkages may cause nonspecific binding at low salt concentrations. [e]The rate of leakage of protein from CNBr-activated agarose is very low (typically <0.02% per day). Leakage is accelerated by alkaline pH, higher temperatures and presence of nucleophiles (e.g. amines such as Tris). The spacer arm of Affigel 10 is attached to the gel by a stable ether linkage, while the spacer arm of Activated CH Sepharose is attached via a labile isourea bond. It is good practice to 'pre-cycle' all affinity columns with the eluting buffer just before use. [f]Spacer arms may give rise to nonspecific adsorption. If the spacer is hydrophobic, nonspecific binding will be increased at high salt concentrations.

Activated succinimide esters coupled to agarose beads are available commercially as "Affigel 10" (Bio-Rad) and "Activated CH Sepharose" (Pharmacia). Affigel 10 is preferable in most situations, because its hydrophilic spacer arm is attached to the gel via a stable ether bond. The spacer arm of Activated CH Sepharose is hydrophobic, and is coupled to the gel via the less stable isourea bond produced by CNBr activation. Hydrophobic spacer arms may give rise to nonspecific binding (Er-El *et al.*, 1972; O'Carra *et al.*, 1973; Lowe, 1979).

Several other activation procedures have been described. Bethel *et al.* (1979) have shown that Sepharose CL-6B may be activated with 1,1′-carbonyldiimidazole (Pierce), producing an imidazolyl carbamate derivative. The activation procedure is simple, and the product reacts smoothly with N-nucleophiles to form a stable bond without additional charge. The activated beads are now available commercially as a stable suspension in dry acetone ("Reacti-Gel"; Pierce). The stability, lack of spacer arms, and high capacity of "Reacti-Gel" overcome many of the problems of other matrices, and it is to be expected that the product will be widely used.

Nilsson and Mosbach (1980) have shown that agarose can be activated with p-toluene-sulphonyl chloride (tosyl chloride), to form corresponding esters (tosylates) which have excellent leaving properties in reactions with nucleophiles. The linkage to protein is very stable, but is charged with neutral pH. A closely related procedure uses tresyl chloride (Nilsson and Mosbach, 1981), and is available as Tresyl-activated Sepharose (Pharmacia).

6.1.2 Stability of Agarose

Native agarose can tolerate undiluted ethanol, methanol, butanol, acetone and dioxane, 80% (v/v) aqueous pyridine and 50% (v/v) dimethyl formamide (Lowe and Dean, 1974), but is dissolved by dimethyl sulphoxide (Lowe, 1979). Freezing of native agarose results in irreversible changes in structure. However, the activation of agarose by CNBr introduces covalent cross-links between the polysaccharide chains, greatly improving its stability. After activation and coupling, the final product is able to withstand high concentrations of salt, urea, guanidine-HCl, sodium dodecyl sulphate, deoxycholate and Triton X-100.

Agarose in which the polysaccharide chains have been cross-linked by 2,3 dibromopropanol is available commercially from Pharmacia as Sepharose CL®. It is highly resistant to disruption by heat, extremes of pH, and organic solvents (Lowe, 1979).

6.1.3 Preparation of CNBr-activated
Agarose

Agarose beads (Sepharose 4B or Sepharose 4B-CL) must be thoroughly washed with distilled water prior to activation. Washing may be carried out on a large sintered glass funnel. Just prior to removal from the funnel, the gel should be washed with two volumes of 2M $NaHCO_3$-Na_2CO_3 buffer, pH $\sim$ 11. The gel is then removed from the funnel, resuspended in an equal volume of buffer, and cooled to 4–5°C in an ice bath.

The reaction is initiated by adding CNBr (100 mg per gram of gel, dissolved in acetonitrile), with constant stirring (March et al., 1974; Nishikawa and Bailon, 1975). Activation takes 10–15 min, after which the gel is washed with ice-cold distilled water on a sintered glass funnel. The liquid should be collected into a side-arm flask containing ferrous sulphate to inactivate residual CNBr and cyanides. Washing after activation must be performed quickly, as the activated groups are prone to hydrolysis, especially at alkaline pH. After the alkaline buffer has been washed out, stability of the gel is enhanced by washing with 1 mM HCl in water. The gel should be used within 10–20 min.

6.1.4 Activation of Agarose by
1,1′-Carbonyldiimidazole

The procedure described is that given by Bethell et al. (1979). Sepharose CL-6B (3 g of moist cake) is washed sequentially with water, dioxane/water, 3:7; dioxane/water, 7:3; and dioxane (20 ml of each), and suspended in 5 ml dioxane. The activating agent, 1,1′-Carbonyldiimidazole (120 mg) is added, and the suspension shaken at room temperature for 15 min. The activated gel is then washed with dioxane (100 ml), and used immediately, although it is stable in anhydrous dioxane. Just prior to coupling with protein, it would seem advisable to reverse the wash procedure and transfer the gel back to water.

The commercial product ("Reacti-Gel"; Pierce) is supplied as a pre-swollen gel in ahydrous acetone, and should be washed in acetone:water (7:3), acetone:water (3:7), and then water, prior to use. Unlike N-hydroxy-succinimide ester activated supports with half-lives of hydrolysis measured in minutes (Chapter 7), gels activated with 1,1′-carbonyldiimidazole require 30 h for complete hydrolysis at pH 8.5.

6.1.5 Activation of Agarose by
p-Toluene Sulphonyl Chloride

The procedure is that of Nilsson and Mosbach (1980). Wet Sepharose CL-6B is transferred into dioxane by washing with 3 × 10 gel volumes of water, water/dioxane (3:1, v/v), water/dioxane (1:3), dioxane, and finally dried dioxane, containing less than 0.01% water. Dry acetone may be used instead of dioxane.

Seven grams of Sepharose is then transferred to a round-bottomed flask containing 1 g *p*-toluene sulphonyl chloride (tosyl chloride) dissolved in 2 ml dried dioxane. Pyridine (1.0 ml) is added dropwise, with stirring. After 1 h reaction at room temperature, the gel is washed twice with 10 volumes dioxane and then gradually transferred back to water by reversing the procedure above.

It was stated that the gels were stored at 4°C in distilled water until used, but no information was given concerning the rate of hydrolysis of the activated gel under these conditions. It would seem prudent to use the gel within an hour or so of activation.

6.1.6 Coupling of Proteins to Activated Gels

The antibody preparation to be coupled to agarose beads need not be purified to homogeneity. For most purposes, ammonium sulphate precipitation, carried out as described in Section 4.2.1, will be sufficient. It is vital to dialyse extensively after ammonium sulphate precipitation, because ammonium ions will inhibit the coupling reaction (see below).

Regardless of the mechanism of activation, the subsequent coupling of proteins occurs by nucleophilic attack on the gel by the ε-amino groups of lysine. The amino groups must be unprotonated; the reaction therefore proceeds most rapidly at slightly alkaline pH. There is also a minor competing hydrolysis of the activated groups on the gel. It is essential to avoid the presence of extraneous nucleophiles. Tris, ammonium sulphate and azide ions will inhibit coupling.

The efficiency of coupling is greatest at slightly alkaline pH (7.5–8.5), but conditions which lead to maximal protein binding may lead to inactivation of antibodies (see Section 6.1.7). Suitable buffers include phosphate-buffered saline, 0.1 M sodium borate or 0.1 M sodium bicarbonate. The reaction is usually completed in 1–2 h at room temperature, or overnight at 4°C, although somewhat longer times are recommended for gels activated by 1,1'-carbonyldiimidazole or tosyl chloride.

The protein-binding capacity of the gels varies depending on the degree of activation, the pH, and the individual protein. CNBr-activated Sepharose 4B will bind 10–15 mg protein per ml of wet gel, and the total mass of antibody should be chosen to exceed this by a small amount. Typical concentrations of protein in the coupling buffer are 2–20 mg/ml, but the important parameter is the ratio of the total protein mass to the mass of activated gel. The kinetics of binding may be followed by removal of small aliquots from the reaction mixture, and measurement of the ultraviolet absorbance at 280 nm after removal of beads by centrifugation.

As soon as the reaction is judged to be complete, it is important to inactivate any remaining activated groups. It is customary to inactivate with 1 M ethanolamine, titrated to pH 8 with HCl, for 1–2 h at room temperature. In some cases, inactivation with ethanolamine may lead to increased non-specific binding (Heinzel *et al.*, 1976), and glycine may be preferred. Alternatively, the reactive groups may be left to hydrolyse for a few days. It is also advisable to wash the gel with several cycles of 0.5 M NaCl, 0.1 M acetate pH ~ 4, followed by 0.5 M NaCl, 0.1 M NaHCO$_3$, pH ~ 8.3, to remove any loosely adsorbed protein.

Coupling of proteins to CNBr-activated Sepharose 4B

Lyophilized cyanogen bromide-activated Sepharose 4B is available from Pharmacia. Provided it is kept dry, it will last for years. The following is a practical procedure for its use.

(1) Calculate the amount of gel needed. Assume that 0.3 g of dry gel will result in 1 ml wet gel, which will in turn bind 10 mg protein.

(2) Weigh out desired amount of dry gel.

(3) Rehydrate gel in 1 mM HCl in a beaker at room temperature for 15 min. Do not use a magnetic stirrer, as it will fragment the beads. Occasionally swirl to mix.

(4) Pour gel slurry into a coarse sintered glass funnel (Schott) attached to a side-arm flask and a water vacuum pump. (It is convenient to have a "vacuum bypass" hole in the rubber stopper of the flask, to control the vacuum by finger pressure).

(5) Wash the gel with ~ 50 volumes 1 mM HCl, *without allowing it to dry out.*

(6) Scoop the gel into a tube containing the protein in an appropriate buffer (typically of 0.1 M NaHCO$_3$).

(7) Immediately cap the tube, and place on a vertical rotating wheel, to give end-over-end-mixing.

(8) Allow coupling to proceed for 1–2 h at room temperature. The progress of coupling may be followed by removing aliquots of the supernatant and measuring the O.D.$_{280}$.

(9) As soon as coupling is more than 90% complete, quench the remaining active sites on the beads by adding one tenth volume 0.1 M glycine or 0.1 M Tris-HCl, pH 8, and hold at room temperature for a further 1–2 h.

(10) Spin out the beads (400 g, 5 min).

(11) Wash the beads, alternating three times between 0.1 M sodium acetate

pH 4.0 plus 0.5 M NaCl, and 0.1 M Tris-HCl, pH 8.0, plus 0.5 M NaCl.

(12) Store the beads in **PBS** plus 0.005% merthiolate.

6.1.7 Optimization of Antibody Activity of Immunoadsorbents

Providing that no extraneous inhibitors are present, the coupling of protein to the gels almost always proceeds without difficulty. Coupling efficiencies of 100% are easily achieved, but are undesirable. A distinction must be made between the efficient coupling of protein, which is easy, and the preservation of maximal antibody-binding activity after coupling, which may present problems.

The commercially available gels are extremely highly activated, and a frequent problem is that the bound protein is attached by so many sites that it is no longer capable of biological activity (Cuatrecasas and Anfinsen, 1971). It is often preferable, then, to minimize multipoint coupling by the following strategies:

(1) The gel may be "offered" a little *more* protein than it is capable of binding. Any unbound protein can easily be recovered and re-used. It is unwise to use a large excess of gel over protein.

(2) The pH of coupling may be as a low as 6.5, increasing the extent of protonation of the ε-amino groups of lysine residues. Coupling of many proteins is still efficient at this pH (Cuatrecasas and Anfinsen, 1971), although some monoclonal antibodies with very acidic isoelectric points may not couple. If difficulty is experienced, raise the pH.

(3) Coupling may be terminated by ethanolamine or glycine as soon as the majority of protein is coupled.

(4) The gel may be "pre-hydrolysed" to reduce the density of activated groups. While this option is theoretically attractive, it may be difficult to guess the extent of hydrolysis achieved.

In the final analysis, each monoclonal antibody may behave differently, and the choice of conditions favouring retention of activity is empirical. Nonetheless, an appreciation of the variables will generally lead to success.

6.1.8 Covalent Binding of Antibodies to Protein A-Sepharose

As discussed in the previous section, the random attachment of antibodies to solid-phase matrices may result in significant loss of binding activity. In contrast, the binding of antibodies via their Fc portions to staphylococcal protein A (Section 4.3.2) leaves the antigen-combining site in the correct orientation for the binding of antigen. Gersten and Marchalonis (1978) have shown that antibodies may be covalently cross-linked to protein A-Sepharose with dimethyl suberimidate, with preservation at antigen-binding activity Schneider *et al.* (1982) have exploited this approach to produce highly active immunoadsorbents. The latter authors used dimethyl pimelimidate, which has a spacer with one extra carbon, and spans 9.2 Å as compared to 8.6 Å for dimethyl suberimidate.

Practical procedure

The following procedure is based on that of Schneider *et al.* (1982). Protein A-Sepharose CL-4B (Pharmacia) is mixed with antibody in 0.1 M borate buffer, pH 8.2, for 30 min at room temperature, and excess antibody removed by washing with the same buffer. The gel is then washed with 0.2 M triethanolamine, pH 8.2, and resuspended in 20 volumes of 10–20 mM dimethyl pimelimidate dihydrochloride (Pierce) freshly made up in the same buffer. The mixture is agitated at room temperature for 45 min, and the reaction terminated by centrifugation and resuspension in an equal volume of ethanolamine, pH 8.2, of the same molarity as the dimethyl pimelimidate. After 5 min, the cross-linked beads are washed three times in borate buffer, pH 8.2, containing 0.02% sodium azide.

The concentration of cross-linking agent was not critical, and antibody activity was preserved over a range of 10–100 mM. Maximal antigen-binding capacity of the columns occurred when the protein A column was 50% saturated with antibody (Schneider *et al.*, 1982).

6.2 Use of Antibody Affinity Columns

Individual monoclonal antibodies may have quite different properties, and it is unlikely that the same conditions of binding and elution will apply in all cases. It is important to examine the conditions for binding and elution for each antibody individually. If possible, it would be preferable to test a number of monoclonal antibodies of the same specificity, and choose the antibody with the most desirable characteristics.

Affinity chromatography on antibody columns may be divided into four equally important phases; pre-cycling, binding, washing and elution.

6.2.1 Pre-cycling the Column

Regardless of the type of linkage of antibody to the column, it should be assumed that slight leakage of antibody may occur during long-term storage. If the antibody is of very high affinity, and the antigen present in very small amounts, leakage might result in total failure of binding to the column. If the antigen emerged bound to antibody, it might not be detected; failure to recover the antigen from the column could lead to the erroneous conclusion that the antigen had been irreversibly bound to the column. In addition, traces of antibody in the antigen solution will degrade the overall degree of purification that may be achieved.

It is therefore vital that antibody columns be washed thoroughly immediately prior to use. Pre-cycling of the column with the eluting buffer, followed by extensive washing in the binding buffer, is strongly advisable. This procedure will remove any loosely bound nonspecifically adsorbed material, and any residual bound antigen from previous uses.

6.2.2 Binding of Antigen

The first requirement is that the antigen be soluble and free of aggregated material or debris which would obstruct the column. The solubilization and handling of membrane antigens is discussed in Section 5.6.2. If there is any doubt concerning solubility or debris, or if the antigen mixture has been frozen, centrifugation at $10\,000\,\mathbf{g}$ or even $100\,000\,\mathbf{g}$ for 10–15 min is advisable before loading the gel. In general, if cell lysates are to be passed over affinity columns, it is not a good idea to use material that has been frozen and thawed. Freezing results in severe agregation (see Turkewitz *et al.*, 1983).

It is customary to perform affinity chromatography in small columns; disposable syringes are ideal. Another excellent and inexpensive column is the Bio-Rad Econo-Column (cat. no. 731-1550), which can accommodate bed volumes from 0.2 ml to 10 ml. The use of columns allows the antigen-containing mixture to percolate slowly through the matrix, and allows optimal chances for interaction. Flow rates of 1–2 ml/min are typical.

Batch procedures are also feasible, but care must be taken to mix in such a way that all the liquid has a chance to interact with the beads. Mixing with a magnetic flea is likely to fragment the beads, and end-over-end mixing on a rotating wheel for several hours is preferable.

It is often helpful to pass the antigen-containing mixture over a "precolumn" of agarose (underivatized or coupled with an irrelevant antibody) to remove any molecules that bind nonspecifically.

The requirements for the buffer in which binding takes place are simple. The pH and salt concentraiton must be such that binding is strong, and if membrane proteins are present, the buffer must contain appropriate amounts of a suitable detergent. Typical loading buffers are phosphate-buffered saline, pH 7.4, or 0.1 M Tris-HCl, pH 8.0.

The volume of antibody-coupled gel should be appropriate to the

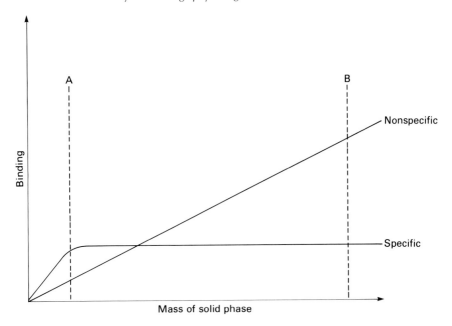

Fig. 6.1 Effect of bed volume of affinity columns on specific and nonspecific binding. If the column is offered a fixed mass of antigen, specific binding will increase with increasing bed volume, until all antigen is bound. In contrast, nonspecific binding may increase in proportion to column size. It follows that the best purification factors will be achieved when the column is close to saturation (line A), rather than when the column is very large (line B).

anticipated mass of antigen. A common mistake is to make the column much too big. Large columns are seldom necessary. Excessively large columns may produce worse results than columns of appropriate size, because any tendency for the matrix to bind nonspecifically will increase linearly with bed volume, while specific binding will increase only until all the antigen is bound (Fig. 6.1).

6.2.3 Washing the Immunoadsorbent: the Problem of Nonspecific Binding

After the antigen-containing mixture has been loaded, unbound material must be removed by washing the gel. In many cases, the gel is simply washed with 10–20 column volumes of the same buffer used for loading. An ultraviolet absorbance monitor will be found extremely useful in deciding when adequate washing has been achieved. In a few cases involving low-affinity antibodies, excessive washing may remove some or all of the bound antigen.

It is important to appreciate that some examples of "nonspecific" binding to affinity columns can have quite well-defined causes. For example, some lectin-like molecules may bind directly to agarose. Many serum proteins (e.g. hormones, low density lipoprotein and transferrin) bind to cells via specific receptors. Transferrin is a very frequent contaminant in immunoglobulin preparations, and is therefore likely to be present on many affinity columns. The possibility of artefacts due to transferrin receptors has been suggested (Goding and Burns, 1981) and a case has been documented (Harford, 1984).

A certain degree of nonspecific binding is inevitable; some is due to properties of the matrix and some to properties of individual molecules in the antigen containing mixture. Regardless of the location of the problem, non-specific adsorption may often be reduced by use of modified wash buffers (see also Section 5.7.3).

Nonspecific binding due to electrostatic effects (i.e. interaction of charged groups on proteins with charged groups on the matrix) are most marked when the total salt concentration is low. Under low salt conditions, the gel may act as an ion exchange resin, and nonspecific binding of proteins of unusually basic or acidic isoelectric points may occur. Because the net charge of proteins varies with pH, nonspecific binding due to electrostatic effects is often pH-sensitive. These considerations suggest that the salt concentration should be kept high (0.3–0.5 M), and that a trial of buffers of different pH may be worthwhile (see Houwen *et al.*, 1975; Zoller and Matzku, 1976; Smith *et al.*, 1978; Schneider *et al.*, 1982).

Another cause of nonspecific binding is the presence of hydrophobic interactions. These are usually fairly minimal when the very hydrophilic agarose beads are used, but may be greatly aggravated by the presence of hydrophobic "spacer arms" (Er-El *et al.*, 1972). Hydrophobic effects are increased at high salt concentrations (> 1 M NaCl). In some cases, non-specific binding due to hydrophobic interactions may be reduced by the presence of detergents (0.5% Triton X-100, 0.5% deoxycholate or 0.1% Tween 20; Smith *et al.*, 1978).

The extent to which increasingly harsh wash buffers may be used will depend on the effect that these conditions have on the conformation of individual antigens and antibodies. In many cases, buffers containing 0.5 M NaCl and/or 0.5% deoxycholate will have no effect on antibody–antigen interactions (e.g. Parham, 1979; Goding and Herzenberg, 1980; Schneider *et al.*, 1982).

In other cases, these relatively mild conditions may cause complete disruption of binding. Monoclonal anti-H-2K^k antibody 11-4.1 (Oi *et al.*, 1978) binds tightly to its antigen in 15 mM phosphate buffer, pH 7, containing 0.5% Nonidet P40, but the interaction is weakened by addition of 0.15 M NaCl, and almost totally disrupted by 0.5 M NaCl or by 0.5% deoxycholate (Herrman and Mescher, 1979). Similar results were obtained with a second anti-H-2 antibody (Stallcup *et al.*, 1981). The disruption of binding by deoxycholate seems to be due to a reversible conformational change in the

antigen, because deoxycholate-treated H-2K^k molecules were more susceptible to digestion by trypsin and chymotrypsin (Herman *et al.*, 1982).

6.2.4 Elution of Antigen from Immunoadsorbents

The bulk of published experience with antibody immunoadsorbents has
involved conventional polyclonal antibodies. The behaviour of such columns
is dominated by the highest affinity subset of antibodies because this subset
must be disrupted before antigen can be released. Elution curves from
polyclonal immunoadsorbents often have sharp leading edges and long trailing edges, indicating that some high-affinity interactions cannot be fully
disrupted. The situation with monoclonal antibodies is completely different.
The homogeneous nature of the interactions means that once appropriate
elution conditions are found, peaks should emerge with minimal trailing. It
is to be expected that elution conditions may often be milder, and recoveries
greater.

In the case of monoclonal antibody 11–4.1, a very minor change in
conditions was sufficient for elution of antigen (Section 6.2.3). In the majority
of cases, however, it may be expected that much harsher conditions will be
required. Nonetheless, it is strongly advisable to try a variety of elution
conditions for each new monoclonal antibody. The most gentle conditions
which are effective for elution should be chosen; this will maximize the
chances of recovering biological activity.

In a few special cases, it may be possible to elute biospecifically. Antibodies to haptens may be eluted with a high concentration of hapten,
providing the affinity is not excessive. Some enzymes undergo conformational changes in response to the binding of cofactors, and it may occasionally
be possible to exploit this property to disrupt antibody binding.

It is often assumed that the highest affinity interactions are the ones that
require the strongest denaturing conditions to disrupt. There is no compelling
theoretical reason why this should always be the case, and there is evidence
that affinity and ease of disruption are not necessarily related (Parham, 1983).

In the great majority of cases, biospecific elution will not be feasible, and
elution will have to depend on the induction of a conformational change by
alteration of pH, dissociating agents such as urea or guanidine, or chaotropic
ions. Antibodies will usually renature after removal of deforming agents
(Section 4.7.1). Table 6.2 lists some common ways in which elution may be
performed.

The most popular method of elution of antibodies or antigens from
immune complexes involves the use of glycine-HCl buffers at pH 2.2–2.8.
Most antibodies will release their antigen under these conditions. If the
antigen is not eluted, a trial of elution at pH 11.5 (Table 6.2) may be
rewarding.

Table 6.2 *Elution of antibodies from immunoadsorbents*

Elution conditions	References	Comments
Glycine-HCl, pH 2.2–2.8	1	Incompatible with deoxycholate. Poor recoveries and aggregation of some membrane antigens.
Propionic acid, 1 M	2	More effective than HCl at same pH, possibly due to slight detergent action. May cause denaturation and irreversible aggregation.
Diethylamine, 0.05 M, pH 11.5	3	Compatible with deoxycholate; often the method of choice for membrane antigens
Ammonia, pH 11	4	
Urea, 2–8 M, pH 7	5	Heating in urea causes carbamylation of proteins.[6]
Guanidine-HCl, 6 M	7	Very strongly denaturing; efficient eluant but may cause severe aggregation.
Sodium thiocyanate, 3.5 M	8	Traces will inhibit iodination and coupling with fluorescein; remove by extensive dialysis.
Magnesium chloride 2–5 M	9	Incompatible with deoxycholate.
Potassium or sodium iodide, 2.5–5 M, pH 7.5–9.0	10	
Ethylene glycol (50%, v/v), pH 11.5	11	Polarity-reducing agent; disrupts hydrophobic interactions.
Dioxane (10%, v/v), at acid pH	11	Polarity-reducing agent; disrupts hydrophobic interactions.
Electrophoresis, isoelectric focusing	12	Avoids denaturing conditions; somewhat slow and cumbersome.

1. Kleinschmidt and Boyer, 1952; numerous other papers.
2. Joniau et al., 1970; Johnson and Garvey, 1977.
3. Letarte-Muirhead et al., 1975; Cresswell, 1977; Brodsky et al., 1979; McMaster and Williams, 1979; Parham, 1979; Sunderland et al., 1979; Schneider et al., 1982; Read et al., 1974.
4. Chidlow et al., 1974.
5. Melchers and Messer, 1970; Pikho et al., 1973; Stenman et al., 1981.
6. Stark et al., 1960; Tollaksen et al., 1981.
7. Dandliker et al., 1968; Weintraub, 1970; O'Sullivan et al., 1979.
8. Dandliker et al., 1968; Zoller and Matzku, 1976; George and Schenck, 1983.
9. Avrameas and Ternynck, 1969; Mains and Eipper, 1976.
10. Avrameas and Ternynck, 1967; Lecomte and Tyrrell, 1976.
11. Hill, 1972; Andersson et al., 1978; Andersson et al., 1979.
12. Brown et al., 1977; Morgan et al., 1978; Haff et al., 1979; Haff, 1981.

Hydrophobic interactions are often important in the binding of antigen to antibody. As mentioned earlier, the slight detergent action of 1 M propionic acid may result in more effective elution than glycine-HCl at the same pH. Elution with propionic acid is relatively harsh, and may result in aggregation and irreversible damage to the antigen. Hydrophobic interactions may also be weakened by the use of polarity-lowering agents such as dioxane (up to 10%) or ethylene glycol (up to 50%) in conjunction with extremes of pH (Table 6.2).

If elution at extremes of pH is not successful in releasing the antigen, or if the antigen or antibody is damaged by these conditions, it is worthwhile to try the use of chaotropic ions. The potency of these ions in disrupting antigen–antibody complexes approximately parallels the Hofmeister series:

$$SCN^- > I^- > ClO_4^- > NO_3^- > Br^- > Cl^- > CH_3COO^-$$
$$> SO_4^{2-} > PO_4^{3-}$$

$$Ba^{++} > Ca^{++} > Mg^{++} > Li^+ > Na^+ > K^+ > Cs^+ > NH_4^+$$

A trial of chaotropic ions should probably commence with NaSCN (3.5 M). Thiocyanate is an extremely potent inhibitor of radioiodination (George and Schenck, 1983), and samples must be dialysed with many changes of buffer for several days before iodination is attempted. $MgCl_2$ (2–4 M) has been used effectively, and is sometimes claimed to be less likely to cause irreversible damage. However, it is not entirely clear whether a lower concentration of the more potent thiocyanate ion would be equivalent.

A third type of eluant includes urea and guanidine-HCl, which are potent denaturants when used at high concentration. Typically, one might elute with 5–8 M urea or 4–6 M guanidine-HCl. Elution with urea or guanidine is extremely effective, but may result in severe damage to the antibodies or antigen. They should probably be reserved for situations in which all other eluants fail.

It is important to remember that the combination of reducing agents with denaturing buffers is likely to cause dissociation of antibody light and heavy chains, and thus destruction of the affinity column. It should also be noted that IgA from BALB/c mice does not possess a disulphide bond between light and heavy chains, and affinity matrices based on BALB/c IgA may not survive the first elution.

In a few cases, binding may be so tight that the necessary elution conditions may destroy the antigen or antibody. The use of monovalent Fab fragments of antibody (Chapter 4) may lower the effective affinity ("avidity") of binding, and facilitate elution in these cases, particularly if the antigen possesses more than one identical antigenic determinant per molecule. The use of a lower degree of substitution of the matrix by antibody may also help.

Gradient elution

Elution of antigen or antibodies by continuous gradients of denaturing agents has been rarely attempted. The wide range of affinities of polyclonal antibodies would resulted in an extremely broad elution profile. However, the homogeneity of monoclonal antibodies might suggest a reconsideration of gradient elution (Stenman *et al.*, 1981). The use of continuous gradients of pH or chaotropic ions might allow even better separations than can be achieved by step gradients. Gradient elution is widely used in other areas of affinity chromatography (Lowe and Dean, 1974; Lowe, 1979).

Affinity chromatography of membrane antigens

The special problems of solubilization and handling membrane antigens have been discussed in Section 5.6. It is essential that all components in the antigen-containing mixture be adequately solubilized, because precipitation on the column will seriously degrade the separation.

The need to maintain solubility means that it is obligatory to use adequate concentrations of a suitable detergent at all stages, including loading, washing and elution. Non-ionic detergents may be used under a wide range of salt concentrations and pH, but deoxycholate will gel or precipitate at a pH below ~ 7.4, and in the presence of divalent cations. The properties of deoxycholate micelles are also subject to large changes depending on the ionic environment (Helenius and Simons, 1975; Helenius *et al.*, 1979). Triton X-100 and Nonidet P-40 absorb light very strongly at 280 nm, while deoxycholate and octyl glucoside do not. It is possible to exchange the detergent by washing the column with buffer containing the new detergent prior to elution, but care must be taken that the antigen remains bound, and is soluble in the new detergent.

Elution at alkaline pH has been used successfully in a number of instances, particularly for cell membrane antigens (Sunderland *et al.*, 1979; Parham, 1979; Parham *et al.*, 1979; Schneider *et al.*, 1982). The choice of alkaline elution conditions for membrane proteins stems partly from compatibility with deoxycholate, and partly from the empirical observation that membrane proteins are less prone to aggregation at alkaline pH (Letarte-Muirhead *et al.*, 1975; Cresswell, 1977; Brodsky *et al.*, 1979; McMaster and Williams, 1979; Sunderland *et al.*, 1979; Parham, 1979; Parham *et al.*, 1979).

A practical example of the purification of a membrane protein by affinity chromatography is given by Stearne *et al.* (1985). Batches of cells were solubilized in 2% Triton X-100 in PBS (50 ml per 10 ml packed cells) for 10 min at 4°C, and debris removed by centrifugation at 800 g for 10 min. The supernatant was then centrifuged at 100 000 g for 60 min in a Beckman SW27 rotor, and passed over a column of transferrin-Sepharose, followed by a column of monoclonal anti-PC-1-Sepharose. The bed volume of the columns was 1.0 ml, and the flow rate 0.7 ml/min. The column was then washed with 20 ml 50 mM Tris-HCl, pH 8.0, containing 0.5 M NaCl with 0.5% Triton X-100. The PC-1 antigen was eluted with 50 mM diethylamine, pH 11.5, containing 0.05% Triton X-100. Preliminary experiments showed that nearly all the antigen was eluted in the second and third 1 ml fractions after application of the elution buffer. The sample was immediately neutralized by adding 200 μl of 1 M Tris-HCl, pH 8.0, and lyophilized. A purification of $\sim$ 20 000-fold was obtained, and the antigen was found to be $\sim$ 50% pure. Purification to homogeneity was achieved by preparative SDS-polyacrylamide gel electrophoresis (see Chapter 8 for details).

Removal of the elution agent

There is evidence that some proteins subjected to denaturing environments may undergo conformational changes that continue for several hours (Shimizu *et al.*, 1974; Porath and Kristiansen, 1975; Tanford, 1969, 1970). The longer that a protein is subjected to these environments, the greater the risk of difficulties in renaturation. The risk of irreversible damage is probably minimized by keeping the sample cold until the denaturing environment is completely removed.

If the protein is eluted by extremes of pH, it is best to neutralize as soon as possible after elution. Rapid removal of the denaturing agent may also be used for other eluants, including thiocyanate, urea and guanidine, although in these cases it is sometimes found that renaturation is more complete if the denaturing agent is removed very slowly over hours to days by dialysis against a series of solutions of decreasing concentration. In general, though, rapid restoration of physiological conditions is best (see Hager and Burgess, 1980).

It is therefore common practice to remove the denaturing agent as soon as possible after the antigen is eluted. If elution has been by pH change, the antigen may be neutralized rapidly by collection into a tube containing 1 M Tris-HCl, pH 7.5–8.0. Neutralization should never be carried out by adding Tris base or NaOH directly to the antigen. Chaotropic ions or urea may be diluted out. The eluted antigen may then be transferred into a more physiological environment by dialysis. It is not uncommon for some aggregation and precipitation to occur at this stage. This is more common when potent denaturants such as urea or guanidine-HCl are used, and may sometimes be minimized by renaturing the protein very slowly by stepwise dialysis in decreasing denaturant concentrations over many hours. The only other solution is to try a different or milder elution procedure, or to centrifuge and discard the aggregates.

Storage of affinity columns

Affinity columns will last virtually indefinitely, providing they are protected from drying, microbial contamination, proteolysis, chemical attack and accumulation of extraneous insoluble material. These requirements are not difficult to meet. Columns should be stored in a neutral or slightly acidic buffer. Phosphate-buffered saline, pH 7.2–7.4, containing 0.005% Merthiolate is suitable. Some authors prefer borate buffers, because they are less likely to support microbial growth. Columns must be tightly sealed to prevent them from drying out. They should be stored at 4°C, but must not be frozen, because freezing causes irreversible disruption to the agarose.

6.2.5 Preparation of Antigen for Protein Sequencing

Although there are now many strategies for gene cloning (Section 5.10), one that is commonly used for low-abundance proteins involves the screening of libraries with oligonucleotides based on amino acid sequence information. Affinity chromatography and preparative SDS-polyacrylamide gel electrophoresis are now very commonly used in the purification of proteins which are present in low abundance. However, the final purification step requires a good deal of care to ensure that the protein is sequenceable.

The first requirement is purity of the protein. Suffice it to say that 10% contamination of an M_r 100 000 protein with an M_r 10 000 peptide represents an equal molar concentration of the impurity, and sequencing would be impossible. In general, the more pure the protein, the less difficulty will be found in obtaining an unambiguous sequence.

The second requirement concerns chemical purity. There are many potential contaminants that may interfere with sequencing. Especially important are aldehydes, which are common contaminants in many organic solvents, and non-volatile amines. The sample should be in a buffer which is completely volatile and contains no non-volatile salts. Suitable solutions include water, aqueous acetic acid, trifluoroacetic acid, ammonia, ammonium bicarbonate and ammonium acetate. The presence of small amounts of SDS is not detrimental, and may help maintain solubility and prevent losses due to adsorption.

If the protein has been purified by preparative SDS-polyacrylamide gel electrophoresis in the final step (Section 8.2), contamination by high molecular weight acrylamide polymers is virtually certain. These cause massive artefacts in sequencing but may be removed by precipitating the protein with 90% methanol.

References

Andersson, K., Benyamin, Y., Douzou, P. and Balny, C. (1978). Organic solvents and temperature effects on desorption from immunoadsorbents. DNP-BSA anti-DNP as a model. *J. immunol. Methods* **23**, 17–21.

Andersson, K. K., Benyamin, Y., Douzou, P. and Balny, C. (1979). The effects of organic solvents and temperature on the desorption of yeast 3-phosphoglycerate kinase from immunoadsorbent. *J. immunol. Methods* **25**, 375–381.

Avrameas, S. and Ternynck, T. (1967). Use of iodide salts in the isolation of antibodies and the dissolution of specific immune precipitates. *Biochem. J.* **102**, 37c–39c.

Avrameas, S. and Ternynck, T. (1969). The cross-linking of proteins with glutaraldehyde and its use for the preparation of immunoadsorbents. *Immunochemistry* **6**, 53–66.

Axèn, R., Porath, J. and Ernback, S. (1967). Chemical coupling of peptides and proteins to polysaccharides by means of cyanogen halides. *Nature* **214**, 1302–1304.

Bethell, G. S., Ayers, J. S., Hancock, W. S. and Hearn, M. T. W. (1979). A novel method of activation of cross-linked agaroses with 1,1'-carbonyldiimidazole which gives a matrix for affinity chromatography devoid of additional charged groups. *J. biol. Chem.* **254**, 2572–2574.

Brodsky, F. M., Parham, P., Barnstable, C. J., Crumpton, M. J. and Bodmer, W. F. (1979). Monoclonal antibodies for analysis of the HLA system. *Immunol. Rev.* **47**, 3–61.

Brown, P. J., Leyland, M. J., Keenan, J. P. and Dean, P. D. G. (1977). Preparative electrophoretic desorption in the purification of human serum ferritin by immunoadsorption. *FEBS Lett.* **83**, 256–259.

Campbell, D. H., Leuscher, E. and Lerman, L. S. (1951). Immunologic adsorbents. I. Isolation of antibody by means of a cellulose–protein antigen. *Proc. natn. Acad. Sci. U.S.A.* **37**, 575–578.

Chaiken, I. M., Wilchek, M. and Parikh, I. (1983). (eds). "Affinity Chromatography" and Biological Recognition. Academic Press, New York.

Chidlow, J. W., Bourne, A. J. and Bailey, A. J. (1974). Production of hyperimmune serum against collagen and its use for the isolation of specific collagen peptides on immunosorbent columns. *FEBS Lett.* **41**, 248–252.

Cresswell, P. (1977). Human B cell alloantigens: separation from other membrane molecules by affinity chromatography. *Eur. J. Immunol.* **7**, 636–639.

Cuatrecasas, P. and Anfinsen, C. B. (1971). Affinity chromatography. *Meth. Enzymol.* **22**, 345–378.

Cuatrecasas, P. and Parikh, I. (1972). Adsorbents for affinity chromatography. Use of N-hydroxysuccinimide esters of agarose. *Biochemistry* **11**, 2291–2299.

Dalchau, R. and Fabre, J. W. (1982). The purification of antigens and other studies with monoclonal antibody affinity columns: the complementary new dimension of monoclonal antibodies. *In* "Monoclonal Antibodies in Clinical Medicine" (A. J. McMichael and J. W. Fabre, eds), pp. 519–556. Academic Press, London and New York.

Dandliker, W. B., de Saussure, V. A. and Levandoski, N. (1968). Antibody purification at neutral pH utilizing immunospecific adsorbents. *Immunochemistry* **5**, 357–365.

Er-El, Z., Zaidenzaig, Y. and Shalteil, S. (1972). Hydrocarbon-coated Sepharoses. Use in the purification of glycogen phosphorylase. *Biochem. biophys. Res. Commun.* **49**, 383–390.

George, S. and Schenck, J. R. (1983). Thiocyanate inhibition of protein iodination by the chloramine-T method and a rapid method for measurement of low levels of thiocyanate. *Anal. Biochem.* **130**, 416–419.

Gersten, D. M. and Marchalonis, J. J. (1978). A rapid, novel method for the solid-phase derivatization of IgG antibodies for immune-affinity chromatography. *J. immunol. Methods* **24**, 305–309.

Goding, J. W. and Herzenberg, L. A. (1980). Biosynthesis of lymphocyte surface IgD in the mouse. *J. Immunol.* **124**, 2540–2547.

Goding, J. W. and Burns, G. F. (1981). Monoclonal antibody OKT-9 recognizes the receptor for transferrin on human acute lymphocytic leukemia cells. *J. Immunol.* **127**, 1256–1258.

Haff, L. A. (1981). An investigation into the mechanism of electrophoretic desorption of immunoglobulin G from protein A-Sepharose. *Electrophoresis* **2**, 287–290.

Haff, L. A., Lasky, M. and Manrique, A. (1979). A new technique for desorbing substances tightly bound to affinity gels: flat bed electrophoretic desorption in Sephadex via isoelectric focusing (FEDS-IEF). *J. biochem. biophys. Methods* **1**, 275–286.

Harford, J. (1984). An artefact explains the apparent association of the transferrin receptor with a *ras* gene product. *Nature* **311**, 673–675.

Hager, D. A. and Burgess, R. R. (1980). Elution of proteins from sodium dodecyl sulfate-polyacrylamide gels, removal of sodium dodecyl sulfate, and renaturation of enzymatic activity: results with sigma subunit of *Escherichia coli* RNA polymerase, wheat germ topoisomerase, and other enzymes. *Anal. Biochem.* **109**, 76–86.

Heinzel, W., Rahimi-Laridjani, I. and Grimminger, H. (1976). Immunoadsorbents: nonspecific binding of proteins to albumin-Sepharose. *J. immunol. Methods* **9**, 337–344.

Helenius, A. and Simons, K. (1975). Solubilization of membranes by detergents. *Biochim. biophys. Acta* **415**, 29–79.

Helenius, A., McCaslin, D. R., Fries, E. and Tanford, C. (1979). Properties of detergents. *Meth. Enzymol.* **56**, 734–749.

Herrmann, S. H. and Mescher, M. F. (1979). Purification of the H-2K^k molecule of the murine major histocompatibility complex. *J. biol. Chem.* **254**, 8713–8716.

Herrmann, S. H., Chow, C. M. and Mescher, M. F. (1982). Proteolytic modifications of the carboxy-terminal region of H-2K^k. *J. biol. Chem.* **257**, 14181–14186.

Hill, R. J. (1972). Elution of antibodies from immunoadsorbents: effect of dioxane in promoting release of antibody. *J. immunol. Methods* **1**, 231–245.

Houwen, B., Goudeau, A. and Dankert, J. (1975). Isolation of hepatitis B surface antigen (HB$_s$Ag) by affinity chromatography on antibody-coated immunoadsorbents. *J. immunol. Methods* **8**, 185–194.

Johnson, G. and Garvey, J. S. (1977). Improved methods for separation and purification by affinity chromatography. *J. immunol. Methods* **15**, 29–37.

Joniau, M., Grossberg, A. L. and Pressman, D. (1970). Arginyl residues in the active sites of antibody against the 3-nitro-4-hydroxy-5- iodophenyl acetyl (NIP) group. *Immunochemistry* **7**, 755–769.

Kleinschmidt, W. J. and Boyer, P. D. (1952). Interaction of protein antigens and antibodies. I. Inhibition studies with the egg albumin-anti-egg albumin-system. *J. Immunol.* **69**, 247–255.

Kowal, R. and Parsons, R. G. (1980). Stabilization of proteins immobilized on Sepharose from leakage by glutaraldehyde cross linking. *Anal. Biochem.* **102**, 72–76.

Lecomte, J. and Tyrrell, D. A. J. (1976). Isolation of antihaemagglutinin antibodies with an influenza A virus immunoadsorbent. *J. immunol. Methods* **13**, 355–365.

Letarte-Muirhead, M., Barclay, A. N. and Williams, A. F. (1975). Purification of the Thy-1 molecule, a major cell-surface glycoprotein of rat thymocytes. *Biochem. J.* **151**, 685–697.

Lowe, C. R. (1979). "An Introduction to Affinity Chromatography." North-Holland, Amsterdam and New York.

Lowe, C. R. and Dean, P. D. G. (1974). "Affinity Chromatography." John Wiley, London and New York.

Mains, R. E. and Eipper, B. A. (1976). Biosynthesis of adrenocorticotropic hormone in mouse pituitary tumor cells. *J. biol. Chem.* **251**, 4115–4120.

March, S. C., Parikh, I. and Cuatrecasas, P. (1974). A simplified method for cyanogen bromide activation of agarose for affinity chromatography. *Anal. Biochem.* **60**, 149–152.

McMaster, W. R. and Williams, A. F. (1979). Identification of Ia glycoproteins in rat thymus and purification from rat spleen. *Eur. J. Immunol.* **9**, 426–433.

Melchers, F. and Messer, W. (1970). The activation of mutant β-galactosidase by specific antibodies. Purification of eleven antibody activatable mutant proteins and their subunits on Sepharose immunosorbents. Determination of the molecular weights by sedimentation analysis and acrylamide gel electrophoresis. *Eur. J. Biochem.* **17**, 267–272.

Mescher, M. F., Stallcup, K. C., Sullivan, C. P., Turkewitz, A. P. and Herrmann, S. H. (1983). Purification of murine MHC antigens by monoclonal antibody affinity chromatography. *Meth. Enzymol.* **92**, 86–109.

Morgan, M. R. A., Johnson, P. M. and Dean, P. D. G. (1978). Electrophoretic desorption of immunoglobulins from immobilised protein A and other ligands. *J. immunol. Methods* **23**, 381–387.

Nilsson, K. and Mosbach, K. (1980). p-Toluenesulfonyl chloride as an activating agent of agarose for the preparation of immobilized affinity ligands and proteins. *Eur. J. Biochem.* **112**, 397–402.

Nilsson, K. and Mosbach, K. (1981). Immobilisation of enzymes and affinity ligands to various hydroxyl group carrying supports using highly reactive sulphonyl chlorides. *Biochem. biophys. Res. Commun.* **102**, 449–457.

Nishikawa, A. H. and Bailon, P. (1975). Affinity purification methods. Improved procedures for cyanogen bromide reaction on agarose. *Anal. Biochem.* **64**, 268–275.

O'Carra, P., Barry, S. and Griffin, T. (1973). Spacer arms in affinity chromatography: the need for a more rigorous approach. *Biochem. Soc. Trans.* **1**, 289–290.

Oi, V. T., Jones, P. P., Goding, J. W., Herzenberg, L. A. and Herzenberg, L. A. (1978). Properties of monoclonal antibodies to mouse Ig allotypes, H-2 and Ia antigens. *Curr. Topics Microbiol. Immunol.* **81**, 115–129.

O'Sullivan, M. J., Gnemmi, E., Chieregatti, G., Morris, D., Simmonds, A. D., Simmons, S., Bridges, J. W. and Marks, V. (1979). The influence of antigen properties on the conditions required to elute antibodies from immunoadsorbents. *J. immunol. Methods* **30**, 127–137.

Parham, P. (1979). Purification of immunologically active HLA-A and -B antigens by a series of monoclonal antibody columns. *J. biol. Chem.* **254**, 8709–8712.

Parham, P. (1983). Monoclonal antibodies against HLA products and their use in immunoaffinity purification. *Meth. Enzymol.* **92**, 110–138.

Parham, P., Barnstable, C. J. and Bodmer, W. F. (1979). Use of a monoclonal antibody (W6/32) in structural studies of HLA-A,B,C antigens. *J. Immunol.* **123**, 342–349.

Parikh, I. and Cuatrecasas, P. (1975). Affinity chromatography in immunology. *Meth. Protein Separation* **1**, 1–44.

Pihko, H., Lindgren, J. and Ruoslahti, E. (1973). Rabbit α-fetoprotein: Immunochemical purification and partial characterization. *Immunochemistry* **10**, 381–385.

Porath, J. and Kristiansen, T. (1975). Biospecific affinity chromatography and related methods. *In* "The Proteins" (H. Neurath and R. L. Hill, eds), Vol. 1, pp. 95–178. Academic Press, New York and London.

Read, R. J. D., Cox, J. C., Ward, H. A. and Nairn, R. C. (1974). Conditions for purification of anti-*Brucella* antibodies by immunoadsorption and elution. *Immunochemistry* **11**, 819–822.

Ruoslahti, E. (1986). "Immunoadsorbents in Protein Purification". *Scand. J. Immunol.* Suppl. **3**.

Schneider, C., Newman, R. A., Sutherland, D. R., Asser, U. and Greaves, M. F. (1982). A one-step purification of membrane proteins using a high-efficiency immunomatrix. *J. biol. Chem.* **257**, 10766–10769.

Secher, D. S. and Burke, D. C. (1980). A monoclonal antibody for large-scale purification of human leucocyte interferon. *Nature* **285**, 446–450.

Shimizu, A., Watanabe, S. Yamamura, Y. and Putnam, F. W. (1974). Tryptic digestion of immunoglobulin M in urea:conformational lability of the middle part of the molecule. *Immunochemistry* **11**, 719–727.

Smith, J. A., Hurrell, J. G. R. and Leach, S. J. (1978). Elimination of nonspecific adsorption of serum proteins by Sepharose-bound antigens. *Anal. Biochem.* **87**, 299–305.

Stallcup, K. C., Springer, T. A. and Mescher, M. F. (1983). Characterization of an anti-H-2 monoclonal antibody and its use in large-scale antigen purification. *J. Immunol.* **127**, 923–930.

Stark, G. R., Stein, W. H. and Moore, S. (1960). Reactions of the cyanate present in aqueous urea with amino acids and proteins. *J. biol. Chem.* **236**, 3177–3181.

Stearne, P. A. van Driel, I. R. Grego, B., Simpson, R. J. and Goding, J. W., (1985). The murine plasma cell antigen PC-1: Purification and partial amino acid sequence. *J. Immunol.* **134**, 443–448.

Stenman, U.-H., Sutinen, M.-L., Selander, R.-K., Tontti, K. and Schröder, J. (1981). Characterisation of a monoclonal antibody to human alpha-fetoprotein and its use in affinity chromatography. *J. immunol. Methods* **46**, 337–345.

Sunderland, C. A., McMaster, W. R. and Williams, A. F. (1979). Purification with monoclonal antibody of a predominant leukocyte-common antigen and glycoprotein from rat thymocytes. *Eur. J. Immunol.* **9**, 155–159.

Tanford, C. (1969). Protein denaturation. *Adv. Protein Chem.* **23**, 121–282.

Tanford, C. (1970). Protein denaturation. Part C. Theoretical models for the mechanism of denaturation. *Adv. Protein Chem.* **24**, 1–95.

Tesser, G. I., Fisch, H. U. and Schwyzer, R. (1974). Limitations of affinity chromatography: solvolytic detachment of ligands from polymeric supports. *Helv. Chim. Acta* **57**, 1718–1730.

Tollaksen, S. L., Edwards, J. J. and Anderson, N. G. (1981). The use of carbamylated charge standards for testing batches of ampholytes used in two-dimensional electrophoresis. *Electrophoresis* **2**, 155–160.

Turkewitz, A. P., Sullivan, C. P. and Mescher, M. F. (1983). Large-scale purification of murine I-A^k and I-E^k antigens and characterization of the purified proteins. *Molec. Immunol.* **20**, 1139–1147.

Weintraub, B. D. (1970). Concentration and purification of human chorionic somato-mammotropin (HCS) by affinity chromatography. Application to radioimmunoassay. *Biochem. biophys. Res. Commun.* **36**, 83–89.

Wilchek, M., Oka, T. and Topper, Y. J. (1975). Structure of a soluble super-active insulin is revealed by the nature of the complex between cyanogen-bromide-activated Sepharose and amines. *Proc. natn. Acad. Sci. U.S.A.* **72**, 1055–1058.

Wofsy, L. and Burr, B. (1969). The use of affinity chromatography for the specific purification of antibodies and antigens. *J. Immunol.* **103**, 380–382.

Zoller, M. and Matzku, S. (1976). Antigen and antibody purification by immunoadsorption: elimination of non-biospecifically bound proteins. *J. immunol. Methods* **11**, 287–295.

7   Immunofluorescence

The use of fluorescent derivatives of antibodies to trace antigen was pioneered by Coons (Coons *et al.*, 1941, 1942; Coons and Kaplan, 1950; Coons, 1961). It was shown that antibodies could be coupled with β-anthracene or fluorescein isocyanate with retention of antigen-binding properties, and that the fluorescent antibodies could be used as very sensitive probes to detect and localize antigen.

Subsequently, Riggs *et al.* (1958) introduced the more stable and convenient fluorescein isothiocyanate (FITC), which has remained the most popular fluorochrome until the present time. One of the main disadvantages of FITC has been its very rapid fading under intense illumination, but this problem is now solved (Johnson and Araujo, 1981; Johnson *et al.*, 1982; Giloh and Sedat, 1982).

Over the years, numerous other fluorochromes have come and gone, with tetramethyl rhodamine isothiocyanate (TRITC) emerging as one of the few of lasting value. In more recent times, a number of useful derivatives of rhodamine with absorption and emission even further into the red region have become available, and the use of the protein phycoerythrin as a fluorescent probe (Oi *et al.*, 1982; Glazer and Stryer, 1984) holds considerable promise.

Immunofluorescence has now made the transition from a tricky and somewhat erratic technique to one of the highest precision. The purity of the fluorochromes and the quality of the optics of fluorescence microscopes have improved enormously. The development of the fluorescence-activated cell sorter (FACS) allows the rapid, sensitive, quantitative and objective analysis of single cells, and also the possibility of cell separation on the basis of membrane antigens. Multi-parameter analysis and sorting is now also a well-established procedure.

As is the case for all procedures in which antibodies are used, the best results will only be obtained if there is an understanding of the basic principles and the important experimental variables. It is the purpose of this chapter to provide a conceptual and practical framework for the optimal use of monoclonal antibodies in immunofluorescence. Methods of tissue preparation and cutting of histological sections will not be explored in detail. An excellent account of this topic is given by Brandtzaeg (1982).

7.1 Principles of Immunofluorescence

When light is absorbed by certain molecules known as fluorochromes, the energy of the photons may be transferred to electrons, which assume a higher energy level. Some of the energy is liberated within 10^{-15} s as heat when the electron returns to the lowest vibrational energy of the excited state; the remainder is released after a few nanoseconds as a photon of lower energy than the initial photon. This phenomenon is called fluorescence, and its efficiency is described by the term *quantum yield* (Crooks, 1978).

The wavelengths which are capable of causing a molecule to fluoresce are known as the excitation spectrum, and the wavelengths of emitted fluorescent light the emission spectrum. The emission spectrum is shifted to a slightly longer wavelength than the excitation spectrum (Stokes' Law), although the two spectra often overlap. For practical purposes, the excitation spectrum is very similar to the absorption spectrum in the visible wavelength range. Spectral data for FITC, TRITC and several other fluorochromes have been summarized by Hansen (1967).

The intensity of fluorescence often varies depending on the physical environment (Crooks, 1978). Some fluorochromes are most highly fluorescent in an aqueous environment (e.g. FITC), while other fluoresce much more intensely in a non-polar environment (e.g. dimethylamino naphthalene). The spectral characteristics of fluorescein are also dependent on pH, and this property has been exploited in the measurement of intracellular hydrogen ion concentration (Ohkuma and Poole, 1978). Fluorochromes which are closely adjacent may interact and transfer energy from one to the other, and may therefore quench each other (Section 7.3.2).

7.1.2 The Fluorescence Microscope

Virtually all modern immunofluorescence microscopy is now carried out using the vertical ("incident" or epi-") illumination system of Brumberg (1959) and Ploem (1967), in which the excitation light reaches the specimen via the objective (Fig. 7.1). The advantages of epi-illumination include much higher intensity of illumination and brighter image, better image quality, ease

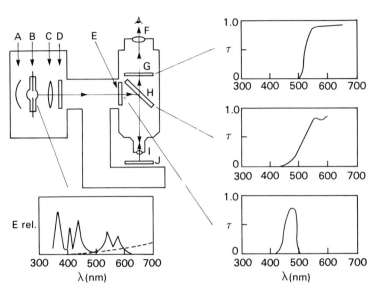

Fig. 7.1 The fluorescence microscope (epi-illumination). Light from the high pressure mercury lamp (B) is concentrated by a mirror (A) and a lens (C), and passes through a heat filter (D), and a barrier filter (E). The barrier filter is usually a bandpass filter designed for optimal excitation but removing the shorter wavelengths that may cause autofluorescence. The light is then reflected by a dichroic mirror (beam splitter, H), and passes through the objective (I) to the specimen (J). The emitted light, which is of longer wavelength, passes through the dichroic mirror and the barrier filter (G), which removes any stray light of wavelengths for excitation. Light then passes through the ocular (F) to the eye. The schematized characteristics of the filters are for FITC.

of usage, and the ability to combine fluorescence simultaneously or in rapid alternation with visible transmission. The combination of immuno-fluorescence with phase contrast transmission microscopy is particularly useful for examination of intact living cells (Nossal and Layton, 1976; Goding and Layton, 1976).

Figure 7.1 shows a typical modern fluorescence microscope. The high-pressure mercury lamp (B) is focused via a curved mirror (A) and a lens (C). The light passes through a heat filter (D) and an excitation filter (E) to dichroic mirror (H), where it is reflected downwards to the objective lens (I), which acts as condenser. Light emitted from the specimen (J) passes back upwards through the objective, but because of its longer wavelength it passes straight through the dichroic mirror. A barrier filter (G) prevents any residual stray excitation light from reaching the eyepiece (F), but freely transmits the emitted fluorescence.

Older instruments, especially those using transmitted light fluorescence, often employed a 200 watt mercury lamp (HBO 200). Newer microscopes with epi-illumination generally employ a 50 watt mercury lamp (HBO 50).

The substantial improvement in filters and the much shorter light path of modern microscopes renders the image as bright or brighter than that obtained with 200 watt lamps.

The mercury lamp has intense peaks of emission at 313, 334, 365, 405, 435, 546 and 578 nm; its output intensity in the range 450–525 nm is much less than that of the peaks. Unfortunately, it is the latter range that is most suitable for excitation of FITC. However, the quantum yield for FITC is very high, and illumination with the mercury lamp is usually quite adequate. Quartz–halogen or high pressure xenon lamps (60–100 W) provide a continuous spectrum of comparable intensity to the mercury lamp in this region (Fig. 7.1; dotted line) and are a viable alternative. They have the advantage that they are less expensive and may be turned on and off whenever desired. Quartz–halogen lamps are not nearly as efficient as mercury lamps in exciting rhodamine derivatives, because the mercury lamp has strong emission peaks at 546 and 578 nm (Fig. 7.1).

The HBO 50 mercury lamp has a maximum life of about 200 h, and towards the end of its life its intensity diminishes. The pressure inside the lamp during operation is 40–70 atmospheres, and if used beyond the recommended life there is a chance of its exploding. Explosion of the lamp is not likely to escape the lamp housing, but will result in considerable damage to the microscope. The lifetime of the lamp is diminished by frequent starting and stopping, and it is recommended that a log book of use be kept, and that once turned on, it be left on for several hours rather than turning it on and off more than once a day (Gardner and McQuillin, 1980).

The numerical aperture (NA) of the objective lens is of prime importance in achievement of maximal fluorescence intensity. The numerical aperture is the sine of the half aperture angle multiplied by the refractive index of the medium filling the space between the specimen and the front lens. Air has a refractive index of 1, so the theoretical maximum NA of an air objective is 1.0. Immersion oil has a refractive index of 1.515, making it possible to achieve a considerable improvement in NA.

In an epi-illumination system, both the intensity of excitation and efficiency of collection of fluorescent light increase as the square of the NA. It would therefore be expected that the observed fluorescence would increase as the fourth power of the NA (Nairn, 1976), and this is the result obtained experimentally (Haaijman and Slingerland-Teunissen, 1978). Objective lenses for immunofluorescence should be chosen for the highest possible numerical aperture.

Gardner and McQuillin (1980) point out that with epi-illumination the most expensive oil immersion lens is not necessarily the most suitable for fluorescence microscopy. Complex apochromatic 50 × objectives with large numbers of lenses have greater internal light scattering than simple fluorite oil immersion lenses, and may produce a worse background and less contrast.

It is preferable to use eyepieces of low magnification (e.g. 8 × rather than 12.5 ×), because fluorescence intensity decreases exponentially with increasing total magnification.

7.1.3 Choice of Fluorochromes

The choice of fluorochrome will be governed by a number of factors. If a single colour is needed, FITC (Fig. 7.2) will usually be the fluorochrome of choice. FITC is inexpensive, has a high quantum efficiency, and is relatively hydrophilic. The rapid fading under the intense ultraviolet illumination of modern fluorescence microscopes can be overcome by phenylenediamine or n-propyl gallate (Section 7.5.4), although these reagents are rather toxic for living cells. The 488 nm line of the argon laser used in the fluorescence-activated cell sorter is ideally suited to excitation of FITC (Table 7.1). The triazine derivative of fluorescein, dichlorotriazinylamino fluorescein (DTAF; Blakeslee and Baines, 1976; Blakeslee, 1977) has very similar optical properties to FITC (Table 7.1), but is considerably more stable. DTAF conjugates

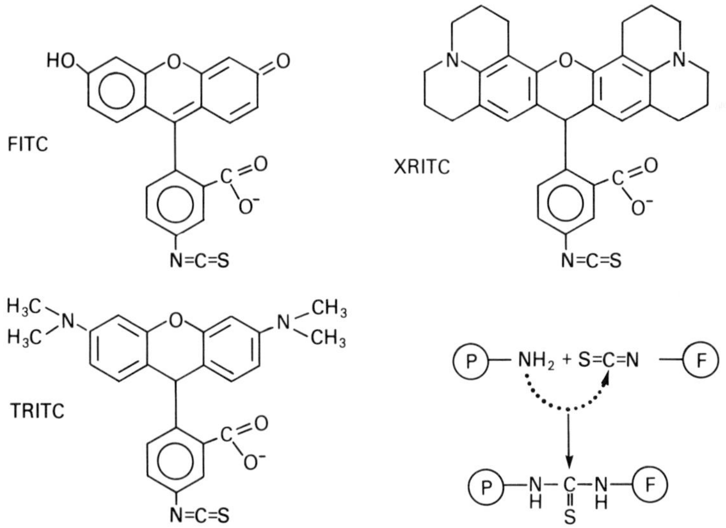

Fig. 7.2 *Structure of commonly used fluorochromes, and mechanism of coupling to protein. The nucleophilic unprotonated ε-amino groups of lysine residues attack the isothiocyanate group, resulting in a thiourea bond.*

Table 7.1 Properties of fluorochromes

Flurochrome	Supplier	Maximum excitation	Emission (nm)	Comments
FITC	RO, MP	495	525 (500–580)	pKa ≃ 5·5. Absorbance and emission maximal at pH > 8.
DTAF	RO	489	515	Similar spectral properties to FITC. Active form more stable
TRITC	RO	554	573	Rather hydrophobic; dissolves easily ir dimethyl sulphoxide.
Texas Red	MP	596	615 (600–680)	Hydrolyses rapidly. Hydrolysis product very soluble in water and not prone to adsorption to protein.
XRITC	RO	582	601	Very hydrophobic; tends to bind noncovalently to protein.
MRITC	RO	540	577	New fluorochrome, more hydrophilic than XRITC.
Phycoerythrin	BD, MP	475–560	576	Protein from red algae. Virtually no emission below 550 nm. Very high absorbance and quantum yield.

The values given may vary by up to 10 nm, depending on whether the fluorochrome is in free solution or bound to protein, on the fluorochrome:protein ratio, and other factors.
RO; Research Organics, 4353 East 49th Street, Cleveland, Ohio 44125.
MP; Molecular Probes, 24750 Lawrence Road, Junction City, Oregon 97448.
BD; Becton Dickinson FACS Systems, 490-B Lakeside Drive, Sunnyvale, California 94086.

may be fractionated by ammonium sulphate precipitation to remove over-conjugated molecules.

The second most popular fluorochrome is tetramethyl rhodamine iso-thiocyanate (TRITC), which is much more highly fluorescent than rhodamine isothiocyanate. TRITC has an absorption and excitation maximum at 550 nm, and an emission maximum at 580 nm. The intense red fluorescence of TRITC is easily distinguished from the green fluorescence of FITC, and for many years these two fluorochromes were the combination of choice for two-colour fluorescence experiments (Nossal and Layton, 1976; Goding and Layton, 1976). Fading of TRITC is much slower than FITC (Giloh and Sedat, 1982).

The use of TRITC is not without its problems, however. It is more hydrophobic than FITC, and therefore has a tendency to bind nonspecifically to proteins and cells. The limited solubility of TRITC in water may be overcome by dissolving it in dimethyl sulphoxide (DMSO) prior to conjugation to antibodies (Bergquist and Nilsson, 1974; Goding, 1976), and it is strongly recommended that this procedure be followed. TRITC dissolves rapidly in DMSO, allowing it to be added to antibodies before significant hydrolysis occurs. The nonspecific adsorption of TRITC to proteins via hydrophobic interactions and subsequent slow release or exchange may cause significant background fluorescence; the use of DMSO as a solvent seems to diminish this problem (Goding, 1976). The hydrophobic nature of TRITC also causes denaturation and precipitation of antibodies if they are too heavily conjugated (Section 7.3). Some of the problems of limited solubility of TRITC may be overcome by a new fluorochrome, morpholinorhodamine isothiocyanate (MRITC; Table 7.1) which is said to be more hydrophilic but to have similar optical properties.

Overconjugation of antibodies with TRITC and other rhodamine derivatives may also lead to a severe reduction in fluorescence intensity due to self-quenching (Section 7.3.2). TRITC has often been used in two-colour immunofluorescence experiments with the fluorescence-activated cell sorter (FACS), but its sensitivity is limited by its relatively poor excitation at the only available lines of the argon laser (488 nm and 514 nm). In spite of all the above, TRITC has proven to be an extremely useful fluorochrome. If attention is paid to these details, excellent results may be obtained.

In the last few years, two new rhodamine derivatives have appeared. These are "XRITC" (Research Organics) and "Texas Red", which is a sulphonyl chloride derivative. The spectral properties of XRITC and Texas Red are very similar (Table 7.1). Maximal excitation of XRITC occurs at 582 nm, and maximal emission at 601 nm, while the corresponding figures for protein-bound Texas Red are 596 nm and 615 nm respectively (Titus et al., 1982). There is very little overlap between the emission spectra of these dyes and that of FITC, so they should be ideal for two-colour fluorescence. Heavily conjugated antibodies tend to precipitate in both cases (Titus et al., 1982).

Table 7.2 Typical filter combinations for epi-illumination

Fluorochrome	Excitation filter	Dichroic mirror	Barrier filter
FITC, DTAF	BP 450–490	FT 510	LP 520
TRITC	BP 546/10	FT 580	LP 590

Mercury lamps provide strong lines at 313, 334, 365, 405, 435, 546 and 578 nm. There is no discrete line in the optimal range for FITC excitation. The filters for TRITC may also be used for Texas Red, XRITC and phycoerythrin, although better results would probably be obtained using an excitation filter which included the 578 nm line, and a dichroic mirror and barrier filter with a slightly longer wavelength.

The filter combination used for TRITC (Table 7.2) allows moderately efficient excitation of XRITC or Texas Red, although the use of the 546 nm mercury line is probably not optimal. A set of filters exploiting the 578 nm line might be preferable. Texas Red and XRITC are not adequately excited by the 488 nm or 514 nm lines available from argon lasers, but excitation with the 568 nm line of krypton lasers is efficient (Titus *et al.*, 1982).

The hydrolysis product of Texas Red is a very water-soluble sulphonic acid derivative, and is thus easily removed with minimal risk of adsorption to proteins. In contrast, removal of the very hydrophobic XRITC and its hydrolysis products is difficult and unreliable. It is claimed that the protein conjugates of Texas Red are more soluble than those of XRITC (Titus *et al.*, 1982). However, it was admitted that protein precipitation occurred at higher conjugation ratios, so the claim for increased solubility of Texas Red conjugates when compared to XRITC conjugates remains unsubstantiated.

Oi *et al.* (1982) have recently demonstrated that phycobiliproteins from red algae have considerable potential as fluorescent probes (see also Glazer and Stryer, 1984). Their molar absorbance coefficients are extremely high because of their multiple bilin chromophores, and they have high quantum yields. R-phycoerythrin would appear to be ideal for use with argon lasers, because it is efficiently excited at 488 nm. The emission spectrum of R-phycoerythrin begins at 550 nm and peaks at about 580 nm, and would seem ideally suited to two-colour fluorescence experiments in conjunction with FITC. The phycoerythrins are highly soluble and stable, and are easily purified. They are available commercially (Molecular Probes, 24750 Lawrence Road, Junction City, Oregon; Becton-Dickinson, 490-B Lakeside Drive, Sunnyvale, California).

Methods for coupling of phycoerythrins to antibodies are still undergoing development. Oi *et al.* (1982) prepared biotinylated phycoerythrin, bound it to avidin and purified the conjugates by high-pressure liquid chromatography. Some biotin-binding sites remained available for binding to biotinylated monoclonal antibodies (see Section 7.4).

Alternatively, phycoerythrin was coupled to antibodies via disulphide bonds. Thiolated phycoerythrin was prepared by treatment with iminothiolane hydrochloride, and antibodies were coupled with protected thiol groups using N-succinimidyl 3-(2-pyridylthio)-propionate (SPDP). The two proteins were mixed to allow formation of disulphide bonds.

Disulphide bonds prepared in this way are not very stable, and it may be worthwhile to explore other coupling procedures. The use of *m*-maleimidobenzoyl N-hydroxysuccinimide ester (MBS) (Kitagawa and Aikawa, 1976; Liu *et al.*, 1979; O'Sullivan *et al.*, 1979; Kitagawa, 1981) allows the formation of stable nonreducible thioether bonds between two different proteins, with minimal like–like cross-linking (Vallera *et al.*, 1982; Volkman *et al.*, 1982). It would seem that MBS or related compounds (Yoshitake *et al.*, 1979; Lee *et al.*, 1980) might be useful in coupling phycoerythrin to monoclonal antibodies (see Youle and Neville, 1980). Molecular Probes offer a detailed protocol on the use of MBS and related compounds for coupling phycoerythrin to antibodies.

Milstein and Cuello (1983) have described a system in which HAT sensitivity was re-introduced into an anti-peroxidase hybridoma. Upon fusion with spleen cells, hybrid antibodies containing one anti-peroxidase arm and one anti-X arm were produced. This procedure allows very simple and efficient coupling of the enzyme to antibodies (Milstein and Cuello, 1984), and could easily be adapted for use with phycoerythrin.

7.1.4 Use of Fluorescent Microspheres

Parks *et al.* (1979) have shown that hybridoma cells may be analysed and fractionated using antigen-coated fluorescent microspheres. The microspheres have the attraction that each sphere contains hundreds of fluorochrome molecules, and the binding of a single particle may be detected with ease (Rembaum and Dreyer, 1980). Higgins *et al.* (1981) have used fluorescent microspheres in a sensitive assay for cell surface antigens.

Hydrophilic fluorescent microspheres containing activated groups for protein coupling are available commercially (Covaspheres; Covalent Technology, 3941 Research Park Drive, Ann Arbor, Michigan 48106). Instructions for use are supplied by the manufacturer (see also Higgins *et al.*, 1981).

7.1.5 Choice of Filters

The choice of filter combinations for immunofluorescence is a large subject, and the range of filters that are commercially available is constantly expanding. The magnitude of the problem can be gauged from the fact that Zeiss offers no less than five different filter combinations for FITC alone. It is therefore possible to give only the most general advice, and the microscope manufacturers should be consulted for further details.

Virtually all modern high-performance filters are of the interference type. Interference filters have much higher transmission, steeper cutoff slopes and

250 Monoclonal Antibodies: Principles and Practice

greater rejection of unwanted wavelengths than the older filters. The barrier filter (Fig. 7.1) usually consists of a long-pass (LP) filter which transmits all wavelengths longer than a certain value (the wavelength at which transmittance is 50%). The excitation filter may consist of a short-pass (KP, German kurzpass) filter in which all wavelengths shorter than a given wavelength are passed. More commonly, the excitation filter is a band-pass (BP) filter which passes a narrow band corresponding to a particular mercury line or portion of the spectrum. Band-pass filters are described by the centre wavelength and the bandwidth (e.g. BP546/10). Band-pass filters may be constructed by combining a long-pass and a short-pass filter. For example, the BP450-490 filter consists of a combination of LP 450 and KP 490.

The other major optical filter is the dichroic mirror or beam-splitter, which is an interference mirror set at 45° to the light path. The dichroic mirror is designed to reflect light of wavelengths shorter than a certain value (i.e. the excitation light), and to freely transmit light of wavelengths longer than this value (i.e. the emission). For example, the FT510 mirror reflects light of wavelength less than 510 nm.

Typical filters for use with the mercury lamp are given in Table 7.2. The excitation filter for FITC passes exciting light in the range 450–490 nm, all of which is reflected to the objective via the FT510 dichroic mirror. Emitted fluorescence (mostly longer than 510 nm) passes through the dichroic mirror. The LP 520 barrier filter provides additional exclusion of the excitation wavelengths.

The corresponding filters for TRITC are BP 546/10 (which selects the 546 nm mercury line), FT580 dichroic mirror and LP 590 barrier filter. As mentioned earlier, the filter set for TRITC is reasonably well suited for Texas Red and XRITC, although better combinations could probably be obtained.

R-phycoerythrin is excited efficiently at 450–490 nm, and emits above 550 nm (Oi et al., 1982; Glazer and Stryer, 1984). The filter combination suggested for FITC would be suitable, because the barrier filter passes all wavelengths above 520 nm.

7.1.6 Direct and Indirect Immunofluorescence

Direct immunofluorescence involves the exclusive use of antibodies which have been covalently coupled with fluorochromes. The specimen is incubated with the labelled antibody, unbound antibody is removed by washing, and the specimen is examined.

In many cases, however, it may be preferred to use an indirect technique, in which the specimen is incubated with an unconjugated antibody, washed, and incubated with a fluorochrome-conjugated anti-immunoglobulin antibody. The second or "sandwich" antibody thus reveals the presence of the first.

A major advantage of indirect immunofluorescence is that one fluorescent anti-immunoglobulin antibody will suffice for many first antibodies; it is not necessary to conjugate each new antibody individually. Indirect immuno-fluorescence is essential if the monoclonal antibody is only available in the form of a culture supernatant, because direct conjugation of supernatants with fluorochromes is unsatisfactory. The indirect technique usually gives brighter fluorescence than the direct, because many second antibodies may bind to the first. Amplifications of six to eight-fold are possible. This may be a decided advantage where monoclonal antibodies are used, becuase their monospecificity results in smaller numbers of binding sites.

The main disadvantage of the indirect technique is that the anti-immunoglobulin sandwich reagent is unable to distinguish between exo-genous and endogenous immunoglobulin. For example, a rabbit anti-mouse immunoglobulin sandwich reagent would detect membrane immunoglobulin on mouse B cells, regardless of whether or not other antibodies are present. The problem is not as severe when mouse monoclonal antibodies are used to stain human cells, because rabbit or goat anti-mouse immunoglobulin will cross-react weakly or not at all with human immunoglobulin. Nonetheless, the possibility of such cross-reactions is a real one, and controls must always be performed in which the first antibody is omitted.

The omission of the first antibody is also a useful control to check for nonspecific binding of the second antibody via Fc receptors. Obviously, such a control does not address the question of Fc receptor binding by the first antibody.

7.1.7 Strategy for Two-colour Fluorescence

It is frequently desirable to examine biological specimens simultaneously for two independent antigens. Two-colour immunofluorescence is not a great deal more difficult than one-colour, but a few simple principles should be observed.

The most common pair of fluorochromes for two-colour fluorescence are FITC and TRITC (e.g. Goding and Layton, 1976). The excitation and emission spectra of this combination overlap somewhat (Fig. 7.3), and care is needed to select filters which provide maximal selectivity (see also Kearney and Lawton, 1975). It may be necessary to choose a somewhat more selective filter combination at the expense of a certain degree of loss of fluorescence intensity. Two-colour immunofluorescence will be greatly facilitated by the recent development of XRITC and Texas Red (Table 7.1, Fig. 7.3), because their emission spectra are much further removed from FITC. If phyco-erythrin were to be used together with FITC, it would be essential to choose barrier filters selective for red and green respectively.

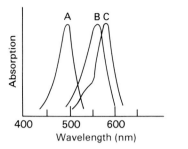 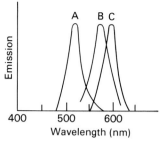

Fig. 7.3 Schematic illustration of the absorption and emission spectra of FITC (A), TRITC (B) and XRITC (C).

The other strategic point that must be considered is that of sandwich reagents. If both antibodies are directly conjugated with fluorochromes, there is no problem. However, if a sandwich procedure is used, the second step reagents must be chosen such that they will only react with the appropriate first step. Anti-immunoglobulin sandwich reagents would bind to both first antibodies. A common strategy is to couple one antibody directly to its fluorochrome, and couple the other with biotin. The biotinylated antibody may then be detected with avidin coupled to a second fluorochrome (Section 7.4).

The opportunities for unexpected artefacts and nonspecificity are greatly increased in two-colour systems, and it is mandatory to include a wide range of controls, such as the omission of each first-stage antibody.

7.2 The Fluorescence-activated Cell Sorter (FACS)

The development of the fluorescence-activated cell sorter (FACS) has been a major contribution to the field of immunofluorescence, and that of cell biology in general. Analysis by the FACS is often known as *flow cytometry*. The principles of operation have been reviewed in detail (Bonner *et al.*, 1972; Herzenberg *et al.*, 1972; Herzenberg *et al.*, 1976; Miller *et al.*, 1981; Loken and Stall, 1982; Kruth, 1982).

A single-cell suspension, labelled with fluorescent antibody or DNA stain, is passed in single file through a narrow laser beam, and the emitted fluorescence is collected by an optical system at right angles to the illumination. The emitted fluorescence of each individual cell is measured and stored in a computer memory. Other parameters, such as low-angle forward light scatter or Coulter volume, may also be measured and recorded on a cell-by-cell basis. Most commercially available machines are also capable of separating the cells into individual fluid droplets which may be electrostatically deflected into tubes, depending on fluorescence, light scatter or a combination of parameters.

The power of the FACS may be exploited in many different ways. Although it was initially envisaged as a preparative machine, experience has shown that the major use in most laboratories is analytical. The FACS can analyse up to 5000 cells per second, and plot any desired combination of parameters. Unlike visual fluorescence microscopy, the readout is rapid, objective and quantitative.

The use of multi-parameter analysis adds enormously to the power of flow cytometry. Simultaneous analysis of surface antigens detected by two different monoclonal antibodies, together with light scatter or Coulter volume, is now routine. Cells may also be separated on the basis of DNA content, or any other parameter which can be measured by fluorescence methods.

It is possible to detect and isolate extremely rare cells. Herzenberg et al. (1979) were able to identify fetal cells in the human maternal circulation. Very rare "class-switch" mutants or variants of myeloma or hybridoma cells may be detected and isolated (Radbruch et al., 1980; Holtkamp et al., 1981; Neuberger and Rajewsky, 1981; Oi et al., 1984). It is possible to use the FACS to sort and clone hybridomas on the basis of their binding of antigen (Parks et al., 1979). Kavathas and Herzenberg (1983) have shown that the FACS may be used in conjunction with monoclonal antibodies to select DNA-transfected mouse L cells which express human surface antigens.

7.2.1 Suitable Fluorochromes for Flow Cytometry

The main constraint on the choice of fluorochromes is the wavelength of the laser emission lines. The commonly used argon laser has a strong line at 488 nm, which is ideally suited to excitation of FITC, but is inefficient for excitation of TRITC (Fig. 7.3). The argon laser also has a strong line available at 514 nm, which may be used to excite either FITC or TRITC. Even at 514 nm, excitation of TRITC is inefficient (Fig. 7.4), but the argon laser does not have any emissions of longer wavelength. Nonetheless, it is possible to perform two-colour fluorescence analyses using FITC and TRITC. Cross-channel spill may be corrected electronically (Loken et al., 1977; Ledbetter et al., 1980a).

The newer rhodamine derivatives XRITC and Texas Red are even less efficiently excited by the argon laser, and are virtually unusable. However, Titus et al. (1982) have shown that excellent two-colour analyses are possible using a combination of FITC and Texas Red in a two-laser system. FITC was excited at 488 nm by an argon laser, while Texas Red was excited at 568 nm by a krypton laser. Unfortunately the krypton laser is expensive and of

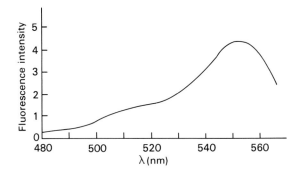

Fig. 7.4 *Excitation spectrum of TRITC. Emission was measured at 575 nm.*

somewhat uncertain reliability. Another possibility is tunable lasers (Hardy *et al.*, 1982a, b), but as yet their use has been limited.

Oi *et al.* (1982) have shown that phycoerythrin and FITC are both excited efficiently by the 488 nm line of the argon lasers and may be used together in two-colour immunofluorescence experiments. In view of the high cost of two-laser systems, it may be anticipated that this system will become very popular.

7.2.2 "Gating Out" Dead Cells

Dead cells may bind large amounts of fluorescent antibody in a nonspecific manner. The presence of dead cells will seriously degrade the precision with which cells may be analysed, particularly when it is desired to identify and sort very rare cells.

It has been shown that the low-angle light scatter correlates well with cell viability (reviewed by Loken and Stall, 1982). Living cells tend to have a larger degree of scatter than dead cells. It is possible to choose a "window" of low-angle light scatter which includes the majority of living cells and excludes dead cells. However, the discrimination achieved by light scatter gating is not absolute.

An attractive alternative involves the use of the DNA stain propidium iodide, which only enters the nucleus of dead cells. Propidium iodide bound to DNA is strongly excited at 488 nm, and emits intense fluorescence at 570 nm (Krishnan, 1975). Addition of 2 μg/ml propidium iodide to the buffer during the final incubation period will label all dead cells. The intensity of fluorescence of dead cells is so great that they may be gated out without affecting the profiles of living cells (Layton, 1980). A stock solution of 100 μg/ml propidium iodide in PBS plus 0.1% azide will last for many months when stored at 4°C. Residual propidium iodide in the medium may stick in the tubing, and give rise to varying degrees of staining of dead cells in later samples. Propidium iodide-treated cells cannot be fixed, since transfer then occurs between labelled and unlabelled cells. Like all DNA stains, propidium iodide may be mutagenic, and should be handled with care.

7.2.3 The Logarithmic Amplifier

The range of fluorescence between the brightest positive and dullest negative cells may easily span two to three orders of magnitude, and it is impossible to display this range on linear coordinates. It is now possible to use amplifiers which directly perform logarithmic transformation of the fluorescence signals. The use of logarithmic presentation is often extremely helpful, because it allows clear-cut distinction of populations of cells which appeared to merge into each other on linear displays (Ledbetter *et al.*, 1980a, b; Hardy *et al.*, 1982a, b).

7.3 Conjugation of Antibodies with Fluorochromes

The conjugation of antibodies with fluorochromes is technically very simple to perform, but the best results will only be obtained if care is taken to follow certain principles. Bright, specific fluorescence is possible only if the antibodies are optimally conjugated.

7.3.1 General Principles

The conjugation of antibodies with the isothiocyanate derivatives of fluorescein or rhodamine proceeds by nucleophilic attack of the unprotonated ε-amino group of lysine on the fluorochrome, resulting in a thiourea bond (Fig. 7.2). Maximal efficiency of conjugation is achieved at pH 9.5, where a large fraction of lysines are unprotonated. Extraneous nucleophiles, such as Tris, amino acids, ammonium ions or azide (Lachman, 1964) will inhibit conjugation.

Susceptibility of fluorochromes to hydrolysis

The isothiocyanate derivatives of fluorochromes are very susceptible to hydrolysis, even by moisture in the air. They must be stored in a dessicator. If stored in the cold, they must be allowed to warm to room temperature before the bottle is opened, to avoid condensation. It is more important that they be kept dry than cold. Almost all preparations of fluorochromes contain a certain proportion of hydrolysed material, which necessitates adding somewhat more total fluorochrome to achieve the desired conjugation ratio.

During conjugation of fluorochromes to proteins, a competing hydrolysis reaction takes place. At high protein concentrations (i.e. > 10 mg/ml), conjugation to protein is strongly favoured, and efficiencies of up to 70% coupling may be achieved. At lower protein concentrations, the competing hydrolysis becomes very significant (The and Feltkamp, 1970a, b). It is perfectly feasible to conjugate antibodies at a protein concentration of 1–2 mg/ml, but it is necessary to add much more fluorochrome. The hydrolysed fluorochrome is easily removed by gel filtration on Sephadex G-25.

Solubility of fluorochromes

Some fluorochromes, notably the rhodamine derivatives, are rather insoluble in water. During attempts to dissolve them, hydrolysis takes place, leading to erratic results. Addition of the fluorochrome to the protein as a solid is not recommended because it will lead to uneven labelling, and in any case does not solve the solubility problem. In addition, it is much easier to deliver a measured volume of a solution than to weigh accurately a very small mass of fluorochrome.

Conjugations will be found to be much easier and predictable if the fluorochrome is made up as a stock solution (10 or 1 mg/ml) in dimethyl sulphoxide, and the desired volume added to the protein dropwise with stirring (Bergquist and Nilsson, 1974; Goding, 1976). Even FITC is more easily handled in this way. The solution should be made up immediately before use, because the dimethyl sulphoxide will usually contain some water. Unlike most organic solvents, dimethyl sulphoxide does not denature proteins when used in low concentrations (1–10% v/v).

Sulphonyl chlorides react with DMSO, and this solvent must not be used with Texas Red. Good results are obtained by adding Texas Red as a powder, perhaps because its hydrolysis product is very hydrophilic (R. Haugland, personal communication). If a solvent is needed, dimethyl formamide or acetonitrile are suitable.

*Achievement of optimal fluorochrome:protein
ratio*

The molar ratio of fluorochrome:protein (F/P) is one of the most important parameters in immunofluorescence. If this ratio is too low, the intensity of fluorescence will be poor. The ratio should certainly not be less than 1.0, because unlabelled antibodies would compete with labelled antibodies for binding sites, reducing the sensitivity. The upper limit is determined by a number of factors.

In the case of fluorescein, conjugation results in a marked lowering of the isoelectric point of the antibody, and overconjugation may produce highly charged acidic species which tend to stick nonspecifically to cells, especially if they are fixed. Optimally FITC-conjugated antibodies have a molar F/P ratio of ~ 2–3 for fixed cells, and ~ 4–6 for intact living cells. Self-quenching due to overconjugation (Section 7.3.2) is not a serious problem with FITC conjugates.

The molar F/P ratio for FITC may be calculated from a formula proposed by The and Feltkamp (1970a, b):

$$\text{F/P ratio} \quad = \quad \frac{2.87 \times OD_{495}}{OD_{280} - 0.35 \times OD_{495}}$$

Similarly, the concentration of IgG may be calculated:

$$[\text{IgG}] \quad = \quad \frac{OD_{280} - 0.35 \times OD_{495}}{1.4} \text{ mg/ml}$$

These formulae make a correction for the contribution of FITC to the total absorbance at 280 nm, and produce a figure that is sufficiently accurate for practical purposes.

Determination of the optimal conjugation ratios for other fluorochromes is not so easy. The various rhodamine derivatives are more hydrophobic than FITC, and even moderately conjugated antibodies tend to precipitate. Precipitation of some of the antibody after conjugation with rhodamine derivatives is not disastrous. The precipitated material probably represents the more heavily conjugated molecules, and the supernatant after centrifugation may contain highly active fluorescent antibodies. An additional problem with rhodamine derivatives is that they are very susceptible to self-quenching if antibodies are overconjugated (see next section). Self-quenching is easily mistaken for inactivation of antigen-binding.

For reasons which will become apparent in the next section, it is not possible to calculate exact molar F/P ratios from the absorption spectra of rhodamine conjugates. The best basis for comparison of conjugation ratios is the ratio of absorbance at the peak in the visible region to the absorbance at 280 nm.

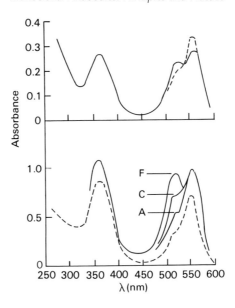

Fig. 7.5 *Effect of close proximity of TRITC molecules to each other.* Upper panel: *absorption spectrum of moderately heavily conjugated TRITC conjugated protein before pronase diges-tion (solid line) and after pronase digestion (dotted line).* Lower panel: *absorption spectrum of free TRITC (dotted line), lightly conjugated protein (A), moderately conjugated protein (C), and heavily conjugated protein (F). Conjugates were diluted such that their absorbances at 550 nm were equal.*

7.3.2 Self-quenching of Rhodamine Derivatives

The absorption spectrum of unbound TRITC in the visible range shows a major peak at 550 nm with a small shoulder at 515–520 nm. However, when TRITC is conjugated to IgG, the shape of the visible absorption peak changes (Fig. 7.5). As the molar F/P ratio increases, the shoulder at 515–520 nm becomes progressively more prominent until it almost reaches the same height as the 550 nm peak. A similar absorption spectrum has been observed for stacked dimers of fluorescein (Forster and Konig, 1957), for fluorescein bound to monoclonal antifluorescein antibody 20-20-3 (Kranz and Voss, 1981) and also for fluorescein in its monomeric protonated form at pH 5.5 (Alexandra *et al.*, 1980). When heavily conjugated TRITC-IgG is digested with pronase, the 515 nm peak decreases and the 550 nm peak increases (Fig. 7.5), suggesting that the spectral changes are due to rho-damine–rhodamine interactions. It is obvious from these results that simple calculations based on spectral data cannot allow accurate assessment of the molar F/P ratios of TRITC conjugates.

Rhodamine–rhodamine interactions have a second very important prac-tical consequence. As the molar F/P ratio increases, the quantum yield of

Table 7.3 Suggested conditions for labelling antibodies with fluorochromes

Fluorochrome	Protein concentration (mg/ml)	Mass of fluorochrome[a] (μg per mg protein)	Ideal absorbance ratio	Conditions
FITC	> 10	10–20	495:280 = 0·5–1·0	pH 9·5, 20°C, 2 h
	3	~ 50	495:280 = 0·5–1·0	pH 9·5, 20°C, 2 h
	1	~ 100	495:280 = 0·5–1·0	pH 9·5, 20°C, 2 h
DTAF	> 10	< 15	495:280 = 0·5–1·0	pH 9·0, 20°C, 2 h
TRITC	> 10	5–15	550:280 = 0·2–0·3	pH 9·5, 20°C, 2 h
XRITC	> 10	5–15	unknown	pH 9·5, 20°C, 2 h
Texas Red	1–2	75–150	596:280 = 0·8–1·0	pH 9·0, 4°C, 1–2 h

[a]The figures given in this table are guidelines only; the mass of fluorochrome may need to be adjusted to achieve the recommended absorbance ratios.

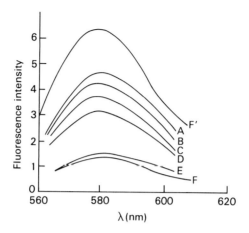

Fig. 7.6 Demonstration of self-quenching of TRITC. A series of conjugates of TRITC to IgG were prepared, with increasing ratios of fluorochrome (A–F), and their concentration adjusted to give equal absorbance at 550 nm. They were then excited at 550 nm, and the fluorescence emission spectrum measured. It is apparent that the quantum efficiency of emission decreases markedly with increasing conjugation ratio. When the most heavily conjugated preparation (F) was treated with pronase, there was a marked increase in quantum yield (F'), showing that self-quenching occurs due to proximity of TRITC molecules to each other. The OD550:OD280 ratios of the various conjugates were as follows: A, 0.27; B, 0.30; C, 0.40; D, 0.49; E, 0.58; F, 0.60.

fluorescence declines drastically (Fig. 7.6). Digestion of heavily conjugated TRITC-IgG with pronase results in a very large increase in fluorescence (Fig. 7.6), indicating that the decline is due to self-quenching by rhodamine–rhodamine interactions.

The foregoing makes it clear that heavily rhodamine-conjugated antibodies may have much weaker fluorescence than more lightly-conjugated antibodies, and practical experience bears this point out. The phenomenon of self-quenching has probably been seen repeatedly by immunologists, but erroneously ascribed to antibody inactivation. Similar phenomena are observed with Texas Red conjugates (Titus *et al.*, 1982).

Recommendations for optimal conjugation ratios are given in Table 7.3.

7.3.3 Practical Procedure

Antibodies for conjugation should be at least partially purified. Ammonium sulphate fractionation (Section 4.2.1) is adequate, providing that it is performed carefully. However, non-immunoglobulin proteins remaining after crude purification may result in higher background staining. In particular, the presence of transferrin might cause artefactual labelling of cells with transferrin receptors (Goding and Burns, 1981). The best results are obtained with highly purified antibodies (see Goding, 1976).

Antibodies to be conjugated with FITC, TRITC or XRITC should be dialysed overnight against pH 9·5 carbonate/bicarbonate buffer (8·6 g Na_2CO_3 and 17·2 g $NaHCO_3$ to 1 litre H_2O), while antibodies to be conjugated with DTAF or Texas Red should be dialysed against 0.025M borate buffer, pH 9·0 (4·76 g $Na_2B_4O_7.10H_2O$ in 1 litre H_2O, titrated to pH 9 with ~ 46 ml 0·1M HCl). In addition to obtaining the optimal pH for conjugation, dialysis removes any inhibitors of conjugation such as amines or azide.

The optical density of the protein at 280 nm should be measured, and the concentration calculated. The concentration of IgG in mg/ml is obtained with sufficient accuracy by dividing the OD_{280} (1 cm cell) by 1·4. The total protein mass should be calculated, and the desired amount of fluorochrome calculated using the guidelines set out in Table 7.3.

The fluorochrome must be allowed to reach room temperature before the bottle is opened, to prevent condensation. The fluorochrome is weighed out and made up to 1·0 or 10·0 mg/ml in dimethyl sulphoxide (except Texas Red; Section 7.3.1), and the desired volume added to the protein dropwise, with stirring.

The reaction is allowed to proceed at room temperature, shielded from light. Thermal movement is quite sufficient, and stirring serves no purpose once the initial mixing has taken place.

After 1–2 h at room temperature, the reaction will be essentially complete. The reaction proceeds somewhat more rapidly at high protein concentrations, and an incubation time of 2–3 h may be desirable if the protein concentration is less than 1–2 mg/ml. If the protein concentration is high ($\geqslant$ 10 mg/ml), the initial fluorochrome: protein ratio should be held at the lower end of the recommended range, and the main risk is one of overconjugation. At low protein concentrations (1–2 mg/ml), overconjugation is not very likely, and much higher initial ratios are needed to achieve adequate conjugation (Table 7.3).

After conjugation, unreacted or hydrolysed dye must be separated from the protein. Gel filtration on Sephadex G-25 in PBS containing 0.1% NaN_3 is convenient and effective. The disposable PD-10 columns (Pharmacia) are ideal. The first coloured band to emerge is the conjugated protein. Removal of free dye by dialysis is very slow and inefficient, and is not recommended. Even small traces of the free dye may cause significant nonspecific fluorescence.

In the older literature, it was frequently recommended that the conjugate be further purified by ion exchange chromatography to remove overconjugated molecules (Cebra and Goldstein, 1965; Goding, 1976). This procedure is seldom used today. Providing that care has been taken in all the aforementioned aspects, ion exchange chromatography is seldom necessary. Ion exchange chromatography will sometimes be required when fixed and permeabilized cells are used.

Principles and practical details of ion exchange chromatography are discussed in Chapter 4. The conjugate should be passed over a Sephadex G-25 or Biogel P-6 column equilibrated with 10 mM Tris-HCl, pH 8.0. (The same procedure can be used to simultaneously remove unbound fluorochrome.) A column of DEAE-Sepharose or DEAE-Sephacel equilibrated with the same buffer will bind virtually all conjugates. As the salt concentration is raised, progressively more heavily conjugated antibodies will be eluted (Cebra and Goldstein, 1965; Goding, 1976).

The absorbance of each conjugate should be measured at 280 nm and at its peak in the visible region. Conjugates are more prone to aggregation than unconjugated antibodies, and are best stored at 4°C, protected from light (Section 4.7).

7.4 The Avidin–Biotin System

When animals are fed on a diet containing raw egg white as their sole source of protein, they develop a condition known as "egg-white injury", characterized by neuromuscular disorders, dermatitis and loss of hair. Investigations by Györgi (1940) established that egg white injury was due to deficiency of the water-soluble vitamin biotin, and subsequently it was shown that egg-white contains a protein which binds biotin with extremely high affinity.

The biotin-binding protein was named "avidin" (reviewed by Green, 1975). Avidin is a tetramer of identical subunits, each of M_r 15 000. Its isoelectric point is 10.5, and its affinity for biotin approximately $10^{15} M^{-1}$. The biotin–avidin complex has been widely used in biology (reviewed by Bayer and Wilchek, 1978; Bayer *et al.*, 1979).

The biotin–avidin system is particularly attractive as a sandwich system used in conjunction with antibodies (Heitzmann and Richards, 1974; Heggeness and Ash, 1977). Biotin is relatively polar, and can be coupled to antibodies under very mild conditions with little disruption to their structure. Avidin may then be used as a stable high-affinity second step reagent which may be coupled with fluorochromes, enzymes, ferritin or other molecules. The use of avidin as a sandwich reagent also avoids the use of anti-immunoglobulin antibodies. Finally, the biotin–avidin system is appealing because only one conjugate need to be prepared and characterized for all affinity systems, and both components are commercially available and inexpensive.

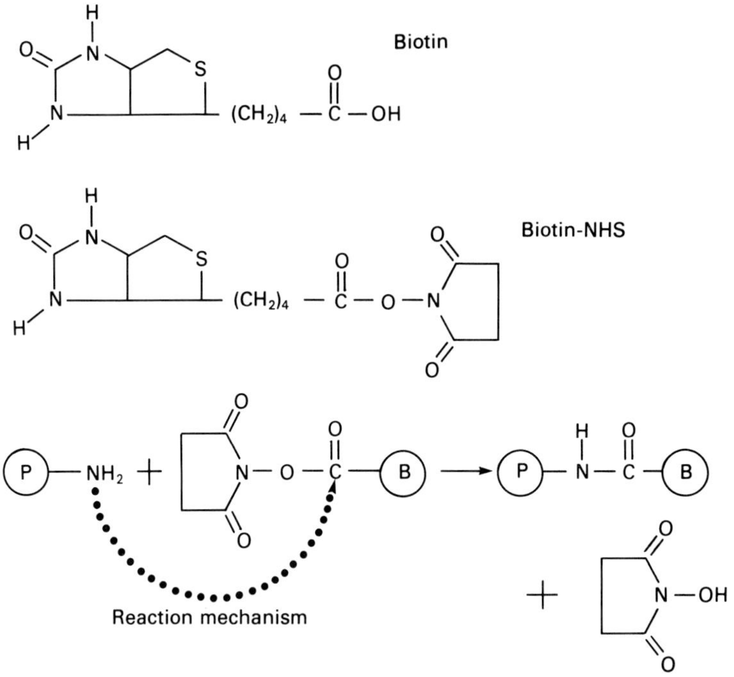

Fig. 7.7 Structure of biotin and its succinimide ester, and mechanism of coupling to proteins. The nucleophilic unprotonated ε-amino groups of lysine residues attack the activated ester, resulting in an amide bond and release of N-hydroxysuccinimide.

7.4.1 Conjugation of Antibodies with Biotin Succinimide Ester

Biotin must be derivatized before it can be coupled to protein; the most convenient method of coupling uses the N-hydroxysuccinimide ester of biotin, which is commercially available from numerous suppliers. Succinimide esters are extremely useful compounds for derivatization of antibodies, because they allow formation of a stable amide bond under very mild conditions (see also Section 5.3.4).

The structures of biotin and its N-hydroxysuccinimide ester are shown in Fig. 7.7. The reaction with proteins involves nucleophilic attack of the unprotonated ε-amino of lysine on the ester, and displacement of N-hydroxysuccinimide. The reaction proceeds most efficiently at slightly alkaline pH. Coupling is inhibited by extraneous amines, Tris or azide.

Succinimide esters are very prone to hydrolysis, and during coupling there is a competing hydrolytic reaction. As is the case with the isothiocyanate

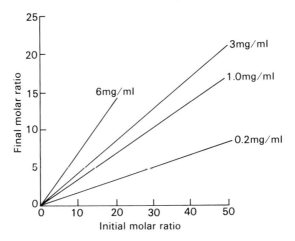

Fig. 7.8 Schematic illustration of the effect of protein concentration on the efficiency of coupling with biotin succinimide ester. At high protein concentrations, the reaction is quite efficient. At low protein concentrations, the competing hydrolysis reaction predominates.

derivatives of fluorochromes (Section 7.3.1), the extent to which coupling and hydrolysis compete depends on the protein concentration.

Figure 7.8 illustrates this point. Bovine IgG was conjugated with the hapten 3-nitro-4-hydroxy-5-iodophenyl-(NIP), using the succinimide ester derivative. Unlike biotin, the NIP group absorbs in the visible range, allowing spectrometric determination of the conjugation ratio. Assuming that the succinimide ester of biotin has a similar degree of reactivity, one may use the curves shown in Fig. 7.8 to make a rough estimate of the likely efficiency of coupling.

Practical procedure

The antibody to be conjugated should be at least partly purified by careful ammonium sulphate precipitation followed by two washes in 40–50% saturated ammonium sulphate (Section 4.2.1). More highly purified antibodies will give better results.

The antibody must then be dialysed overnight against $0.1M$ $NaHCO_3$, pH 8.0–8.3. If precipitation with ammonium sulphate has been used, it is advisable to change the dialysis fluid once or twice. Following dialysis, the IgG concentration should be measured from the absorbance at 280 nm (Section 7.3.3), and the protein concentration adjusted to 1.0 mg/ml by dilution with $0.1M$ $NaHCO_3$.

The biotin succinimide ester must be warmed to room temperature before the bottle is opened. The ester is then weighed out, and dissolved in dimethyl sulphoxide to 1·0 mg/ml immediately before use. The ester is freely soluble in dimethyl sulphoxide, which is important because any delays in dissolving it in water will result in hydrolysis. The half-life of succinimide esters in 0·1M NaHCO$_3$ is of the order of minutes.

The ester solution is then added to the antibody, and mixed immediately. If the conditions of pH and protein concentration given above are followed strictly, it will be found that 120 μl of the ester solution per ml of antibody will result in optimal conjugation. Sometimes it may help to vary the ratio of biotin:protein in the range 60 μl/ml to 240 μl/ml. Underconjugation results in weak staining; overconjugation results in damage to the antibody and loss of specificity.

The mixture should be held at room temperature for 1–2 h, by which time the reaction will have gone to completion. The biotin-conjugated protein should then be dialysed overnight against PBS with 0.1% sodium azide, and stored at 4°C. It is best not to freeze conjugated proteins, as they are prone to aggregation.

Avidin conjugated with FITC or TRITC is available from Vector Laboratories, 1479 Rollins Road, Burlingame, California 94010. Alternatively, avidin may be purchased from Sigma or other suppliers, and conjugated using the procedures given in Section 7.3.3. Optimally conjugated FITC-avidin has an $OD_{496}OD_{280}$ ratio of 1·4–1·6, while optimally conjugated TRITC-avidin has an $OD_{550}:OD_{280}$ ratio of about 0.5.

7.4.2 Problems with the Avidin–Biotin System

When used to label intact living cells, the biotin–avidin system is capable of excellent results. The "background" nonspecific binding is very low, and the fluorescence is bright. However, the extremely basic nature of avidin (pI = 10.5) may cause it to bind electrostatically to acidic structures. When FITC-avidin is used to stain permeabilized and fixed cells, marked binding to condensed chromatin is observed (Heggeness, 1977). The chromosomes are beautifully outlined, and banding of *Drosophila* salivary gland chromosomes is vividly illustrated.

The nonspecific binding of avidin to DNA may be diminished by raising the salt concentration (0·3M KCl; Heggeness, 1977), and may also be diminished by competition with a large excess of the basic protein cytochrome C. A combination of KCl (0·3–0·5M) and cytochrome C (1 mg/ml) during staining lowers the background considerably. Finn *et al.*, (1980) have shown that the nonspecific binding of avidin may also be diminished by exhaustive succinoylation of lysine groups. Alternatively, it is possible to use anti-biotin antibodies (Barger, 1979). Monoclonal antibodies to biotin would be ideal.

An alternative to avidin is *streptavidin*, a biotin-binding protein from *Streptomyces*. Streptavidin has four identical chains of similar molecular weight to those of avidin, but amino acid analysis shows that streptavidin has only half the number of basic amino acids and the same number of acidic amino acids (Green, 1975). Streptavidin would therefore be expected to have a much less basic isoelectric point, and show corresponding less nonspecific binding. So far, relatively few papers have appeared on streptavidin (Hofman *et al.*, 1980; Finn *et al.*, 1981). The protein is available commercially from Bethesda Research Laboratories, Zymed Laboratories and from Amersham, already conjugated with fluorochromes or enzymes.

A second potential problem with the avidin–biotin system concerns the fact that *most tissue culture media contain biotin*. It is therefore important to wash the cells in a buffer lacking biotin prior to use of avidin, and to avoid the use of tissue culture medium at any stage during staining. Failure to observe this point may result in very erratic results.

7.5 Staining Cells with Fluorescent Antibodies

The staining of cells for immunofluorescence is very simple. Cells are held with the antibody for 30–60 min, washed and examined. Providing the antibodies have the correct specificity and are not under- or overconjugated, and providing the microscope is suitable, little difficulty will be experienced at this stage.

If cells bearing Fc receptors are present, it is strongly advisable to de-aggregate all antibodies just prior to staining. De-aggregation should be at 100 000 g. The Beckmann Airfuge is ideal, because its small tubes and rapid acceleration allow short centrifugations. Typically, antibodies are de-aggregated at 20–25 psi for 5–10 min, and the top half of the liquid used. The bottom half may be saved and re-used.

Alternatively, binding to Fc receptors may be abolished by use of Fab or F(ab')₂ fragments (Chapters 4 and 8), but these should be used for both first and second steps. The binding of the second step reagent via Fc receptors may be suspected if controls omitting the first antibody are not totally negative. Protocols for the generation of F(ab')₂ and Fab fragments of sheep and goat antibodies are given by Davies *et al.* (1978) and Mage (1980). Fragmentation of rabbit antibodies is very simple, and suitable procedures are given by Stanworth and Turner (1978). The generation of fragments of sheep, goat and rabbit IgG is discussed in Chapter 8.

It is strongly advisable to titrate all reagents, and to use concentrations which are slightly higher than those needed to cause maximal fluorescence. Use of higher concentrations is wasteful, and results in poorer signal:noise ratio. The logic of Figure 6.1 is applicable to any affinity system, including immunofluorescence.

The kinetics of binding of individual monoclonal antibodies to cells varies considerably. In many cases, as little as 15 min incubation will be sufficient to acheive saturation. However, the occasional monoclonal antibody may take much longer (see Chapter 2). If precise quantitation of the intensity of fluorescence is needed, it is strongly recommended that the incubation times be held constant from one experiment to the next.

Antibodies should be diluted in buffers containing irrelevant protein, such as 5% fetal calf serum or 1% bovine serum albumin. As a general rule, it is advisable to include 0.1% sodium azide in all buffers. This will discourage microbial growth and inhibit metabolism of the cells to be stained. The staining of membrane antigens of living, metabolically active cells may result in redistribution, endocytosis or shedding of antigen–antibody complexes (Taylor *et al.*, 1971).

If indirect immunofluorescence is to be used, some thought should be given to the quality of the sandwich reagent. It makes no sense to use an extremely specific monoclonal antibody for the first step, and a poorly defined second step. The amplification given by polyclonal second step antibodies may be very useful in increasing the brightness, but care should be taken to use the optimal dilution. Whenever possible, affinity-purified second antibodies are preferred, because they will have the least background.

7.5.1 Membrane Immunofluorescence

The membranes of intact, living cells are impermeable to antibodies. If the living cells are kept cold, labelling will be restricted to the membrane. The use of azide to inhibit cellular metabolism is not as effective as keeping the cells cold. It is possible, however, for antibodies to enter the cell by pinocytosis if the cell is metabolically active (Taylor *et al.*, 1971). It is claimed that auto-antibodies may reach the nucleus of the cell by this route (Alarcon-Segovia, 1979), although these results are not widely accepted.

It should be noted that dead cells often take up large amounts of fluorescent antibody in a nonspecific manner. Care should be taken to ensure that the cells are highly viable, and dead cells should be excluded from any count. Dead cells are usually distinguishable from living cells under phase contrast. They are a dull grey colour, while living cells are usually bright, refractile and smooth. The use of phase contrast visible illumination in conjunction with immunofluorescence is strongly recommended.

Practical procedure

(1) Prepare cell suspension, and wash × 2–3 in **PBS** containing 0·1–1·0%

bovine serum albumin and 0·1% azide ("medium"). All steps should be carried out at 4°C.

(2) Count cells; adjust to 10^7/ml.

(3) To 100 μl cells, add desired volume of first antibody. Leave on ice for 30–90 min.

(4) Resuspend cells in 1–5 ml medium; centrifuge at 400 g for 5 min (= wash).

(5) Repeat washing (step 4).

(6) Resuspend in 100 μl medium; add desired volume of second antibody. Leave on ice 30–90 min.

(7) Wash as before.

(8) Resuspend in 20–30 μl medium containing 10% glycerol and 10–100 μg/ml phenylenediamine to prevent fading (Johnson and Araujo, 1981; see Section 7.5.4). The absorption and emission of FITC is markedly pH-dependent, and the mounting fluid should be neutral or slightly alkaline for maximal sensitivity. Place on a glass slide, and add coverslip. Seal edges with nail polish.

(9) Examine immediately.

Cells may be fixed with 1% paraformaldehyde in 0.85% NaCl after staining, and examined immediately or kept at 4°C for at least a week (Lanier and Warner, 1981). It is also possible to fix cells with paraformaldehyde prior to staining (Biberfeld *et al.*, 1974; Smit *et al.*, 1975; Nossal and Layton, 1976; Goding and Layton, 1976), although Lanier and Warner were not able to achieve good results using this approach.

7.5.2 Cytoplasmic Fluorescence

Reaction of antibodies with the cytoplasmic components of cells requires that they be fixed and made permeable to proteins. There are a large number of different ways of fixing cells, and it may be necessary to adapt the fixation procedure for each individual problem. In many cases, fixation and permeabilization are performed simultaneously by the use of organic reagents such as ethanol, methanol, acetone, or acetic acid. A variety of more sophisticated procedures are available. If the antigen to be detected by a monoclonal antibody is destroyed by one method of fixation, a method based on a different principle should be tried.

In general, cytoplasmic staining is more prone to problems of nonspecific binding than is the case with living cells. It may be necessary to wash for prolonged periods (30–120 min) between steps. It is often recommended that antibodies with lower F/P ratios should be used, and removal of over-conjugated molecules by ion exchange chromatography may sometimes be necessary. Absorption of conjugates with "acetone liver powder" is a time-honoured but poorly understood procedure which may lower the background (Nairn, 1976). It is one of the last of the "black magic" methods of the 1950s to survive into the 1980s, but may still be found useful as a last resort.

Cells may be grown on coverslips and processed *in situ*, while single-cell suspensions may be deposited onto slides as smears or using a cytocentrifuge (25 000 cells per slide in 100 μl of 50% fetal calf serum). Plasma cells may be air-dried and stored for long periods dessicated at $-20°C$. Other cells may require different handling.

Fixation by organic solvents

The simplest fixation procedure is a brief dip of the slide into acetone at $-20°C$ (Gutman and Weissman, 1972; Rouse *et al.*, 1979). Alternatively, the slides may be fixed in 95% ethanol, 5% acetic acid at $-12°C$ for 15 min (Kearney and Lawton, 1975). The exact temperature is not critical. A third procedure involves fixation in absolute methanol for 15 min (Goldstein *et al.*, 1982).

Whichever method is chosen, it is advisable to wash the slide thoroughly in PBS after fixation, and to keep it moist until staining. If the slide is allowed to dry out after fixation, the subsequent nonspecific staining may be severe.

Fixation by formaldehyde with subsequent permeabilization

Lazarides (1976) fixed cells in 3·5% formaldehyde in PBS for 30 min at room temperature, followed by three washes in PBS. The cells were then permeabilized by treatment with acetone (3 min in 50% acetone/water at 4°C; 5 min in pure acetone; 3 min in 50% acetone/water; 3 min in PBS). After brief drying, cells were exposed to antiserum.

Heggeness *et al.* (1977) fixed in 3% formaldehyde in PBS for 20–45 min at 20°C, rinsed in PBS and quenched any remaining aldehyde groups by washing in PBS containing 0·1M glycine. After a further rinse with PBS, cells were permeabilized by treatment with 0·1% Triton X-100 in PBS, followed by washing in PBS.

In one of the most elaborate fixation procedures, Osborn *et al.* (1978) treated cells with a "stabilization buffer" containing 0·1M piperazine-N, N'-bis[2-ethane sulphonic acid], pH 6·9, 1 mM EGTA, 2·5 mM GTP and 4% polyethylene glycol 6000. Cells were treated with two changes of stabilization buffer (30 s at 20°C), followed by 4 min in the same buffer plus 0·2% Triton X-100. The cytoskeletons were then washed twice with stabilization buffer, and fixed in the same buffer with 1% glutaraldehyde for 10 min. Remaining aldehyde groups were reduced with sodium borohydride (0·5 mg/ml in PBS; two changes of 4 min each), followed by three washes in PBS.

Treatment of cells with glutaraldehyde usually results in severe auto-fluorescence, but the reduction of aldehyde groups by sodium borohydride was apparently sufficient to abolish the problem.

Staining procedure

(1) Without allowing them to dry, transfer the rack of fixed slides into a dish containing PBS + 1% BSA, and wash for about 1 h, stirring gently with a magnetic flea. Change the medium a few times during washing.

(2) Place the slides horizontally in a humidified plastic box, and add 10–20 μl of appropriately diluted first antibody. Leave at 20°C for at least 30 min.

(3) Wash off excess antibody with PBS from a squirt bottle, then wash in PBS/BSA as in step 1.

(4) Repeat step 2, using second antibody.

(5) Repeat step 3.

(6) Add one drop of mounting medium, followed by a coverslip. Mounting medium may consist of 50% glycerol in PBS, or (preferably) 5% w/v n-propyl gallate in glycerol to prevent fading (Giloh and Sedat, 1982; Section 7.5.4). As mentioned previously, the pH of the mounting medium should be neutral or slightly alkaline.

(7) Seal edges of coverslip with nail polish.

7.5.3 Histological Sections

The processing of tissues for histology is described in detail by Pearse (1980), Nairn (1976), Sternberger (1979) and Brandtzaeg (1982). Tissue for frozen sections should be cut into 3–4 mm cubes, and placed in an aluminium foil "boat" on a dry-ice–isopentane mixture or a slurry of semi-solid isopentane in liquid nitrogen. The specimen is then transferred to the pre-cooled chuck of the cryostat, held in a vertical position. The block is frozen onto the chuck by a drop or two of saline of gelatin solution. The chuck is then mounted in the machine, and 4–6 micron sections cut and transferred immediately onto absolutely clean glass slides. In some cases, air-drying for 20 min is the only fixation needed. In others, additional fixation in acetone or methanol may be required. Fixation must be optimized individually for each antigen.

In some instances, it is also possible to process paraffin-type embedded sections for immunofluorescence (Sainte-Marie, 1982; Nairn, 1976; Wick *et al.*, 1978), but many antigenic determinants may be destroyed in the fixation process. A thoughtful and rational account of tissue fixation is given by Brandtzaeg (1982).

7.5.4 Photobleaching and its Prevention

The intense illumination of fluorochromes results in rapid fading of the image. The problem is particularly severe for FITC, but also occurs at a slower rate when TRITC is used. It is claimed that Texas Red is more resistant to photobleaching than TRITC (Titus *et al.*, 1982).

Until recently, little could be done to prevent fading, and it had to be accepted as a fact of life. However, it has now been shown that *p*-phenylenediamine is effective in retarding fading of FITC when added to the specimen in the mounting buffer (Johnson and Araujo, 1981; Johnson *et al.*, 1982). The *o*- and *p*-isomers appear to be equally effective, and the effective concentration may be as little as $1-10\,\mu g/ml$ (J.W. Goding, unpublished). Giloh and Sedat (1982) subsequently made a detailed and quantitative study of photobleaching, and found that n-propyl gallate (0·1–0·25M, in glycerol) was effective for both FITC and TRITC. It appears that molecular oxygen or oxygen-induced free radicals may be involved in photobleaching.

Even in the absence of phenylenediamine or n-propyl gallate, photobleaching is a slow process, with half-times measured in seconds. The duration of exposure of cells to laser light in the fluorescence-activated cell sorter is measured in microseconds, and fading is not a problem in flow cytometry.,

7.6 Nonspecific Fluorescence

Specificity in biological systems is seldom absolute, and nowhere is this more true than in immunofluorescence. The various factors that tend to degrade specificity usually conspire to produce artefactual positive results (Winchester *er al.*, 1975; Goding, 1978), and it is absolutely crucial that rigorous negative controls be included in every experiment.

The causes of nonspecific fluorescence are legion, and include inadequate removal of unconjugated fluorochrome, excessively high F/P ratios, binding of aggregated IgG to Fc receptors, fluorochrome-conjugated non-immunoglobulin contaminants such as albumin and transferrin, dead cells in membrane-staining experiments, contaminating antibodies (including antibodies against calf serum or albumin), inadequate washing, autofluorescence, and light scattering by lenses.

Prevention of nonspecific fluorescence depends on the recognition that it is occurring (not always a trivial point), and the diagnosis of its cause.

7.6.1 Problems Due to the Antibody Preparation

If the antibody contains aggregates, binding to Fc receptors may occur. This problem may be made worse by the use of harsh purification procedures (e.g. elution from affinity columns with strongly denaturing buffers), or by multiple freeze–thaw cycles. Some antibodies (e.g. mouse IgG2b and IgG3) are intrinsically more prone to aggregation than others. The solution is to prevent aggregation if possible, to de-aggregate before use (Section 7.5), or to make Fab or F(ab')$_2$ fragments (Chapter 4).

Contaminating antibodies are not a problem when hybridoma supernatants are used, but the serum of hybridoma-bearing mice will always contain small amounts of "natural antibodies" against almost any antigen. If the serum from hybridoma-bearing mice is used at the optimal dilution (typically $1:10^{4-5}$), these contaminating antibodies are unlikely to be a problem. Purification by ion-exchange chromatography with careful gradient elution will also diminish the proportion of irrelevant antibodies.

A more serious problem concerns the sandwich anti-immunoglobulin reagents for indirect immunofluorescence. If these are not first-rate, they will degrade the specificity of staining. It should be remembered that antibodies against bovine serum albumin (Sidman, 1981) or fetal calf serum components (Johnsson *et al.*, 1976) are common in anti-immunoglobulin sera, and may cause severe nonspecific fluorescence.

A third problem with the antibody preparation concerns the presence of non-immunoglobulin contaminant proteins. These are almost always more acidic than immunoglobulin. Conjugation with fluorochromes makes them even more acidic, and therefore prone to nonspecific electrostatic interactions.

Transferrin is a frequent contaminant in immunoglobulin preparations, and fluorochrome-labelled transferrin may cause artefacts by binding to transferrin receptors on proliferating cells (Goding and Burns, 1981). Similarly, antibodies to tranferrin are present in many anti-immunoglobulin antisera, and may bind to cell-bound transferrin. Low density lipoprotein also binds to cellular receptors, and could probably cause similar problems.

Some commercial antisera have had soluble antigens added to them to "absorb out" unwanted antibodies. This practice virtually guarantees that the antisera will contain antigen–antibody complexes which will bind to Fc receptors. The consumer should make certain that any absorption was done using immobilized antigen. Even if the free antigen does no harm on its own, unexpected reactions may occur when mixtures are used (e.g. in two-colour fluorescence). Liquid-phase absorption is not an acceptable practice in the 1980s.

Most of these problems are avoided by use of good quality antibodies, preferably highly purified before conjugation, and use of antibodies at optimal dilution. If necessary, anti-immunoglobulin sandwich reagents may be affinity-purified on immobilized immunoglobulin.

7.6.2 Problems Due to Conjugation

The presence of unconjugated flourochrome in the antibody preparation is a potent source of nonspecific fluorescence. Removal of free fluorochrome by dialysis is very slow and inefficient, and gel filtration should always be used. There must be a clear area of gel lacking colour between the protein and the free dye. If there is not, the column is not big enough.

A second problem concerns loose adsorption of free dye to protein. This problem is more severe with the more hydrophobic dyes such as TRITC and XRITC, which tend to bind to protein and gradually leach off during staining. The result is a very uniform nonspecific fluorescence. The problem is not usually encountered with FITC or Texas Red, because their hydrolysis products are very hydrophilic. Solving this problem is not easy; it is minimized by using highly purified IgG for conjugation (albumin binds many hydrophobic small molecules noncovalently) and by ensuring that the dye is dissolved in dimethyl sulphoxide before use. Dialysis of conjugates against PBS containing 10% dimethyl sulphoxide may help (see Goding, 1976).

Aggregation of IgG may occur during conjugation, for a variety of reasons. The older practice of dissolving fluorochromes in acetone before addition to the antibody is a potent cause of aggregation, as is the adjustment of pH of antibody solutions by direct addition of NaOH. Aggregation may also occur if an excessive F/P ratio is used, and is particularly prone to occur with the more hydrophobic rhodamine derivatives.

7.6.3 Problems Due to the Antigen

If fluorescent anti-immunoglobulin is used, any immunoglobulin present will stain, regardless of its source. For example, roughly half of spleen cells and 10–20% of peripheral blood lymphocytes have membrane immunoglobulin (mostly IgM and IgD). Some cells may possess cytophilic immunoglobulin adsorbed from serum. Staining of immunoglobulins is avoided by using directly conjugated antibodies, or by use of the avidin–biotin system (Section 7.4). B cells expressing membrane IgG are rare, and anti-γ antibodies may often be used in situations where more broadly reactive anti-immunoglobulin antibodies would give excessively high background (Goding and Layton, 1976).

Some tissues or cells may autofluoresce under the near-ultraviolet light used in fluorescence microscopy. The problem may be lessened by use of good quality band-pass filters in the excitation path. Autofluorescence is often a more yellow colour than the fluorescence of fluorescein. In some cases, counter-staining with other dyes may be used to disguise or eliminate autofluorescence (Nairn, 1976; Gardner and McQuillin, 1980).

Cells grown in tissue culture may show autofluorescence, especially when used in the FACS. It is suspected that this is partly due to components of the tissue culture medium, notably riboflavin and phenol red.

7.6.4 Problems Due to Staining Technique

The problem of nonspecific staining of dead cells in membrane immuno-fluorescence has already been discussed (Sections 7.2.2 and 7.5.1). In general, it is wise to include "carrier" protein in all buffers, to saturate nonspecific protein-binding sites. Suitable proteins include bovine serum albumin (0·1–1·0%) or fetal calf serum (1–10%), but the possibility that one or other antibody might cross-react with the carrier protein (Section 7.6.1) should not be forgotten.

Inadequate washing between steps may also result in nonspecific fluor-escence due to free conjugate or resultant antigen–antibody complexes. The amount of washing that is necessary will be kept to a minimum if all reagents are used at their optimal dilutions (Section 7.5). If a single-cell suspension is used, two washes are usually sufficient between steps. On the other hand cytoplasmic fluorescence of fixed cells or histological sections may require washes over a period of 30–120 min to remove nonspecifically bound anti-body.

Apart from nonspecific staining of the specimen, inadequate washing may give rise to a very uniform fluorescent background over the entire field. A similar problem may occur due to light scattering in the microscope, especially if objective lenses with large numbers of elements (apochromatic) are used (Gardner and McQuillin, 1980). This problem is easily revealed by examining the background with a blank slide on the stage.

Very little experimentation has been carried out on the composition of the wash buffers (see Section 5.7.3). In some cases, nonspecific binding of anti-body may be due to electrostatic effects. This is particularly likely for anti-bodies heavily conjugated with FITC, and a trial of wash buffers with added NaCl (up to 0.5M) or of different pH (5–9) may be rewarding.

7.7 Lack of Staining

In some cases, immunofluorescence with monoclonal antibodies may be weak or totally negative. Assuming that the antibodies can be proven to be active prior to conjugation, it is worth considering whether the conjugation has destroyed activity.

Inactivation of polyclonal antisera by conjugation with fluorochromes is extremely unlikely, because it would require the simultaneous destruction of hundreds of different binding sites. In contrast, inactivation of monoclonal antibodies by conjugation is likely to be an "all-or-none" process. In practice, most monoclonal antibodies may be coupled with fluorochromes or biotin without damage, but an occasional one is totally destroyed.

Virtually all the commercially available fluorochromes utilize lysine residues for coupling. It is fortunate that lysine does not often seem to be a crucial residue in antigen-combining sites. It would probably be possible to label monoclonal antibodies by partial reduction followed by reaction with iodoactamidofluorescein (Molecular Probes, Junction City, Oregon), but this approach has seldom been used.

If it is proven that the antibody is inactivated by coupling with fluoro-chromes, a trial of coupling with biotin is worthwhile. Even though lysine residues are involved in both cases, it may be found that the biotin-conjugated antibodies retain activity. If this approach also fails, the main alternative is to use unconjugated monoclonal antibodies followed by fluorescent anti-immunoglobulin.

Other problems that may be traced to the antibody include a fluoro-chrome: protein ratio that is too low (Table 7.3) or too high (Section 7.3.2).

Yet another cause of failure to detect fluorescence is destruction of the antigen by fixation. In many cases, cells fixed with acetone (Rouse et al., 1979) or methanol (Goldstein et al., 1982) still react with monoclonal anti-bodies. There is evidence that high concentrations of aldehyde fixatives may result in destruction of individual antigenic determinants (Gatti et al., 1974), but such instances are probably uncommon. If it is suspected that fixation has destroyed the antigenic determinant recognized by a particular monoclonal antibody, the empirical trial of a few alternative methods of fixation is the only possible approach, apart from using a different antibody (see Brandtzaeg, 1982, for a detailed discussion of fixation methods).

Another cause of unexpected absence of staining is the presence of biotin in tissue culture medium, when the biotin–avidin system is used.

Finally, it should be remembered that many monoclonal antibodies are of low affinity, and may be removed by excessive washing. A trial of fewer washes, longer incubation periods with antibody, and shorter delays during processing, is indicated if this problem is suspected.

REFERENCES

Alarcón-Segovia, D., Ruíz-Arguelles, A. and Llorente, L. (1979). Antibody penetration into living cells. II. Antiribonucleoprotein IgG penetrates into T$_\gamma$ cells causing

their deletion and the abrogation of suppressor function. *J. Immunol.* **122**, 1855–1862.

Alexandra, I., Kells, D. I. C., Dorrington, K. J. and Klein, M. (1980). Non-covalent association of heavy and light chains of human immunoglobulin G: studies using light chain labelled with a fluorescent probe. *Molec. Immunol.* **17**, 1351–1363.

Barger, M. (1979). Antibodies that bind biotin and inhibit biotin-containing enzymes *Meth. Enzymol.* **62**, 319–326.

Bayer, E. A. and Wilchek, M. (1978). The avidin-biotin complex as a tool in molecular biology. *Trends biochem. Sci.* **3**, N257–259.

Bayer, E. A., Shutelsky, E. and Wilchek, M. (1979). The avidin-biotin complex in affinity cytochemistry. *Meth. Enzymol.* **62**, 308–315.

Bergquist, N. R. and Nilsson, P. (1974). The conjugation of immunoglobulins with tetramethyl rhodamine isothiocyanate by utilization of dimethylsulfoxide (DMSO) as a solvent. *J. immunol. Methods* **5**, 189–198.

Biberfeld, P., Biberfeld, Z., Molnar, Z. and Fagraeus, A. (1974). Fixation of cell-bound antibody in the membrane immunofluorescence test. *J. immunol. Methods* **4**, 135–148.

Blakeslee, D. (1977). Immunofluorescence using dichlorotriazinylaminofluorescein (DTAF). II. Preparation, purity and stability of the compound. *J. immunol. Methods* **17**, 361–364.

Blakeslee, D. and Baines, M. G. (1976). Immunofluorescence using dichlorotriazinylaminofluorescein (DTAF). I. Preparation and fractionation of labelled IgG. *J. immunol. Methods* **13**, 305–320.

Bonner, W. A., Hulett, H. R., Sweet, R. G. and Herzenberg, L. A. (1972). Fluorescence activated cell sorting. *Rev. Sci. Instrum.* **43**, 404–409.

Brandtzaeg, P. (1982). Tissue preparation methods for immunochemistry. *In.* "Techniques in Immunocytochemistry" (G. R. Bullock and P. Petrusz, eds), Volume 1, pp 1–75, Academic Press, London.

Brumberg, Ye. M. (1959). Fluorescence microscopy of biological objects using light from above. *Biophysics* **4**, 97–104.

Cebra, J. J. and Goldstein, G. (1965). Chromatographic purification of tetramethyl-rhodamine-immune globulin conjugates and their use in the cellular localization of rabbit γ-globulin polypeptide chains. *J. Immunol.* **95**, 230–245.

Coons, A. H. (1961). The beginnings of immunofluorescence. *J. Immunol.* **87**, 499–503.

Coons, A. H. and Kaplan, M. H. (1950). Localization of antigen in tissue cells. II. Improvements in a method for the detection of antigen by means of fluorescent antibody. *J. exp. Med.* **91**, 1–13.

Coons, A. H., Creech, H. J. and Jones, R. N. (1941). Immunological properties of an antibody containing a fluorescent group. *Proc. Soc. exp. Biol (N.Y.)* **47**, 200–202.

Coons, A. H., Creech, H. J., Jones, R. N. and Berliner, E. (1942). The demonstration of pneumococcal antigen in tissues by the use of fluorescent antibody. *J. Immunol.* **45**, 159–170.

Crooks, J. E. (1978). "The Spectrum in Chemistry." Academic Press, London, New York and San Francisco.

Davies, M. E., Barrett, A. J. and Hembry, R. M. (1978). Preparation of antibody fragments: conditions for proteolysis compared by SDS-gel electrophoresis and quantitation of antibody yield. *J. immunol. Methods* **21**, 305–315.

Finn, F. M., Titus, G., Montibeller, A. and Hofman, K. (1980). Hormone-receptor studies with avidin and biotinyl insulin-avidin complexes *J. biol. Chem.* **255**, 5742–5746.

Finn, F. M., Iwata, N., Titus, G. and Hofman, K. (1981). Hormonal properties of avidin-biotinylinsulin and avidin-biotinylcorticotropin complexes. *Hoppe-Seyler's Z. Physiol. Chem.* **362**, 679–684.

Forster, Th. and Konig, E. (1957). Absorption Spektren und Fluoreszenzeigenschaften Konzentrierter Losungen organischer Farbstaffe. Z. Electrochem. 61, 344–348.

Gardner, P. S. and McQuillin, J. (1980) "Rapid Virus Diagnosis. Application of Immunofluorescence", 2nd ed. Butterworth, London.

Gatti, R. A., Ostborn, A. and Fagraeus, A. (1974). Selective impairment of cell antigenicity by fixation. J. Immunol. 113, 1361–1368.

Giloh, H. and Sedat, J. W. (1982). Fluorescence microscopy: reduced photobleaching of rhodamine and fluorescein protein conjugates by n-propyl gallate. Science 217, 1252–1255.

Glazer, A. N. and Stryer, L. (1984). Phycofluor probes. Trends biochem. Sci. 9, 423–427.

Goding, J. W. (1976). Conjugation of antibodies with fluorochromes: modifications to the standard methods. J. immunol. Methods 13, 215–226.

Goding, J. W. (1978). Allotypes of IgM and IgD receptors in the mouse: a probe for lymphocyte differentiation. Contemp. Topics Immunobiol. 8, 203–243.

Goding, J. W. and Layton, J. E. (1976). Antigen-induced co-capping of IgM and IgD-like receptors on murine B cells. J. exp. Med. 144, 852–857.

Goding, J. W. and Burns, G. F. (1981). Monoclonal antibody OKT-9 recognizes the receptor for transferrin on human acute lymphocytic leukemia cells. J. Immunol. 127, 1256–1258.

Goldstein, L. C., McDougall, J., Hackman, R., Meyers, J. D., Thomas, D. and Nowinski, R. C. (1982). Monoclonal antibodies to cytomegalovirus: rapid identification of clinical isolates and preliminary use in diagnosis of cytomegalovirus pneumonia. Infection and Immunity 38, 273–281.

Green, N. M. (1975). Avidin. Adv. Protein Chem. 29, 85–133.

Gutman, G. and Weissman, I. L. (1972). Lymphoid cell architecture. Experimental analysis of the origin and distribution of T-cells and B-cells. Immunology 23, 465–479.

Györgi, P. (1940). A further note on the identity of vitamin H with biotin. Science 92, 609–610.

Haaijman, J. J. and Slingerland-Teunissen, J. (1978). Equipment and preparative procedures in immunofluorescence microscopy: Quantitative studies. In "Immunofluorescence and Related Staining Techniques" (W. Knapp, K. Holubar and G. Wick, eds), pp. 3–10. Elsevier/North Holland, Amsterdam and New York.

Hansen, P. A. (1967). Spectral data of fluorescent tracers. Acta histochem. Suppl. 7, 167–180.

Hardy, R. R., Hayakawa, K., Haaijman, J. and Herzenberg, L. A. (1982a). B-cell subpopulations identified by two-colour fluorescence analysis. Nature 297, 589–591.

Hardy, R. R., Hayakawa, K. and Herzenberg, L. A. (1982b). B-cell subpopulations identifiable by two-color fluorescence analysis using a dual-laser FACS. Ann. N.Y. Acad. Sci. 399, 112–121.

Heggeness, M. H. (1977). Avidin binds to condensed chromatin. Stain Technology 52, 165–169.

Heggeness, M. H. and Ash, J. F. (1977). Use of avidin–biotin complex for localization of actin and myosin with fluorescence microscopy. J. Cell. Biol. 73, 783–789.

Heggeness, M. H., Wang, K. and Singer, S. J. (1977). Intracellular distributions of mechanochemical proteins in cultured fibroblasts. Proc. natn. Acad. Sci. U.S.A. 74, 3883–3887.

Heitzmann, H. and Richards, F. M. (1974). Use of the avidin–biotin complex for specific staining of biological membranes in electron microscopy. Proc. natn. Acad. Sci. U.S.A. 71, 3537–3541.

Herzenberg, L.A., Sweet, R. G. and Herzenberg, L. A. (1976). Fluorescence-activated cell sorting., *Scient. Am.* **234**, 108–117.

Herzenberg, L. A., Bianchi, D. W., Schroder, J., Cann, H. M. and Iverson, G. M. (1979). Fetal cells in the blood of pregnant women: Detection and enrichment by fluorescence-activated cell sorting. *Proc. natn. Acad. Sci. U.S.A.* **76**, 1453–1455.

Higgins, T. J., O'Neill, H. C. and Parish, C. R. (1981). A sensitive and quantitative fluorescence assay for cell surface antigens. *J. immunol. Methods* **47**, 275–287.

Hofmann, K., Wood, S. W., Brinton, C. C., Montibeller, J. A. and Finn, F. M. (1980). Iminobiotin affinity columns and their application to retrieval of strept-avidin. *Proc. natn. Acad. Sci. U.S.A.* **77**, 4666–4668.

Holtkamp, B., Cramer, M., Lemke, H. and Rajewsky, K. (1981). Isolation of a cloned cell line expressing variant H-2K^k using fluorescence-activated cell sorting. *Nature* **289**, 66–68.

Johnson, G. D. and Araujo, G. M. (1981). A simple method of reducing the fading of immunofluorescence during microscopy. *J. immunol. Methods* **43**, 349–350.

Johnson, G. D., Davidson, R. S., McNamee, K. C., Russell, G., Goodwin, D. and Holborow, E. J. (1982). Fading of immunofluorescence during microscopy: a study of the phenomenon and its remedy. *J. immunol. Methods* **55**, 231–242.

Johnsson, M. E., Bergquist, N. R. and Grandien, M. (1976). Antibodies to calf serum as a cause of unwanted reaction in immunofluorescence. *J. immunol. Methods* **11**, 265–272.

Kavathas, P. and Herzenberg, L. A. (1983). Stable transformation of mouse L cells for human membrane T cell differentiation antigens, HLA and β_2-microglobulin: selection by fluorescence-activated cell sorting. *Proc. natn. Acad. Sci. U.S.A.* **80**, 524–528.

Kearney, J. F. and Lawton, A. R. (1975). B lymphocyte differentiation induced by lipopolysaccharide. I. Generation of cells synthesizing four major immunoglobulin classes. *J. Immunol.* **115**, 671–676.

Kitagawa, T. (1981). *In* "Enzyme Immunoassay" (E. Ishikawa, T. Kawai and K. Miyai, eds), pp. 81–89. Igaku-Shoin, Tokyo and New York.

Kitagawa, T. and Aikawa, T. (1976). Enzyme coupled immunoassay of insulin using a novel coupling reagent. *J. Biochem (Tokyo)* **79**, 233–236.

Kranz, D. M. and Voss, E. W. (1981). Partial elucidation of an anti-hapten repertoire in BALB/c mice: comparative characterization of several monoclonal anti-fluorescyl antibodies. *Mol. Immunol.* **18**, 889–898.

Krishnan, A. (1975). Rapid flow cytofluorometric analysis of mammalian cell cycle by propidium iodide staining *J. Cell Biol.* **66**, 188–193.

Kruth, H. S. (1982). Flow cytometry: rapid biochemical analysis of single cells. *Anal. Biochem.* **125**, 225–242.

Lachman, P. J. (1964). The reaction of sodium azide with fluorochromes. *Immunology* **7**, 507–510.

Lanier, L. L. and Warner, N. L. (1981). Paraformaldehyde fixation of hematopoietic cells for quantitative flow cytometry (FACS) analysis. *J. immunol. Methods* **47**, 25–30.

Layton, J. E. (1980). Anti-carbohydrate activity of T cell-reactive chicken anti-mouse immunoglobulin antibodies. *J. Immunol.* **125**, 1993–1997.

Lazarides, E. (1976). Actin, α-actinin, and tropomyosin interaction in the structural organization of actin filaments in nonmuscle cells. *J. Cell. Biol.* **68**, 202–219.

Ledbetter, J. A., Rouse, R. V., Micklem, H. S. and Herzenberg, L. A. (1980a). T cell subsets defined by expression of Lyt-1,2,3 and Thy-1 antigens. Two-parameter immunofluorescence and cytotoxicity analysis with monoclonal antibodies modifies current views. *J. exp. Med.* **152**, 280–295.

Ledbetter, J. A., Goding, J. W., Tokuhisa, T. and Herzenberg, L. A. (1980b). Murine

T-cell differentiation antigens detected by monoclonal antibodies. *In* "Monoclonal Antibodies. Hybridomas: A New Dimension in Biological Analyses", (R. H. Kennett, T. J. McKearn and K. B. Bechtol, eds), pp. 235–249. Plenum Press, New York and London.

Lee, A. C. J., Powell, J. E., Tregear, G. W., Niall, H. D. and Stevens, V. C. (1980). A method for preparing β-hCG COOH peptide-carrier conjugates of predictable composition. *Mol. Immunol.* **17**, 749–756.

Liu, F.-T., Zinnecker, M., Hamaoka, T. and Katz, D. H. (1979). New procedures for preparation and isolation of conjugates of proteins and a synthetic copolymer of D-amino acids and immunochemical characterization of such conjugates. *Biochemistry* **18**, 690–697.

Loken, M. R. and Stall, A. M. (1982). Flow cytometry as an analytical and preparative tool in immunology. *J. immunol. Methods* **50**, R85–R112.

Loken, M. R., Parks, D. R. and Herzenberg, L. A. (1977). Two-color immunofluorescence using a fluorescence-activated cell sorter (FACS). *J. Histochem. Cytochem.* **25**, 899–907.

Mage, M. G. (1980). Preparation of Fab fragments from IgGs of different animal species. *Meth. Enzymol.* **70**, 142–150.

Miller, R. G., Lelande, M. E., McCutcheon, M. J., Stewart, S. S. and Price G. B. (1981). Usage of the flow cytometer-cell sorter. *J. immunol. Methods* **47**, 13–24.

Milstein, C. and Cuello, A. C. (1983). Hybrid hybridomas and their use in immunocytochemistry. *Nature* **305**, 537–540.

Milstein, C. and Cuello, A. C. (1984). Hybrid hybridomas and the production of bi-specific monoclonal antibodies. *Immunol. Today* **5**, 299–304.

Nairn, R. C. (1976) "Fluorescent Protein Tracing", 4th ed. Livingstone, Edinburgh and London.

Neuberger, M. S. and Rajewsky, K. (1981). Switch from hapten-specific immunoglobulin M to immunoglobulin D secretion in a hybrid mouse cell line. *Proc. natn. Acad. Sci. U.S.A.* **78**, 1138–1142.

Nossal, G. J. V. and Layton, J. E. (1976). Antigen-induced aggregation and modulation of receptors on hapten-specific B lymphocytes. *J. exp. Med.* **143**, 511–528.

Ohkuma, S. and Poole, B. (1978). Fluorescence probe measurement of the intralysosomal pH in living cells and the perturbation of pH by various agents. *Proc. natn. Acad. Sci. U.S.A.* **75**, 3327–3331.

Oi, V. T., Glazer, A. N. and Stryer, L. (1982). Fluorescent phycobiliprotein conjugates for analyses of cells and molecules. *J. Cell. Biol.* **93**, 981–986.

Oi, V. T., Vuong, M., Hardy, R., Reidler, J., Dangl, J., Herzenberg, L. A. and Stryer, L. (1984). Correlation between segmental flexibility and effector function of antibodies. *Nature* **307**, 136–140.

Osborn, M., Webster, R. E. and Weber, K. (1978). Individual microtubules viewed by immunofluorescence and electron microscopy in the same P_tK2 cell. *J. Cell Biol.* **77**, R27–34.

O'Sullivan, M. J., Gnemmi, E., Morris, D., Chieregatti, G., Simmonds, A. D., Simmons, M., Bridges, J. W. and Marks, V. (1979). Comparison of two methods of preparing enzyme-antibody conjugates: application of these conjugates for enzyme immunoassay. *Anal. Biochem.* **100**, 100–108.

Parks, D. R., Bryan, V. M., Oi, V. T. and Herzenberg, L. A. (1979). Antigen-specific identification and cloning of hybridomas with a fluorescence-activated cell sorter. *Proc. natn. Acad. Sci. U.S.A.* **76**, 1962–1966.

Pearse, A. G. (1980). "Histochemistry, Theoretical and Applied", Vol. 1, 4th ed. Churchill, London.

Ploem, J. S. (1967). The use of a vertical illuminator with interchangeable dichroic mirrors for fluorescence microscopy with incident light. *Z. Wiss. Mikroscopie* **68**, 129–142.

Radbruch, A., Liesegang, B. and Rajewsky, K. (1980). Isolation of variants of mouse myeloma X63 that express changed immunoglobulin class. *Proc. natn. Acad. Sci. U.S.A.* **77**, 2909–2913.

Rembaum, A. and Dreyer, W. J. (1980). Immuno-microspheres: reagents for cell labeling and separation. *Science* **208**, 364–368.

Riggs, J. L., Seiwald, R. J., Burckhalter, J. H., Downes, C. M. and Metcalf, T. G. (1958). Isothiocyanate compounds as fluorescent labeling agents for immune serum. *Am. J. Pathol.* **34**, 1081–1098.

Rouse, R. V., van Ewijk, W., Jones, P. P. and Weissman, I. L. (1979). Expression of MHC antigens by mouse thymic dendritic cells. *J. Immunol.* **122**, 2508–2515.

Sainte-Marie, G. (1962). A paraffin embedding technique for studies employing immunofluorescence. *J. Histochem. Cytochem.* **10**, 250–256.

Sidman, C. L. (1981). Lymphocyte surface receptors and albumin. *J. Immunol.* **127**, 1454–1458.

Smit, J. W., Meijer, C. J. L. M., Décary, F. and Feltkamp-Vroom, T. M. (1975). Paraformaldehyde fixation in immunofluorescence and immunoelectron microscopy. *J. immunol. Methods* **6**, 93–98.

Stanworth, D. R. and Turner, M. W. (1978). Immunochemical analysis of immunoglobulins and their sub-units. *In* "Handbook of Experimental Immunology", (D. M. Weir, ed), 3rd ed., Vol. 1, pp. 6.1–6.102. Blackwell, Edinburgh and Oxford.

Sternberger, L. A. (1979). "Immunocytochemistry." John Wiley, New York.

Taylor, R. B., Duffus, W. P. H., Raff, M. C. and De Petris, S. (1971). Redistribution and pinocytosis of lymphocyte surface immunoglobulin induced by anti-immunoglobulin antibody. *Nature (New Biol.)* **223**, 225–229.

The, T. H. and Feltkamp, T. E. W. (1970a). Conjugation of fluorescein isothiocyanate to antibodies. I. Experiments on the conditions of conjugation. *Immunology* **18**, 865–873.

The, T. H. and Feltkamp, T. E. W. (1970b). Conjugation of fluorescein isothiocyanate to antibodies. II. A reproducible method. *Immunology* **18**, 875–881.

Titus, J. A., Haugland, R., Sharrow, S. O. and Segal, D. M. (1982). Texas Red, a hydrophilic, red-emitting fluorophore for use with fluorescein in dual parameter flow microfluorometric and fluorescence microscopic studies. *J. immunol. Methods* **50**, 193–204.

Vallera, D. A., Youle, R. J., Neville, D. M. and Kersey, J. H. (1982). Bone marrow transplantation across major histocompatibility barriers. V. Protection of mice from lethal graft-vs.-host disease by pretreatment of donor cells with monoclonal anti-Thy-1.2 coupled to the toxin ricin. *J. exp. Med.* **155**, 949–954.

Volkman, D. J., Ahmad, A. A., Fauci, A. S. and Neville, D. M. (1982). Selective abrogation of antigen-specific human B cell response by antigen-rich conjugates. *J. exp. Med.* **156**, 634–639.

Weber, K., Bibring, T. and Osborne, M. (1975). Specific visualization of tubulin containing structures in tissue culture cells by immunofluorescence. *Exp. Cell. Res.* **95**, 111–120.

Wick, G., Baudner, S. and Herzog, F. (1978). "Immunofluorescence." Die Medizinische Verlags gesellschaft, Marburg/Lahn.

Winchester, R. J., Fu, S. M., Hoffman, T. and Kunkel, H. G. (1975). IgG on lymphocyte surfaces: technical problems and the significance of third cell population. *J. Immunol.* **114**, 1210–1212.

Yoshitake, S., Yamada, Y., Ishikawa, E. and Masseyeff, R. (1979). Conjugation of glucose oxidase from *Aspergillus niger* and rabbit antibodies using N-hydroxy-succinimide ester of N-(4-carboxycyclohexyl-methyl)-maleimide. *Eur. J. Biochem.* **101**, 395–399.

Youle, R. J. and Neville, D. M. (1980). Anti-Thy-1.2 monoclonal antibody linked to ricin is a potent cell-type-specific toxin. *Proc. natn. Acad. Sci. U.S.A.* **77**, 5483–5486.

8   Generation of Conventional Antibodies

It may seem somewhat paradoxical to end a book on monoclonal antibodies by describing the production of conventional polyclonal antibodies. However, there are many reasons for doing so.

The production of monoclonal antibodies involves a great deal of work. A suitable screening assay must be developed before the fusion, and hundreds or thousands of tests will have to be performed before the prized clone is immortalized. The sheer work and time involved in "cell farming" is considerable. In comparison, the preparation of antibodies with nothing more than antigen, a rabbit, and a syringe, might be seen as a technological breakthrough! For many purposes, conventional antibodies will do the job adequately, with much less work.

In addition, there are some cases where the extreme monospecficity of monoclonal antibodies may be a liability rather than an asset, and it would seem that these problems will be with us for some time to come. Most involve experiments in which the antigen is not in its native conformation.

A common problem concerns the isolation of proteins from cell-free translation systems. Unless microsomal membranes are added, membrane and secretory proteins synthesized in cell-free systems will not be glycosylated, and will retain a "leader" sequence which is normally removed as the nascent chain enters the lumen of the endoplasmic reticulum. The majority of membrane and secretory proteins are glycosylated, and it is known that glycosylation influences the conformation of proteins. Similarly, the cell-free translation of a single subunit of a multimeric protein may result in a product which is different in conformation to that of the native, fully assembled protein. In each of these cases, a particular monoclonal antibody may or may not recognize the antigen. It may sometimes be possible to choose or make a monoclonal antibody specially for the purpose, but this is not always feasible or desirable.

For similar reasons, polyclonal antibodies might also be preferred for the detection of genes cloned in bacteria. If cloned sequences could be identified by antibodies, the uncertainties of "plus–minus" screening would be eliminated, as would the need to perform hundreds or thousands of cell-free translations and immunoprecipitations (Section 5.10). However, most of the current expression vectors synthesize the cloned gene product as part of a fused polypeptide. On theoretical grounds, it would be expected that only a minority of the original antigenic determinants would be detectable, and experience has borne this out. Although a number of genes have been cloned using antibodies to identify clones (Section 5.10), the majority of these have involved the use of polyclonal antibodies. The construction of improved expression vectors (Young and Davis, 1983), or the use of the fluorescence-activated cell sorter to identify gene expression in transfected eucaryotic cells (Sections 5.10 and 7.2) may make screening by antibody more feasible in the future (Kemp *et al.*, 1983).

For all these reasons, polyclonal antibodies will continue to have a place for a long time to come. One possible future scenario might involve the purification of a protein by affinity chromatography with monoclonal antibodies, and the subsequent generation of highly specific polyclonal antibodies, which would in turn be used to identify the gene after cloning in bacteria.

8.1 Strategies for the Preparation of Highly Specific Polyclonal Antibodies

8.1.1 Dose of Antigen

In the older literature, it was common to use 1–10 mg antigen for each immunization, but experience indicates that much lower doses (10–100 μg) are often sufficient (Hurn and Chantler, 1980; Vaitukaitis, 1981). In some instances, even lower doses may be used. Johansson *et al.* (1979) were able to generate highly specific antisera to adenovirus with as little as 50 ng of antigen coupled to affinity beads. Specific antisera against membrane IgD could be generated by six injections of 2×10^7 spleen cells (Goding *et al.*, 1976). Assuming 10^5 IgD molecules per cell, the dose of antigen was only 0.25 μg per injection. In general, the lower doses of antigen lead to higher-affinity antibodies.

If the antigen is readily available and extremely pure, higher doses (1–2 mg) may result in brisker and stronger responses. However, the risk of production of antibodies to impurities increases with dose. An old adage amongst immunologists is to "Always remember that the rabbit is a better immunologist than you are."

8.1.2 Form of Antigen

The form of antigen and use of adjuvants is discussed in detail in Chapters 2 and 3. A high degree of aggregation favours good responses, and the use of Freund's adjuvant is virtually universal. Molecules of very low molecular weight (< 1000) are generally very poorly immunogenic, but may evoke strong responses when coupled to an immunogenic larger molecule. The small molecule is known as a "hapten", and the larger molecule a "carrier" or "Schlepper" (Yiddish). A large number of drugs and hormones may be used as haptens. Sometimes, even quite large molecules are poorly immunogenic, but good responses may be achieved by treating them as haptens and coupling them to strongly immunogenic carriers. Suitable carriers include keyhole limpet haemocyanin, bovine serum albumin, ovalbumin or fowl immunoglobulin. (In many cases, one may wish to avoid bovine serum albumin because it is a component of fetal calf serum and many buffers.) The chemistry of coupling depends on the availability of suitable groups on the hapten (see Erlanger, 1980; Bauminger and Wilchek, 1980; Reichlin, 1980).

8.1.3 Antigen Purity

The purity of antigen is crucial for generation of specific antisera (see also Section 8.2.9). As a general rule, there should be no more than 1–2% contaminants. Antibodies to contaminants may still occur at this level. Methods of antigen purification could include any of the procedures outlined in Chapters 3–6, but will have to be individualized for each case. For best results, at least two procedures which frationate on the basis of different parameters should be used sequentially. The greatest purity will be obtained by combinations of high resolution methods such as isoelectric focusing, chromatofocusing, high performance liquid chromatography, affinity chromatography or polyacrylamide gel electrophoresis (see Scopes, 1982).

8.1.4 Immunization with Proteins Purified by Polyacrylamide Gel Electrophoresis

In 1974, Stumph and colleagues showed that SDS-treated proteins were capable of eliciting strong antibody responses, and that the resulting antibodies reacted with the native protein. Subsequently, the extreme resolving power of SDS-polyacrylamide gel electrophoresis was used to purify proteins for immunization to produce many highly specific antisera (Tjian *et al.*, 1975; Springer *et al.*, 1977; Dahl and Bignami, 1977; Lane and Robbins, 1978; Carrol *et al.*, 1978; Granger and Lazarides, 1980; Boulard and Lecroisey, 1982).

In most cases, the Coomassie blue-stained protein band was excised, and the gel crushed and emulsified in complete Freund's adjuvant (Section 3.2.1). Acrylamide is said to act as an adjuvant in its own right (Weintraub and Raymond, 1963), but it should be noted that antibodies may also be formed against the acrylamide itself, and against Coomassie blue (Granger and Lazarides, 1980).

8.2 Preparative SDS-polyacrylamide Gel Electrophoresis

Sometimes, the escape of antigen from the acrylamide is too slow to allow sufficient stimulation. If this is suspected, the protein may be eluted electrophoretically prior to injection. Stephens (1975) has described a simple method for electrophoretic elution into a dialysis sac. Figure 8.1 shows a modified version (see also Stearne *et al.*, 1985).

The polyacrylamide gel may be either one- or two-dimensional, exactly as described in Chapter 5. Molecular weight standards run at the sides of the gel may help identify the desired band. Gels may be stained for 5 min in Coomassie blue, followed by destaining in ethanol–acetic acid until bands are visible (Chapter 5), or they may be "stained" by precipitating the SDS-protein complexes with ice-cold 0.25 M KCl until the bands are clearly visible by oblique lighting (Hager and Burgess, 1980). The desired band is then cut with a scalpel, and equilibrated with elution buffer (see below) plus 5 mM dithiothreitol for 30–60 min. (Losses due to diffusion in this time are negligible). The function of the dithiothreitol is to ensure that the protein does not form a large oxidized disulphide-bonded polymer that is trapped in the gel.

The acylamide gel slice is then loaded into the elution tube (Fig. 8.1), and the tank and tube filled with elution buffer. The elution buffer may be 0.1% SDS in 50 mM NH_4HCO_3 (volatile buffer suitable for protein sequencing) or 50 mM $NaHCO_3$. SDS running buffer (1x; Table 5.2) may also be used.

Elution is at 50 V for 1–2 days. The buffer in the tank should be replaced every 24 h to prevent pH changes. If the gel was stained with Coomassie blue, the dye will be observed to elute from the gel slice and concentrate in a narrow band at the bottom of the tube (Fig. 8.1, I). Note that the dye is not covalently linked to the protein, and elutes from the gel at a much faster rate than the protein.

When elution is complete, there will be ~ 200 µl of 10% SDS in the

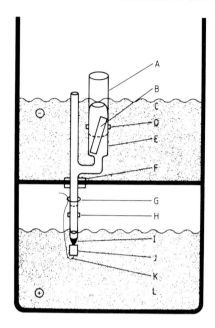
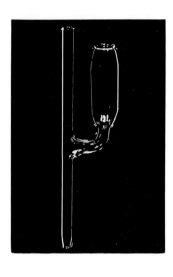

Fig. 8.1 Apparatus for elution of proteins from polyacrylamide gel slices. A standard tube gel tank is used, but with a modified glass tube (right). A,dialysis tubing, 25 mm flat width, to prevent entry and concentration of macromolecular contaminants from the upper tank buffer; B, gel slice; C, tank buffer; D, Silastic tubing, 12.7 mm inside diameter, Cat. No. 601–625; E, elution tube; F, rubber grommet; G, rubber band; H, Silastic tubing, 6.4 mm inside diameter, Cat. No. 601–441; I, eluted protein; J, Spectrapor clip, Cat. No. 132734; K, dialysis tubing, 10 mm flat width; L, tank buffer. The straight portion of the tube is 110 mm in length and 7 mm in diameter. The wide section is 40 mm in length and 16 mm in diameter. Dotted line indicates the upper edge of dialysis tubing. The lower end of the dialysis tubing is held above the buffer by a rubber band (G), so even if clip J leaks, the sample will remain inside the dialysis tubing. See text for further details. From Stearne et al. (1985).

bottom of the tube. The build-up of SDS is caused by the trapping of SDS micelles ($M_r \sim 20\,000$) by the lower dialysis membrane, and can be seen by a sharp change in refractive index. If Coomassie blue is present, it will become concentrated in the region of concentrated SDS. Even though the Coomassie blue is a small molecule, it does not pass through the dialysis membrane because it becomes inserted into the SDS micelles. The dye remains trapped even if no protein is present.

The build-up of such high SDS concentrations should not be seen as being a problem. On the contrary, the increased density of the SDS-enriched layer stabilizes against convection during elution and removal of the sample. It is this dense layer that allows most of the buffer inside the tube to be removed at the end of elution without disturbing the protein.

Recovery of the eluted protein is achieved by gently removing the liquid above the SDS-enriched layer with a long Pasteur pipette. Virtually all this liquid can be removed without danger of disturbing the protein layer. Finally, a fresh Pasteur pipette is used to remove the protein.

Recovery of protein is usually better than 90%, even for submicrogram amounts of protein. The elution system is virtually leak-proof, because the direction of the electric field is always away from the seals.

The protein may be recovered from the SDS and contaminating acrylamide polymers by precipitation with methanol (Stearne *et al.*, 1985). The protein is transferred to a siliconized Corex tube, and 9 volumes of methanol (pre-cooled to − 20°C) added and mixed. The tube is kept at − 20°C overnight, and then centrifuged at 10 000 rpm in a Sorvall HB-4 swing-out rotor at − 5°C. The protein is precipitated as a compact transparent or slightly milky gelatinous pellet, leaving the SDS and acrylamide in solution. It may then be recovered for amino acid sequencing or emulsified in Freund's adjuvant for immunization (Section 3.2.1).

[The above protocol was worked out after much trial and error. Of many organic solvents tried, only methanol was capable of keeping such large amounts of SDS in solution. Methanol also has the advantage that it is available commercially in high purity without contamination by aldehydes, which is particularly important if the protein is to be sequenced. It is essential to keep the sample cold at all times, because precipitation of microgram amounts of protein by organic solvents is more efficient at low temperatures. The temperature should not be lower than − 20°C, however, because the SDS may precipitate. If the above protocol is followed exactly, recovery of microgram amounts of protein is usually more than 90%. Occasional very hydrophobic or low molecular weight proteins may fail to be precipitated].

8.3 Immunization

8.3.1 Choice of Species

Any species other than that of the antigen may be used, but in practice the commonly used recipients are goat, sheep and rabbit. It is widely believed that larger animals need more antigen, but there is little hard evidence (Hurn and Chantler, 1980). Goats, sheep and rabbits will all respond vigorously to 50–100 μg of protein emulsified in complete Freund's adjuvant, especially when given repeatedly. Sheep and goats may be preferred for their large size (Steward-Tull and Rowe, 1975), but it has been shown that rabbits may be bled of 100 ml at weekly intervals with no mortality and only minimal haematological disturbances (Nerenberg *et al.*, 1978).

Rabbits are notoriously variable in their immune responsiveness between individuals. If rabbits are used as recipients, a minimum of three should be injected, and the sera tested individually. One has the impression that the responsiveness of goats and sheep is more uniform, and that it may often be possible to obtain a good antiserum from a single randomly chosen individual.

8.3.2 Immunization Protocol

Many different immunization protocols have been used, and there is little but anecdotal evidence to form a basis for comparison. In general, good results will be obtained by distributing 0.5–2.0 ml of the antigen, emulsified in complete Freund's adjuvant, over a number of sites. Freund's adjuvant is a potent inflammatory stimulus, and subcutaneous or intramuscular injections probably cause the least distress. The popular use of foot-pad injections has not been justified for effectiveness by a controlled trial, and is unnecessarily cruel to the animal. Similarly, the use of intradermal injections results in skin breakdown and ulcers which take weeks to heal. The dangers of Freund's adjuvant to laboratory personnel should also be remembered (Section 3.2.1).

In order to obtain a strong antibody response, it will usually be necessary to boost at least once, and possibly several times. It is customary to boost in incomplete Freund's adjuvant (i.e. lacking the tubercle bacilli) to avoid severe hypersensitivity reactions. However, many workers boost using complete Freund's adjuvant without encountering this problem. Boosing is also quite effective using water-soluble antigen without adjuvant, possibly because the existing antibody causes the formation of antigen–antibody complexes which bind avidly to Fc receptor-bearing antigen-presenting cells.

The dose of the boosting antigen is not critical, and 50–200 μg per injection are usually adequate. The frequency and timing of booster injections may also be varied over a wide range. Typically, one might boost at 3–4 weeks after the priming dose, and perform a test bleed 5–7 days layer. Subsequent boosts might be at intervals of 3–6 weeks, depending on the strength of the response. Bleedings may be taken 5–7 days after boosts, but the titre will usually remain high for several weeks. When a satisfactory response has been achieved, it is advisable to kill bleed the animal to obtain a large and uniform pool of serum.

8.3.3 Bleeding Rabbits

The rabbit should be wrapped up firmly in a tea-towel with its head protruding, and one ear gently warmed by placing it over a low-wattage (10–25 W) light bulb attached to a goose-neck reading lamp support without the shade. Once the vessels are dilated, a small transverse cut in a marginal vein will usually allow 40–50 ml blood to be collected in 5–10 min.

Alternatively, blood may be collected with ease by vacuum aspiration from a nicked ear-vein (Nerenberg et al., 1978). It is not necessary to heat the ear or to use xylol or other irritants. A side-arm flask is connected to a water-pump, and the neck of the flask is placed over the ear and pressed gently against the head. Collection of blood into the flask is rapid and painless. Finally, the central ear artery may be punctured with a hubless

18-gauge needle (Gordon, 1981). In my experience, this method is less reliable, and in addition arterial puncture is more painful than venous.

Anaesthetized rabbits may also be bled by cardiac puncture with an 18-gauge needle attached to a 50 ml syringe. In skilled hands, the mortality from cardiac puncture is very low.

8.3.4 Bleeding Sheep and Goats

It is easiest to bleed sheep and goats if two people are present. One person places the sheep on its rump, and holds it from behind. The other person feels for the jugular vein, using the anterior edge of the sternomastoid muscle as a landmark. The vein is usually made visible if its lower end is gently obstructed by finger pressure. A 12-gauge needle is inserted by pushing upwards through the skin over the vein, and will be felt to pop into the vein with a sudden release of resistance. Bleeds of 200–300 ml may be performed without risk (see Steward-Tull and Rowe, 1975).

The same general procedure is used for goats, but the goat is held against a fence and is bled standing up.

8.3.5 Collection of Serum

Blood collected into glass or plastic containers will clot rapidly. However, the maximum amount of serum is obtained by incubating at 37°C for an hour, and then leaving the blood at 4°C overnight to allow the clot the retract. The serum is recovered by centrifugation (1000 g for 10 min). It is important to be sure that there are no red cells present in the serum, because freezing of red cells will cause haemolysis.

Serum may be stored frozen at -20°C or below. Alternatively, it may be kept at 4°C as a slurry in 50% saturated ammonium sulphate, or may be lyophilized and stored at 4°C (see Section 4.7).

8.4 Purification and Fragmentation of Rabbit, Sheep and Goat IgG

8.4.1 Binding of Rabbit, Sheep and Goat IgG to Staphylococcal Protein A

The binding of IgG to protein A has been discussed in Section 4.3.2 (see also Goding, 1976, 1978; Langone, 1982). Rabbit antisera have the distinct advantage that all their IgG binds to protein A at pH 7.4, and all elutes at pH 4.0. This fact may be used to purify rabbit IgG, and to separate Fab and

F(ab')$_2$ fragments of rabbit IgG from Fc or undigested IgG (Goding, 1976, 1978). Affinity chromatography on protein A is the method of choice for rabbit antisera.

Sheep and goats have two IgG subclasses. The major subclass (IgG1) binds very weakly to protein A at alkaline pH, and virtually not at all at neutral or acid pH (Delacroix and Vaerman, 1979; Duhamel *et al.*, 1980). The minor IgG2 subclass (10–20% of total IgG) binds firmly to protein A.

8.4.2 Purification of Sheep and Goat IgG by Ion Exchange Chromatography

The purification of IgG from sheep and goat serum is best performed by ion exchange chromatography (Section 4.2.4). After precipitation in 40% saturated ammonium sulphate, the IgG is resuspended in **PBS** and dialyzed overnight against 10 mM Tris-HCl, pH 8.0. It is then passed over a column of DEAE-Sephacel equilibrated with the same buffer. Any "dropthrough" material will be pure IgG (those IgG molecules with the most basic isoelectric points). The remaining IgG (the majority) may be eluted with a salt gradient (0–250 mM NaCl in 10 mM Tris-HCl pH 8.0). The first peak to emerge will be IgG2, and it will be immediately followed by a peak containing IgG1. At this point, the IgG should be about 90% pure. Further purification may be achieved by gel filtration (Section 4.2.5).

8.4.3 Production of Fab and F(ab')$_2$ Fragments of IgG from Rabbits, Goats and Sheep

The production of Fab fragments of IgG from rabbits, goats and sheep is quite straightforward. The basic principles and procedures described in Section 4.5.1 may be applied with little modification (see also Mage, 1980). The IgG is purified by careful ammonium sulphate precipitation (Section 4.2.1), and dialysed against 0.1 M Tris-HCl, 1 mM EDTA, pH 8.0. Further purification is usually unnecessary, but may be by ion exchange chromatography or gel filtration (Chapter 4).

Digestion is carried out in 0.1 M Tris-HCl, 1 mM EDTA pH 8.0 (or PBS plus 1 mM EDTA) plus a small amount of reducing agent (25 mM mercaptoethanol or 1–2 mM dithiothreitol). An enzyme:substrate ratio of 1:100 is customary, but 1:1000 may be sufficient. After incubation at 37°C for 1 h, the reaction is terminated by addition of an excess of iodoacetamide. The Fab fragment may be separated from the Fc by ion exchange chromatography (Section 4.5.1; Mage, 1980).

The production of F(ab')$_2$ fragments must be individualized depending on the species. Rabbit IgG is easily digested in pH 4–4.5 acetate buffer at 37°C overnight, using an enzyme:substrate ratio of 1:100 (Stanworth and Turner, 1978). Sheep and goat IgGs are rather resistant to pepsin, but adequate digestion may be achieved at pH 4.0–4.5 using an enzyme:substrate ratio of 1:50 at 37°C for 48 h. Alternatively, the cleavage of sheep IgG with trypsin may be used (Davies et al., 1978).

Peptic digestion results in extensive degradation of the Fc, and simple dialysis against PBS at pH 7.4 will irreversibly terminate the reaction and remove most of the Fc products. A fragment of the Fc (pFc′) consisting of a noncovalent dimer of the C_H3 domains (total M_r 27 000) may be removed by gel filtration on Sephacryl S-200 or S-300.

Whichever method is chosen, it is strongly advisable to check the nature and completeness of digestion by SDS-polyacrylamide gel electrophoresis.

8.4.4 Assessment of the Specificity of Polyclonal Antisera

The concentration of total IgG in serum ranges from 5–20 mg/ml. A very strong polyclonal antiserum might contain 1–3 mg/ml of specific antibody, or occasionally even more. More commonly, the antibody level may be 50–200 μg/ml, and an antiserum may be adequate for some purposes with even lower levels.

One cannot assume that because the antigen was "pure", the antiserum will be specific. There are many reasons why this need not be the case (Chapter 2). The principles of antigen analysis outlined in Chapter 5 may be applied with equal effectiveness to the analysis of antibodies.

If an antiserum is to be used in cell-binding assays, immunofluorescence or radioimmunoassay, the results of a crude test of specificity such as gel diffusion (Ouchterlony analysis) may be very misleading. The specificity of an antiserum must be tested in a system which is at least as sensitive as the one in which it is to be used.

8.5 Specific Antibodies from Nonspecific Antisera

Even when the antigen has been purified with great care, some impurities are certain to remain. There is no such thing as absolute purity, and antibodies against contaminants are an ever-present risk.

In addition, many occasions will arise in which immunological cross-reactions occur. Antisera against IgG are virtually certain to cross-react with other immunoglobulin classes, because the light chains are shared. Similarly, different glycoproteins often possess similar or identical carbohydrate moieties. Baird and Raschke (1982) have shown that chicken anti-mouse immunoglobulin cross-reacts with the envelope protein gp 70 of murine leukaemia virus, possibly through carbohydrate sharing (Layton, 1980).

Sometimes, these problems may be overcome by passing the antiserum over columns of immobilized antigen. For example, anti-IgG may be depleted of antibodies to light chains and thus rendered specific for γ heavy chains by passage over a series of columns containing other classes of immunoglobulin (see Chapter 6 for a detailed discussion of affinity chromatography). Conversely, the desired antibodies may be selectively enriched by affinity chromatography on immobilized antigen (Chapter 6).

All of the above presupposes that the antigen, contaminants, or cross-reacting substances are available in sufficient quantity and purity to allow the construction of suitable affinity columns. Specific antibodies may be affinity-purified on a micro-scale from nonspecific antisera by eluting antibodies from Western blots. The antigen-containing mixture is subjected to SDS-polyacrylamide gel electrophoresis, and the resolved proteins transferred electrophoretically to nitrocellulose. The paper is then cut into sections corresponding to the desired bands, and incubated with antiserum. Specific antibodies are eluted by 0.2 M glycine-HCl pH 2.2, and rapidly neutralized (Olmsted, 1981; Talian et al., 1983; Coudrier, 1983; Smith and Fisher, 1984). Recovery of antibody is facilitated by "carrier" protein such as BSA or gelatin in the elution buffer. This technique promises to be extremely useful for production of small quantities of highly specific polyclonal antibodies, and might be ideal as a source of antibodies for screening of cloned genes.

Finally, it is sometimes possible to identify antigens by Western blotting using nonspecific antisera. The trick is to exploit the fact that antibodies are symmetrical and bivalent. The crude antigen-containing mixture is fractionated by polyacrylamide gel electrophoresis, transferred electrophoretically to nitrocellulose, and probed with nonspecific antibodies. The region of the membrane containing the desired antigen is identified by probing the membrane with labelled or enzymically-active antigen, which binds to the "free arms" of the relevant antibodies (Muilerman et al., 1982; van der Meer et al., 1983).

References

Baird, S. M. and Raschke, W. C. (1982). Murine T-lymphoma "immunoglobulin" is identical to leukemia virus gp 70. Mol. Immunol. **19**, 1045–1050.

Bauminger, S. and Wilchek, M. (1980). The use of carbodiimides in the preparation of immunizing conjugates. Meth. Enzymol. **70**, 151–159.

Boulard, Ch. and Lecroisey, A. (1982). Specific antisera produced by direct immunization with slices of polyacrylamide gel containing small amounts of protein. J. immunol. Methods **50**, 221–226.

Carroll, R. B., Goldfine, S. M. and Mehero, J. A. (1978). Antiserum to poly-acrylamide gel-purified simian virus 40 T antigen. Virology **87**, 194–198.

Coudrier, E., Reggio, H. and Louvard, D. (1983). Characterization of an integral membrane glycoprotein associated with the microfilaments of pig intestinal micro-villi. *EMBO J.* **2**, 469–475.

Dahl, D. and Bignami, A. (1977). Effect of sodium dodecyl sulfate on the immuno-genic properties of the glial fibrillary acidic protein. *J. immunol. Methods* **17**, 201–209.

Davies, M. E., Barrett, A. J. and Hembry, R. M. (1978). Preparation of antibody fragments: conditions for proteolysis compared by SDS slab-gel electrophoresis and quantitation of antibody yield. *J. immunol. Methods* **21**, 305–315.

Delacroix, D. and Vaerman, J. P. (1979). Simple purification of goat IgG1 and IgG2 subclasses by chromatography on protein A-Sepharose at various pH. *Molec. Immunol.* **16**, 837–840.

Duhamel, R. C., Meezan, E. and Brendel, K. (1980). The pH-dependent binding of goat IgG1 and IgG2 to protein A-Sepharose. *Molec. Immunol.* **17**, 29–36.

Erlanger, B. F. (1980). The preparation of antigenic hapten-carrier conjugates: A survey. *Meth. Enzymol.* **70**, 85–104.

Goding, J. W. (1976). Conjugation of antibodies with fluorochromes: modifications to the standard methods. *J. immunol. Methods* **13**, 215–226.

Goding, J. W. (1978). Use of staphylococcal protein A as an immunological reagent. *J. immunol. Methods* **20**, 241–253.

Goding, J. W., Warr, G. W. and Warner, N. L. (1976). Genetic polymorphism of IgD-like cell surface immunoglobulin in the mouse. *Proc. natn. Acad. Sci. U.S.A.* **73**, 1305–1309.

Gordon, L. K. (1981). A reliable method for repetitively bleeding rabbits from the central artery of the ear. *J. immunol. Methods* **44**, 241–245.

Granger, B. L. and Lazarides, E. (1980). Synemin: a new high molecular weight protein associated with desmin and vimentin filaments in muscle. *Cell* **22**, 727–738.

Hager, D. A. and Burgess, R. R. (1980). Elution of proteins from dodecyl sulfate-polyacrylamide gels, removal of sodium dodecyl sulfate, and renaturation of enzymatic activity: results with sigma subunit of *Escherichia coli* RNA poly-merase, wheat germ topoisomerase and other enzymes. *Anal. Biochem.* **109**, 76–86.

Hurn, B. A. L. and Chantler, S. M. (1980). Production of reagent antibodies. *Meth. Enzymol.* **70**, 104–142.

Johansson, M. E., Wadell, G., Jacobsson, P. A. and Svensson, L. (1979). Preparation of specific antisera against adenoviruses by affinity bead immunization (ABI). *J. immunol. Methods* **26**, 141–149.

Kemp, D. J., Coppel, R. L., Cowman, A. F., Saint, R. B., Brown, G. V. and Anders, R. F. (1983). Expression of *Plasmodium falciparum* blood-stage antigens in *Es-cherichia coli*: detection with antibodies from immune humans. *Proc. natn. Acad. Sci. U.S.A.* **80**, 3787–3791.

Lane, D. P. and Robbins, A. K. (1978). An immunochemical investigation of SV40 T antigens. 1. Production, properties and specificity of a rabbit antibody to purified simian virus 40 large-T antigen. *Virology* **87**, 182–193.

Langone, J. J. (1982). Protein A of *Staphylococcus aureus* and related immuno-globulin receptors produced by streptococci and pneumonococci. *Adv. Immunol.* **32**, 157–252.

Layton, J. E. (1980). Anti-carbohydrate activity of T cell-reactive chicken anti-mouse immunoglobulin antibodies. *J. Immunol.* **125**, 1993–1997.

Mage, M. G. (1980). Preparation of Fab fragments from IgGs of different animal species. *Meth. Enzymol.* **70**, 142–150.

Muilerman, H. G., ter Hart, H. G. J. and Van Dijk, W. V. (1982). Specific detection of inactive enzyme protein after polyacrylamide gel electrophoresis by a new enzyme-immunoassay method using unspecific antiserum and partially purified active enzyme: application to rat liver phosphodiesterase I. *Anal. Biochem.* **120**, 46–51.

Nerenberg, S. T., Zedler, P., Prasad, R., Biskup, N. S. and Pedersen, L. (1978). Hematological response of rabbits to chronic, repetitive, severe bleedings for the production of antisera. *J. immunol. Methods* **24**, 19–24.

Olmsted, J. B. (1981). Affinity purification of antibodies from diazotized paper blots of heterogeneous protein samples. *J. biol. Chem.* **256**, 11955–11957.

Reichlin, M. (1980). Use of glutaraldehyde as a coupling agent for proteins and peptides. *Meth. Enzymol.* **70**, 159–165.

Scopes, R. K. (1982). "Protein Purification: Principles and Practice." Springer-Verlag, New York.

Smith, D. E. and Fisher, P. A. (1984). Identification, developmental regulation, and response to heat shock of two antigenically related forms of a major nuclear envelope protein in *Drosophila* embryos: Application of an improved method of affinity purification of antibodies using polypeptides immobilized on nitrocellulose blots. *J. Cell Biol.* **99**, 20–28.

Springer, T. A., Kaufman, J. F., Siddoway, L. A., Mann, D. L. and Strominger, J. L. (1977). Purification of HLA-linked B lymphocyte alloantigens in immunologically active form by preparative sodium dodecyl sulfate-gel electrophoresis and studies on their subunit association. *J. biol. Chem.* **252**, 6201–6207.

Stanworth, D. R. and Turner, M. W. (1978). Immunochemical analysis of immunoglobulins and their subunits. *In* "Handbook of Experimental Immunology" (D. M. Weir, ed), 3rd ed., Vol. 1, pp. 6.1–6.102. Blackwell, Edinburgh and Oxford.

Stearne, P. A., van Driel, I. R., Grego, B., Simpson, R. J. and Goding, J. W. (1985). The murine plasma cell antigen PC-1: purification and partial amino acid sequence. *J. Immunol.* **134**, 443–448.

Stephens, R. E. (1975). High resolution preparative SDS-polyacrylamide gel electrophoresis: fluorescent visualization and electrophoretic elution-concentration of protein bands. *Anal. Biochem.* **65**, 369–379.

Steward-Tull, D. E. S. and Rowe, R. E. C. (1975). Procedures for large-scale antiserum production in sheep. *J. immunol. Methods* **8**, 37–45.

Stumph, W. E., Elgin, S. C. R. and Hood, L. E. (1974). Antibodies to proteins dissolved in sodium dodecyl sulfate. *J. Immunol.* **113**, 1752–1756.

Talian, J. C., Olmsted, J. B. and Goldman, R. D. (1983). A rapid procedure for preparing fluorescein-labelled specific antibodies from whole antiserum: its use in analyzing cytoskeletal architecture. *J. Cell Biol.* **97**, 1277–1282.

Tjian, R., Stinchcomb, D. and Losick, R. (1974). Antibody directed against bacillus subtilis σ factor purified by sodium dodecyl sulfate slab gel electrophoresis. *J. biol. Chem.* **250**, 8824–8828.

Vaitukaitis, J. L. (1981). Production of antisera with small doses of immunogen: Multiple intradermal injections. *Meth. Enzymol.* **73**, 46–52.

van der Meer, J., Forssers, L. and Zabel, P. (1983). Antibody-linked polymerase assay on protein blots: a novel method for identifying polymerases following SDS-polyacrylamide gel electrophoresis. *EMBO J.* **2**, 233–237.

Weintraub, M. and Raymond, S. (1963). Antiserums prepared with acrylamide gel used as an adjuvant. *Science* **142**, 1677–1678.

Young, R. A. and Davis, R. W. (1983). Efficient isolation of genes by using antibody probes. *Proc. natn. Acad. Sci. U.S.A.* **80**, 1194–1198.

Glossary

Adjuvant substance which promotes immune responses.

Allelic exclusion expression of only one allele (maternal or paternal) in an individual cell; a characteristic feature of immunoglobulin synthesis in lymphocytes.

Allotype allelic form.

Amphiphatic consisting of one hydrophilic portion and one hydrophobic portion. Amphiphatic molecules form micelles and membranes in water.

Antibody antigen-specific molecule synthesized in response to stimulation; consists of light and heavy chains.

Antigen any substance which elicits a specific immune response.

Antigenicity degree to which an antigen stimulates an immune response (in this sense, synonymous with *Immunogenicity*); degree to which an antigen reacts with particular antibody or antibodies (in this sense, *not* synonymous with *Immunogenicity*).

Antigen-combining site that portion of the antibody molecule which combines with antigen.

Antigenic competition concept that when an animal is immunized with two antigens at the same time, the response to each is diminished. The validity of the concept is questionable.

Antigenic determinant small site on antigen to which antibody binds; each antigen may have many antigenic determinants.

Avidity strength of binding of antibody to antigen; takes into account both affinity and valence.

B lymphocyte lymphocyte expressing immunoglobulin; produced in the bone marrow.

Class of antibody classification of antibody structure on the basis of the constant portion of the heavy chain; there are five classes, IgM, IgD, IgG, IgA, and IgE.

Clone group of cells with common ancestor; also used as verb to describe the growth of cells from a single ancestor; also used to describe the process of isolation and replication of individual genes.

Complement   group of plasma proteins which interact with antibodies resulting in cell destruction and other effects.

Critical micelle concentration   concentration above which the monomer concentration of detergent remains constant.

Cross-reaction   reaction of an antiserum with a molecule not present in the immunizing preparation; usually a manifestation of structural similarity.

Cryoglobulin   immunoglobulin which precipitates in the cold (without antigen).

D gene   diversity-generating gene element; a part of the immunoglobulin heavy chain gene complex; encodes portion of third hypervariable region and is contained in or close to antigen-combining site.

Denaturation   change in the conformation of a protein to a form that is different to the *Native* conformation; may be partially or fully reversible; proteins may be denatured by many conditions including heat, extremes of pH, chemical modification, organic solvents, urea, and certain ions and detergents.

Detergent   amphipathic molecule which forms small micelles in aqueous solution; often used for solubilization of lipids and integral membrane proteins.

Domain   structural unit of a protein, consisting of compact folded region, and usually encoded for by a single exon. Some authors use the term to describe two closely juxtaposed *Homology Units* of immunoglobulin heavy and/or light chains.

Dynamic range   ratio of the strongest possible signal to the weakest detectable.

Electrophoresis   technique of separation of molecules on the basis of their mobility in an electric field.

Enhancer   gene segment that causes increased transcription of adjacent gene, works regardless of orientation and is only minimally affected by its position in relation to the gene that it controls.

Epitope   chemically defined antigenic determinant.

Euglobulin   protein which precipitates at low ionic strength.

Exon   gene segment that is present in mature messenger RNA; often encodes discrete protein domain, but does not always code for protein (see *Intron*).

Fab fragment   proteolytic fragment of immunoglobulin containing antigen-combining site; univalent; consists of intact light chain disulphide-bonded to N-terminal fragment (Fd) of heavy chain.

F(ab')$_2$ fragment   proteolytic fragment of immunoglobulin containing two antigen-combining sites; contains intact light chains and N-terminal portion of heavy chains (Fd').

Fc fragment   homogeneous C-terminal portion of immunoglobulin heavy chain.

Fc receptor   molecule which binds to Fc portion of immunoglobulins.

Fluorography   exposure of photographic film by light; as opposed to *Autoradiography*, in which exposure is due to direct ionizing radiation.

Freund's adjuvant   commonly used adjuvant consisting of an emulsion of the antigen in saline and a mixture of an emulsifying agent (e.g. Arlacel A) in mineral oil with killed mycobacteria (complete Freund's adjuvant) or without mycobacteria (incomplete Freund's adjuvant).

Fv fragment   small proteolytic fragment of antibody containing one antigen-combining site; consists of variable domains of heavy and light chains.

Gamma globulin   obsolete term for serum proteins of low electrophoretic mobility; virtually synonymous with *Immunoglobulin*.

Genetic polymorphism   presence of allelic forms.

Haplotype   set of allelic forms of closely linked genes; usually inherited *en bloc*.

Hapten   substance that can combine with antibody, but is not immunogenic unless coupled to an immunogenic "carrier" molecule. Haptens are usually (but not always) low molecular weight (< 1000), while carriers are usually proteins.

HAT selection   technique in which mutant cells are unable to grow in a medium containing hypoxanthine, aminopterin and thymidine; hybridization to cells lacking the mutation allows growth.

Heavy chain   component polypeptide of immunoglobulins; heavy chains are always glycosylated, and have molecular weights from 50 000–85 000.

Heterokaryon   multinucleate cell containing at least two different types of nuclei.

Hinge   portion of immunoglobulin molecule between Fab and Fc; generally open and flexible conformation, and often susceptible to proteolytic attack.

Homology unit   segment of immunoglobulin polypeptide chain consisting of ~ 110 amino acids, and containing an intra-chain disulphide bond; thought to reflect evolution of immunoglobulins by a series of gene duplications.

Hybridoma   hybrid word combining elements of Greek and Latin; strictly speaking, the use of "-oma" should be confined to tumours in animals, but the word is generally used to describe any continuously growing cell line which is a hybrid between a malignant cell and a normal cell.

Hydrophilic   literally, water-loving; polar or ionic species freely soluble in water.

Hydrophobic   literally water-fearing; substance which is poorly soluble in water due to its non-polar nature.

Hypervariable region   portion of immunoglobulin light or heavy chain containing largest degree of variation between molecules; the intact immunoglobulin molecule is folded such that the hypervariable portions are part of the *Antigen-combining Site*.

Immunogenicity   degree to which an antigen is capable of eliciting an immune response.

Immunoglobulin   group of molecules consisting of κ or λ light chains and μ, δ, γ, ε or α heavy chains; all antibodies are immunoglobulins, but not all immunoglobulins have known antibody properties.

Integral membrane protein   membrane protein which interacts strongly with the lipid bilayer, and can only be solubilized by detergents; contains hydrophobic portion embedded in lipid bilayer.

Intron   gene segment which is transcribed into messenger RNA precursor but is absent from mature mRNA; introns are excised from messenger RNA during its maturation; their function is not known, but occasionally they contain *Enhancer* segments. Introns are also known as *Intervening Sequences*.

Isoelectric focusing   electrophoretic technique in which an electric field sets up a stable pH gradient; proteins move to the unique point where their net charge is zero; the technique is simple, yet capable of extremely high resolution. Separation is based on isoelectric point (pH at which net charge is zero).

Isotype   group of heavy or light chains with similar or identical constant region sequence; sometimes used synonymously with *Class* or *Subclass*. The term is also sometimes used to describe families of variable region sequences.

J chain   small, highly acidic glycosylated polypeptide disulphide-bonded to heavy chains of polymeric immunoglobulins (IgM and polymeric IgA); J chain is now thought to be intimately involved in interaction with *Secretory Piece* in the transport of polymeric immunoglobulins across epithelia.

J gene   short region of DNA in heavy and light chain gene clusters; encodes for amino acids at junction of variable constant regions; J genes are intimately involved in joining of variable and constant regions.

Leader sequence   short and relatively hydrophobic N-terminal sequence of secretory and membrane proteins which guides them across the membrane of the endoplasmic reticulum; virtually always removed by proteolytic cleavage in the lumen of the endoplasmic reticulum.

Lectin   carbohydrate-binding protein.

Light chain   polypeptide constituent of immunoglobulins, of molecular weight 22 000–25 000; usually not glycosylated; may be subdivided into κ and λ subsets.

Lymphocyte   small, round cell with scanty cytoplasm and round nucleus, involved in immunity; may be subdivided into T (thymus derived) and B (bone-marrow derived).

Macrophage   large vacuolated cell with irregular outline and specialized for phagocytic function.

Malignant   capable of forming rapidly growing tumours in animals.

Micelle   aggregate of amphipathic molecules in water; the hydrophobic portions face inwards, while the hydrophilic portions face outwards. The lipid bilayer of cell membranes is closely related to micelles in structure; the main difference being that micelles are small and curved, while membranes are large and planar.

Microcurie   unit of radioactivity; 2.2×10^6 disintegrations per minute.

Mycoplasma   diverse family of very small organisms capable of passing through a 0.45 μm filter, but capable of growth on artificial media.

Myeloma   tumour consisting of malignant form of plasma cell.

Native   conformation in which protein is synthesized or exists in nature; see *Denaturation*.

Non-equilibrium pH gradient electrophoresis   form of electrophoresis closely related to isoelectric focusing, but in which proteins do not stop moving; useful for analysis of basic proteins. The separation is based on net charge or isoelectric point.

Ouchterlony analysis   form of analysis in which antigen and antibody are allowed to diffuse through agar gel; the presence of a reaction is indicated by the formation of visible precipitation lines. Synonymous with *Double Diffusion*. A test based on the same principle was described at the same time by Oudin.

Peripheral membrane protein   membrane protein which may be released and solubilized by minor changes in pH or ionic strength, and does not require detergents to maintain solubility.

Phage   shorthand expression for bacteriophage; a virus that grows in bacteria.

Plasma   portion of blood remaining after removal of cells and platelets; in order to collect plasma, agents such as heparin or EDTA must be used to prevent clotting.

Plasma cell   antibody-secreting cell with eccentric nucleus and large amount of basophilic cytoplasm; the term is now often applied to all antibody-secreting cells, even though many do not possess classical plasma cell morphology.

Plasmid   relatively small circular DNA molecule capable of autonomous self-replication in bacteria.

Plasmacytoma   malignant tumour of plasma cells; synonymous with *Myeloma*.

Polymorphism   literally, many shapes; see *Genetic Polymorphism*.

Pronase   mixture of proteases from *Streptomyces griseus*.

Protein A   protein of molecular weight 42 000, made by most strains of *Staphylococcus aureus*; binds certain IgG subclasses in certain species.

Receptor   molecule which binds another molecule with high affinity and specificity; most receptors are proteins; in some cases, binding is followed by particular biological consequences.

Secretory piece   glycosylated polypeptide of molecular weight 50 000–80 000; bound to secretory IgA; a proteolytic fragment of the receptor for IgA on secretory epithelial cells.

Serum   non-cellular components of blood which remain after clotting.

Signal:noise ratio   ratio of desired information (signal) to undesired background (noise). The signal:noise ratio is thus dependent on the signal level, which is variable, and the noise level, which is more or less constant.

Subclass   group of antibodies with very similar characteristics (e.g. IgG2a, IgG2b). See also *Class* and *Isotype*.

Titre   maximum dilution of antibody at which reaction with antigen can still be detected; an approximate measure of antibody concentration.

T lymphocyte   thymus-derived lymphocyte; the main role of T cells is to regulate the activities of other cells, notably B cells; a subset of T cells is also capable of killing other cells by direct contact (the ultimate in regulation).

Tunicamycin   antibiotic which inhibits the glycosylation of asparagine residues.

Variable region   N-terminal domain of antibody heavy and light chains; contains *Antigen-combining Site*.

Western blot   electrophoretic technique in which proteins are separated in a poly-acrylamide gel, and then transferred electrophoretically to a nitrocellulose membrane. The membrane is then probed with antibodies.

Index